Praise for *Vegan's Daily Companion*:

"From the exquisite photographs to the reader-friendly, daily-message format, *Vegan's Daily Companion* may be the most complete guide to a cruelty-free, go-green, love-your-body, and heal-the-planet lifestyle ever written. I want one copy for my kitchen and another for my coffee table."
> — Victoria Moran, author of *The Love-Powered Diet* and *Creating a Charmed Life*

"An unfettered, unabashed daily affirmation of the joy of being vegan. An invitation and a promise, a process and a guide for creating a compassionate world. And some darn good recipes, too!"
> — Carol J. Adams, author of *The Sexual Politics of Meat*

"As a vegan advocate for nearly two decades, I was pleasantly surprised to learn a wealth of brand new and fascinating information in this completely unique book that combines practical tips and insightful wisdom for eating healthfully and living joyfully. Full of stunning photos and interesting facts about animals in history and literature, this is a fantastic resource for vegans as well as for curious, compassionate non-vegans."
> — Melanie Joy, Ph.D., author of *Why We Love Dogs, Eat Pigs, and Wear Cows*

QUARRY

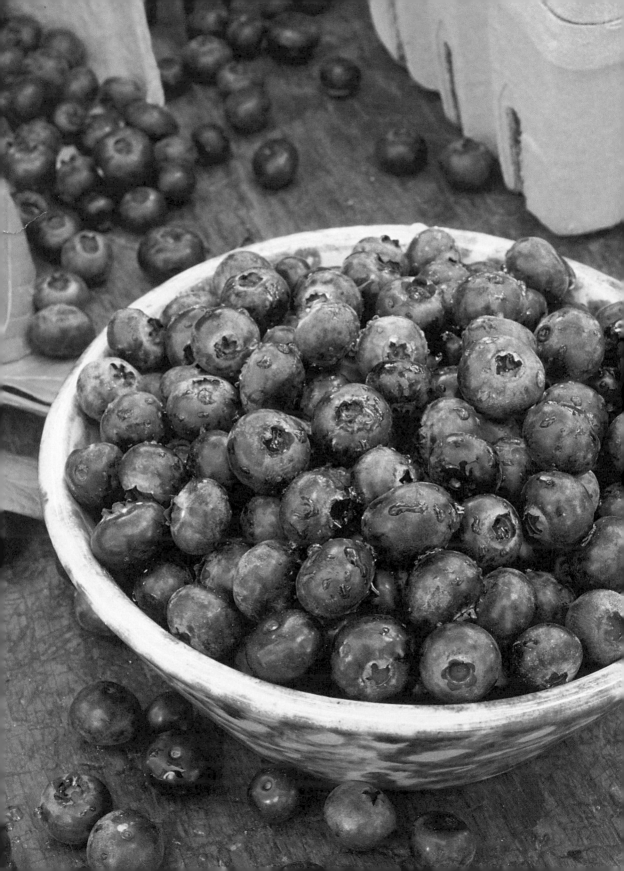

BEVERLY MASSACHUSETTS

VEGAN'S
DAILY COMPANION

QUARRY BOOKS

365 DAYS OF **INSPIRATION** FOR COOKING, EATING, AND **LIVING COMPASSIONATELY**

COLLEEN PATRICK-GOUDREAU

First published in the United States of America by
Quarry Books, a member of
Quayside Publishing Group
100 Cummings Center
Suite 406-L
Beverly, Massachusetts 01915-6101
Telephone: (978) 282-9590
Fax: (978) 283-2742
www.quarrybooks.com

Library of Congress Cataloging-in-Publication Data

Patrick-Goudreau, Colleen.
 Vegan's daily companion : 365 day of inspiration for cooking, eating, and living compassionately / Colleen Patrick-Goudreau.
     p. cm.
Includes index.
ISBN-13: 978-1-59253-679-5
ISBN-10: 1-59253-679-4
1. Vegan cooking. 2. Cookbooks. I. Title.
TX837.P3378 2011
641.5'636--dc22

                                                              2010046878

ISBN-13: 978-1-59253-855-3
Digital edition published 2011
eISBN-13: 978-1-61058-015-1

10 9 8 7 6 5 4 3 2

Design: Rita Sowins / Sowins Design
Contributing cover photographs: Kathy Stevens (lower left); Connie Pugh (upper right)

Printed in China

TO THOSE WHO SPEAK ON BEHALF OF THE ANIMALS AND LIVE BY THEIR VALUES OF COMPASSION. YOU ARE MY INSPIRATION.

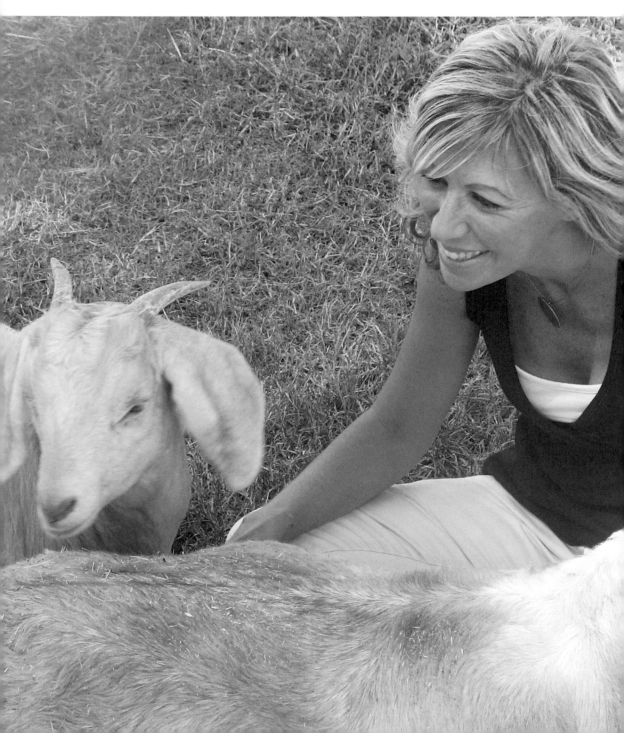

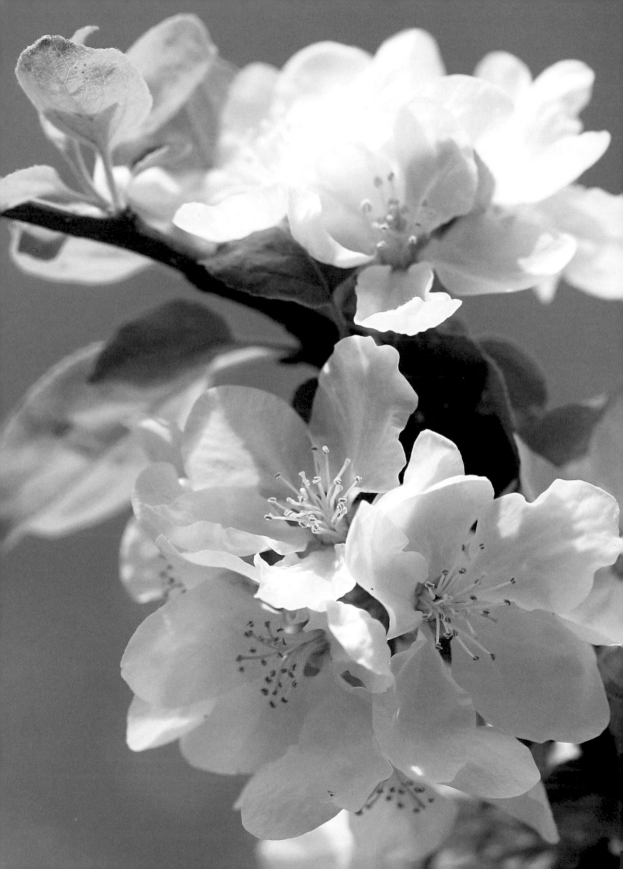

Contents

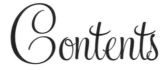

A YEAR IN THE LIFE OF A JOYFUL VEGAN

 MONDAY / **FOR THE LOVE OF FOOD**

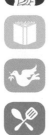 TUESDAY / **COMPASSIONATE COMMUNICATION**

WEDNESDAY / **OPTIMUM HEALTH FOR BODY, MIND, AND SPIRIT**

THURSDAY / **ANIMALS IN THE ARTS: LITERATURE AND FILM**

FRIDAY / **STORIES OF HOPE, RESCUE, AND TRANSFORMATION**

SATURDAY + SUNDAY / **HEALTHFUL RECIPES**

INTRODUCTION

The word *vegan* was coined in 1944 by British activist Donald Watson (1910–2005), the founder of the first vegan organization. Watson crafted the word *vegan* from the beginning and the end of the word "**veg** etari **an**," because he was frustrated the word *vegetarian* had come to include dairy products and eggs. He defined veganism as "a philosophy and way of living which seeks to exclude—as far as is possible and practical—all forms of exploitation of and cruelty to animals for food, clothing, or any other purpose."

Watson's definition is a profound statement in a world where the pursuit of pleasure is considered a right rather than a privilege, and it provides the perfect framework for those who want to live an intentional life based on consciousness and kindness.

But I think Watson would agree with my perception that being vegan is not about attaining an impossible level of purity in order to become a *100 percent certified vegan*. There is no such thing—the world is just too imperfect for that, as Watson indicates in his definition.

Rather, being vegan is a means to an end, not an end in itself. For me, the ultimate goal is unconditional, unfettered, unabashed compassion, and being vegan is an easy and effective step toward attaining that goal.

Although Watson coined the term *vegan* less than a century ago, the principle of compassion has been a guiding force in all the world's religions and secular philosophies for centuries. The idea of nonviolence, of ahimsa—causing no harm—is certainly not a new idea, and veganism is simply an extension of that principle.

Being vegan is about living my life with integrity and compassion, knowing that every decision I make is done so with the intention of not contributing to violence toward and exploitation of human and nonhuman animals where I have the power to do so. This intention guides my every action and shaped the content for this book.

The problem isn't that we wake up in the morning wanting to contribute to cruelty or violence. The problem is we don't wake up in the morning wanting to create more compassion, peace, and nonviolence. If that were on our to-do list every day, imagine what we could accomplish. Imagine what our world would be like.

May our daily choices be a reflection of our deepest values, and may we use our voices to speak for those who need us most, those who have no voice, those who have no choice. It's up to each one of us to create the world we want to live in; if not you, then who? If not now, then when?

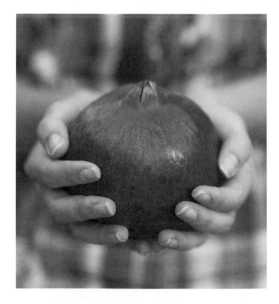

This book is organized as a day minder, with entries creating a complete year's worth of information. Each of the year's fifty-two weeks has six entries.

You can start reading this book from the beginning, following the days of the week through the calendar year, or reading one entry a day (except for Saturday and Sunday, which are combined). You can also read from the middle of the book, the end, or skip around from week to week as inspiration strikes. The most important thing to remember is that you can use this book however you want.

A YEAR IN THE LIFE OF A JOYFUL VEGAN

MONDAY / **FOR THE LOVE OF FOOD**
A celebration of familiar as well as new foods to spark enthusiasm for eating healthfully.

TUESDAY / **COMPASSIONATE COMMUNICATION**
Techniques and tactics for speaking on behalf of veganism effectively and compassionately.

WEDNESDAY / **OPTIMUM HEALTH FOR BODY, MIND, AND SPIRIT**
Care and maintenance for becoming and remaining a joyful vegan.

THURSDAY / **ANIMALS IN THE ARTS: LITERATURE AND FILM**
Inspiration across the ages that reflects our consciousness of and relationship with nonhuman animals.

FRIDAY / **STORIES OF HOPE, RESCUE, AND TRANSFORMATION**
Heartening stories of people who have become awakened and animals who have found sanctuary.

SATURDAY + SUNDAY / **HEALTHFUL RECIPES**
Favorite recipes to use as activism and nourishment.

KALE

Without exaggeration, kale is one of the most nutrient-dense foods on the planet: low in calories, low in fat, high in protein per calorie, high in dietary fiber, high in iron and calcium, and super high in phytochemicals.

The curly varieties tend to have a very thick stem from which the leaves grow, and I do prefer to remove the leaves from the stem before using. For flat-leaf varieties, there is no need.

When choosing kale, avoid leaves that have begun to turn yellow. Store kale—and all greens—in the crisper drawer in the refrigerator, preferably in a plastic bag. Kale kept in warm temperatures for too long will wilt and lose its flavor, and the nutrients will begin to deteriorate.

Ideas for your daily dose of kale:

* Sauté kale with fresh garlic, olive oil, and salt, and squeeze on a little lemon juice before serving.

* Steam chopped kale. Toss with a chopped apple, balsamic vinegar, and chopped walnuts (raw or toasted).

* Throw chopped kale in at the last minute of cooking pasta. Drain, transfer to a large bowl, and toss with toasted pine nuts, chopped olives, salt, and olive oil.

* Add chopped kale to any soup or stew.

* Add chopped (and lightly sautéed) kale to pizza on top of your favorite marinara sauce.

* Add kale to a fruit smoothie, or make a green smoothie with kale, frozen bananas, and apple juice.

If you're trying kale for the first time and find it bitter, just give it time. You can also try cutting the bitterness by adding something acidic, such as lemon juice, vinegar, or orange juice.

COMPASSIONATE ALTERNATIVE: **KILL TWO BIRDS WITH ONE STONE**

Most of us grew up with the expression "to kill two birds with one stone," which means "to achieve two objectives with a single effort." Ovid, the Roman poet who lived from about 43 BCE to 17 CE, used a similar expression in Latin nearly 2,000 years ago. It's a perfect time to put this violent idiom to rest.

Instead, try: "to cut two carrots with one knife." With practice, it becomes as natural to say as the outdated "kill two birds with one stone." Besides spreading nonviolent language, the best part about saying it will be watching people stop you in midsentence and say, "What did you just say? Nice!" It never fails to make people smile and think twice about the violence of the original phrase.

We can still say what we mean without promoting violence toward animals.

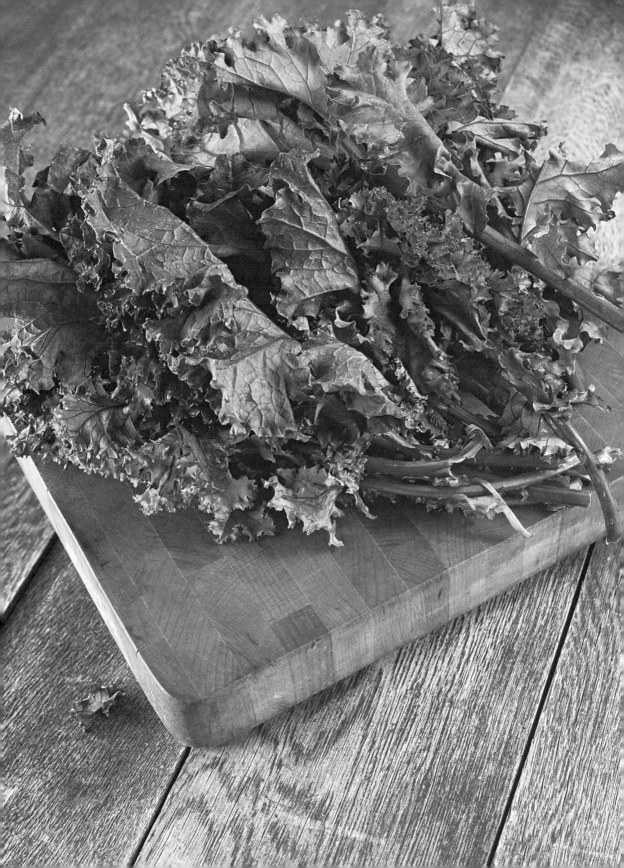

LAUGHING

When you're aware of the suffering so many billions of animals endure every day, it's easy to get swallowed up by the sorrow it induces. Consciously choosing to laugh can be very therapeutic, and though we know this intuitively, research supports this as well. Laughter:

* lowers blood pressure

* relaxes the body and muscles

* boosts the immune system by decreasing stress hormones and increasing infection-fighting antibodies

* triggers the release of endorphins, the body's natural "feel-good" chemicals

Although other benefits may not be able to be measured, we know laughter brings people together, attracts us to others, defuses tension and conflict, and strengthens relationships.

Some activists feel guilty for laughing when they're aware of so much misery, but the animals aren't going to be helped by our being miserable. To have the energy and the stamina to do this work for the rest of our lives, we need to be as strong and healthy as possible, and laughter is one thing that helps us cope.

Choosing to laugh doesn't undermine the serious work we have to do. It enables us to do it.

Molly, a rescued goat at Farm Sanctuary

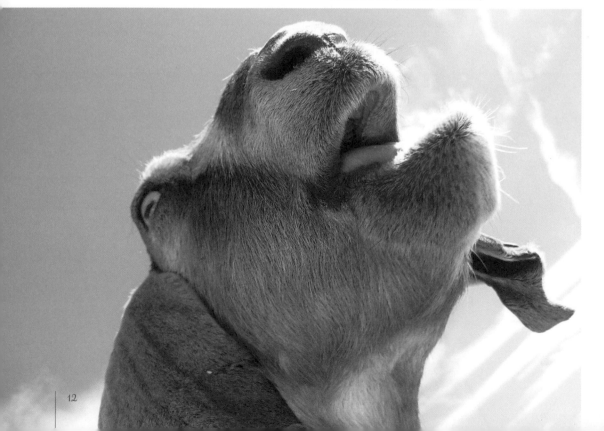

"A DOG'S TALE"
BY MARK TWAIN

An avid supporter of animal advocacy, Mark Twain spoke openly about his antivivisection stance.

"A Dog's Tale," written in 1903, is a first-person narrative told by a beloved and loyal house dog who recounts her early days as a pup, the painful and inexplicable separation from her mother, and life in her new home with Mr. Gray, a "renowned scientist," his "sweet and lovely" wife, and their children.

As fiercely protective and loving as her own mother, she is overcome with joy when her own puppy is born and displays equal affection for her as well as for the Grays' toddler. Risking her life when a fire breaks out, she drags the screaming baby out of her crib to safety, only to be met with cruel admonitions and a severe beating by Mr. Gray, who thought she was attacking the child. Distraught and injured, she hides away for several days until her maternal instincts drive her back to her puppy.

A warm reunion with Mrs. Gray, her children, and the servants make life sunny once again—but not for long. Mr. Gray's "distinguished" scientific colleagues return to the house laboratory again and again, discussing "optics, as they called it, and whether a certain injury to the brain would produce blindness or not."

Proud when the scientists summon her puppy but naive to their intentions, our canine narrator finds that they've used her puppy in their cruel experiment. Trying in vain to comfort her as she dies in her arms, she never leaves her puppy's side, breaking the hearts of the servants, who witness her inconsolable grief.

WINCHESTER, THE MIRACLE CAT

A young lady emailed us about a cat she had found. She wrote:

> I'm writing about my cat. Well, he's not really mine, but I'm his. He wandered into my yard a couple weeks ago, after an obvious accident, or some sort of attack. He was so skinny and obviously starving, and I couldn't turn him away. I went into the house and got some food; he's been on my front porch ever since.
>
> I'm a teenager living at home and I will be leaving soon, and cannot take him with me. He has an old injury to his leg that the vet said is too old to fix, and he will always be lame. He only has three teeth; well, that's all I could see but his mouth is swollen, so they could be hiding.
>
> I kept him alive when he was about to die, but I can't give him a good life. I hope you can take him or find a good home for him.

Her note almost brought tears to our eyes. We emailed her the same day and said we could take him, but we asked her to drive the cat straight to our vet.

Our vet called right after they did the exam. "Did you know this cat has been shot four times?"

The X-rays revealed what happened: Lodged in his abdomen was a .22 bullet. Another bullet had pierced his back and stopped just $5/8$ inch (15 mm) from his spine. One bullet had ripped through his rear leg, leaving no fragments behind. And the fourth bullet had hit him in the front of his mouth, shattering some teeth and ricocheting out through his neck. Other smaller bullet fragments were scattered around his body.

Our vet was as astonished as we were. We hadn't even seen him yet, but we knew what to name him: Winchester. After a week in the hospital, Winchester came home to the sanctuary. Our vets saved for us the bullet they took from his abdomen. They decided it was safer to leave the bullet near his spine alone, rather than risk opening him up to remove it.

This small, loving guy is one of the most affectionate cats we've ever known. It takes us twice as long to clean the cat house every Saturday morning, because Winchester is constantly circling our feet, rubbing against our ankles, wanting to be picked up and loved. Winchester also eagerly rolls over on his back to have his tummy scratched.

Thanks to his own incredible will to live—and a young lady with a big heart—Winchester survived. Now he'll never be in harm's way again and has found a forever home with one of our volunteers.

—*Rolling Dog Ranch Animal Sanctuary, Lancaster, New Hampshire (U.S.)*

MASSAGED KALE SALAD (A.K.A. ARI'S SPECIAL K)

Thanks to podcast listener-turned-friend, awesome voice-for-the-animals Ari Solomon, for this delicious recipe!

1 bunch curly kale
½ cup (92.5 g) cooked quinoa
½ yellow or white onion, thinly sliced
1 carrot, peeled and grated
½ avocado, cubed
2 tablespoons (30 ml) apple cider vinegar
2 to 4 tablespoons (30 to 60 ml)
   fresh lemon juice
1 tablespoon (11 g) Dijon mustard
1 teaspoon (3 g) garlic powder
⅛ teaspoon sea salt
½ cup (75 g) halved cherry tomatoes

Rinse the kale, and pull the leaves away from the stem. Place in a salad bowl, along with the quinoa, onion, carrot, and avocado.

Add the apple cider vinegar, lemon juice, mustard, garlic powder, and sea salt. With both hands, firmly massage all the ingredients together. Don't be afraid to get your hands dirty! Do this for about a minute or two until you can't see the avocado chunks anymore; they should spread over the salad and act as an "oil."

Along with your massage, the lemon juice and apple cider vinegar help tenderize the kale. Add the tomatoes, and gently toss to combine with the rest of the salad.

Yield: 4 servings

Oil-free, wheat-free, soy-free

DATES

Dates are nature's candy. The most well-known cultivars are the Deglet Noor and the Medjool, both of which will make you swear off artificial candy and refined sweeteners. The smaller Deglet Noor dates are more common, though the larger Medjool dates have great texture and sweetness.

∗ All dates have a large pit in the center, unless they are pitted. Always pit them before you eat them.

∗ Add dates to your fruit smoothies. They may not puree completely, but you can enjoy the

little chewy bits floating in the fruity goodness.

∗ Use date sugar (made from ground, dehydrated dates) instead of cane or beet sugar. It can be used in equal parts for sugar in most baking recipes, but because the tiny pieces tend not to dissolve very well, it's not ideal as a sweetener for beverages.

∗ Dates make a wonderful low-calorie snack, and they provide all the sweetness we need— from nature.

COMPASSIONATE LANGUAGE: **ACCEPTABLE ANIMAL IDIOMS**

There are some idioms in particular that—though they involve animals—are not derived from violent imagery and don't necessarily merit alternatives.

One is "to have an albatross hanging around one's neck," which refers to some unfortunate person who is forced to carry a burden. Literature lovers know that it comes from Samuel Taylor Coleridge's poem "The Rime of the Ancient Mariner," in which the character who shot an albatross is obliged to carry the bird hung around his neck.

> God save thee, ancient Mariner
> From the fiends that plague thee thus
> Why look'st thou so?—With my cross-bow
> I shot the ALBATROSS.

> Ah. well a-day. what evil looks
> Had I from old and young
> Instead of the cross, the Albatross
> About my neck was hung.

In the poem, an albatross starts to follow a ship, which is seen as a good omen. When a sailor shoots the albatross, he is punished by being forced to wear the albatross around his neck as a reminder of his disgrace.

Because the bird is a symbol of the sailor's shame, I don't necessarily think the expression itself is one that denigrates birds in general—or albatrosses in particular. If you prefer a different expression, however, you can say that something is a "burden on your shoulders" or a "weight around your neck."

RECEIVING LESSONS AND GIFTS

I heard someone say once that all our life experiences are either lessons or gifts—that we either learn from our daily experiences or they are simply blessings to be treasured and appreciated. I like that. It means that every moment is an opportunity to grow or to be grateful (or both!). It means that every encounter we have holds within it the potential to become better people or to just make someone happy (or both!).

As much as we are each recipients, so, too, are we each bestowers. We never know what impact we have on another, but we can be sure we do influence those around us.

I really don't know of a more powerful experience than to plant seeds that will change the course of another's life. The humility is not knowing whom we actually touch. The power is knowing that we unmistakably do.

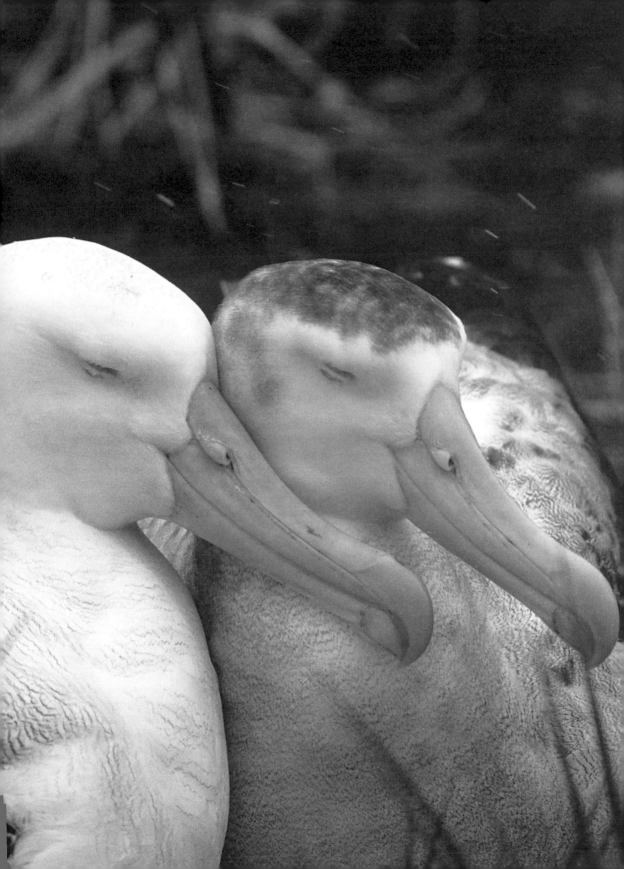

"PIG"
BY ROALD DAHL

Known mostly for his children's stories, Roald Dahl also wrote a number of rather macabre short stories for adults. Reminiscent of a Brothers Grimm fairy tale, "Pig" opens with a happy couple welcoming home their newborn son, whom they name Lexington. Twelve days after his birth, he's orphaned when the police mistake his parents for robbers and shoot them dead.

Sent to live with his Aunt Glosspan in the isolated countryside, Lexington is raised a "strict vegetarian," since Glosspan "regarded the consumption of animal flesh as not only unhealthy and disgusting, but horribly cruel."

Teaching him about the inherent violence of meat production, she home schools her nephew in several subjects, including cooking, in which he becomes quite expert. Lexington leaves for the city when his ninety-year-old aunt dies, instructed by her in a letter to see her lawyer, who will provide him with the money he needs to pursue his cooking ambitions. Eating in a restaurant for the first time, he is served pork and finds it delicious.

Eager to learn more about this discovery, Lexington meets the chef, who tells him it starts with "a properly butchered pig," so he ventures to a slaughterhouse to see how it's done.

When he arrives, he's led to the "shackling area," where screaming pigs are grabbed, looped about the ankle with a chain, and then dragged up through a hole in the roof. While Lexington is watching, a chain is slipped around his ankle, and before he can comprehend what is happening, he's being dragged along in the same manner. Mirroring the procedures of a modern-day slaughterhouse, he next arrives at the "sticker," who treats Lexington as just another nameless, faceless victim in the industry of meat production.

Colleen with Cesak, a rescued pig living the good life at Farm Sanctuary

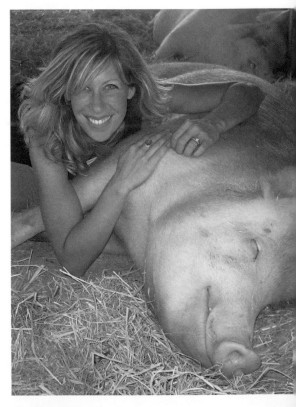

FROM BULLFIGHT SPECTATOR TO VEGAN ACTIVIST

In the summer of 1992, I joined two friends in Pamplona for the annual foolishness known as "the Running of the Bulls." This was something I had long wanted to do, and I was thrilled to be sprinting up a cobblestone street with hundreds of other people from around the world.

After the run, my friends and I wandered back to the bullring. Dozens of bull-runners were chasing several bulls around the arena, smacking them with newspapers. These bulls would die in the afternoon bullfights. The spectators cheered as men poked and teased these noble animals, mocking them in their fate. Whatever excitement I had felt earlier was now eclipsed by contrition. These bulls, I realized, wanted to live as much as I do. Am I the only person to travel to Spain, run with the bulls, and then feel shame?

That morning, I began to extend my circle of compassion—though I still had a long way to go.

I gradually gave up eating animal flesh while examining the role compassion played in my life. I worked for and wrote about human rights, which eventually led me to read *Diet for a New America* by John Robbins. I was horrified to learn how hens and cows are treated in the egg and dairy industries.

When I discovered there was a sanctuary not far from my home where I could visit farmed animals rescued from abuse, I signed up for a tour. I was profoundly moved by each animal's story, and I went vegan that day.

My reverence for all life has become my guiding principle. It informs every aspect of my existence, including my choices about work, entertainment, home decor, health care, fashion, and, of course, diet. I have found my core belief surprisingly simple to adhere to. They are not sacrifices. If compassion is my religion, these are the actions I use to celebrate it. These are my rituals. For me, living fully awake means embracing all species with the same level of respect and kindness.

Being a joyful vegan doesn't take willpower— just a willingness to try new things and choose mercy over misery.

—Mark Hawthorne is an extraordinary writer and activist. Find his work at strikingattheroots .com. Striking at the Roots: A Practical Guide to Animal Activism is his first book.

PINE NUT–ANISE COOKIES

A favorite recipe from *The Joy of Vegan Baking* (originally based on a recipe from *The Millennium Cookbook*), these are elegant cookies that beg to be served with tea or coffee.

> 3 cups (375 g) unbleached all-purpose flour
> ¼ teaspoon salt
> 1½ teaspoons (7 g) baking powder
> 1 tablespoon (8 g) anise seeds
> 1 cup (135 g) pine nuts, toasted
> ¾ cup plus 2 tablespoons (275 g) pure maple syrup
> ½ cup (120 ml) canola oil
> ¼ cup (60 ml) water
> 2 tablespoons (30 ml) anise extract
> 1 teaspoon (5 ml) vanilla extract

Preheat the oven to 350°F (180°C, or gas mark 4). Line 2 baking sheets with parchment paper or lightly grease with canola oil.

In a large bowl, combine the flour, salt, baking powder, anise seeds, and pine nuts. In a small bowl, stir together the maple syrup, oil, water, anise extract, and vanilla extract.

Pour the wet mixture into the dry mixture and stir until just combined. Form a ball with 2 tablespoons (35 g) of dough and place on the prepared pan. Press with your hand to a thickness of about ⅓ inch (1 cm). Repeat, and place the cookies 3 inches (7.5 cm) apart on the sheet. Bake for 20 to 30 minutes, or until the cookies are golden brown.

Let cool on a wire rack.

Yield: 1 ½ to 2 dozen cookies

*Soy-free

Originally published in *The Joy of Vegan Baking*

WALNUTS

Of all the nuts I eat, I eat walnuts the most frequently. They're great:

* in oatmeal
* in a salad
* as a snack
* in granola or trail mix
* sautéed with veggies
* toasted, coarsely chopped, and sprinkled on top of soup or pasta
* mixed with chopped fruit and served with nondairy yogurt

They are also a wonderful source of omega-3 fatty acids. Just ¼ cup (25 grams) provides 90.8 percent of the Daily Value for these essential fats. And for the protein-obsessed, that same ¼ cup (25 grams) provides almost 4 grams of protein, so they're a good nut to have around. (Stored in the refrigerator or freezer, they stay fresh longer.)

ANSWERING THE SAME QUESTIONS AGAIN AND AGAIN

Every day, whether it's via email, in lectures or classes, or on the street, I'm asked questions about veganism and animal rights that I've been asked countless times. They may be questions that have answers that seem obvious to me. They may be questions whose answers can easily be found with a little research. They may be one of the more commonly asked questions that every vegan gets.

However many times I've heard it, I try and treat each question as if I'm being asked for the very first time; in fact, I really am being for the very first time—by the person asking it. Each interaction—whether with a group of people or an individual—*is* unique.

People choose to be vegan for a variety of reasons, and not everyone wants to have to answer to people about their choices. To avoid this, many vegans choose not to disclose the fact that they're vegan at all, or they answer flippantly, or they get annoyed that they have to answer the same question that has been debunked and demystified for several decades, such as, "Where do you get your protein?"

Frankly, I believe we have a responsibility to respond to every question we get with grace, humility, and truth, even to a question we've heard a million times. That may be the first time that person is asking that question. You may be the first vegan he's ever met. The fact that he's even asking a question means that he wants to engage in a dialogue, and it provides you with a wonderful opportunity to express the joys and benefits of living compassionately.

Whether we like it or not, if we're the vegan someone comes to, we represent *all vegans*. He may write off veganism altogether if he finds that we're just not interested in talking about it or if we make him feel silly or self-conscious for asking questions.

If, instead, we treat a question as if we're hearing it for the first time, and our answer is genuine and enthusiastic, the person asking feels engaged and empowered. In some ways, the specific question he's asking is less important than the way we answer it.

The point is to have a dialogue with someone who is curious or ignorant about what might be commonplace for us. Aim to engage people—not alienate them.

BEING SILENT

Busy though I am, I lead a very quiet life, but being quiet is not necessarily the same as being silent. Despite all the time I spend alone, I also live in a continual cycle of speech. As much as I love to talk about living a compassionate, healthful life, speech is exhausting—not only for the person talking but also for those listening.

Consciously choosing to be silent is at once powerful and calming. Although I often fall short, my goal is to be silent one day a week. It's not always possible to anticipate disruption, but I try to choose a day of the week when I'm pretty sure I'll be uninterrupted.

I don't choose weekend days as one of my "silent days," because that's the time I want to spend with my husband and friends. I give my husband a warning when I'll be silent the following day so he doesn't expect me to talk the next day when we wake.

When I'm absolutely forced to break my silence, I keep it brief, and then continue being silent for the rest of the day.

I find great clarity and stillness on my days of silence, and I find that I'm more attuned to everything around me. My silence makes me a better observer, but the benefits are not felt only on the silent days themselves. They spill into the subsequent days as well.

Try it. On the first day you break your silence, you may find that you're more thoughtful in the words you choose and the things you say. You may be much more aware of how much energy it takes to talk, especially if you're not really saying anything at all. How often do we talk just to fill up the quiet space? How often do we waste our breath talking about nonsense—or talking about someone else—for no reason other than we think we have to talk if someone else is in the room?

In the days following your silent day, you may be less apt to want to use your breath on meaningless chitchat, and you may take much greater care in choosing just the right words to convey what you mean to say.

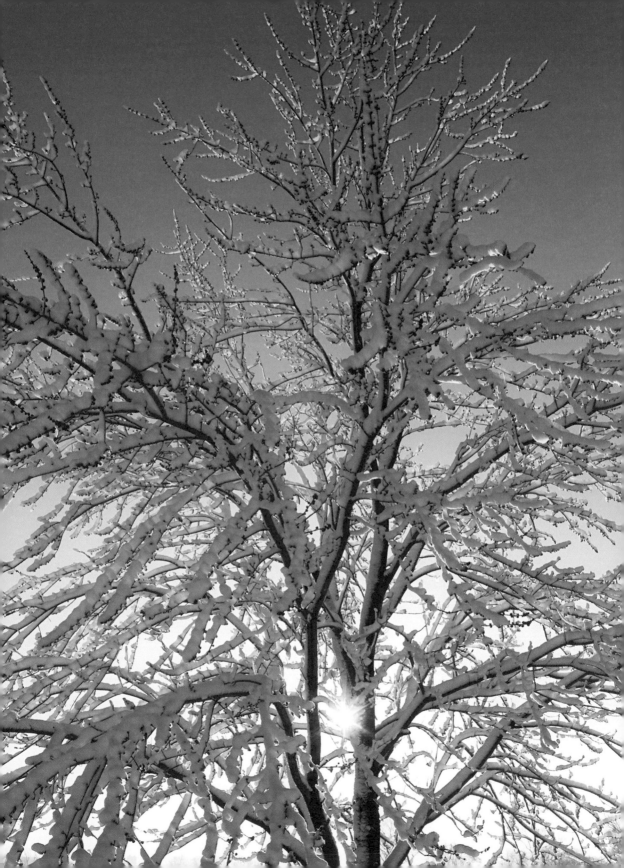

"THE ANARCHIST—HIS DOG"
BY SUSAN GLASPELL

"The Anarchist—His Dog" was written in 1912 by Susan Glaspell, a best-selling novelist and a Pulitzer Prize–winning playwright, who lived from 1876 to 1948. She was heavily involved in social justice issues and progressive causes, which is reflected in her plays and stories.

This story, set in a working-class American city in the early twentieth century, follows Freddie "Stubby" Lynch, a poor paper boy who befriends a stray dog who follows him along his route. At first, he acts tough and unmoved, all the while masking his desperate desire to make this dog his own.

He begs his mother to let him keep this "stocky, shapeless, squint-eyed yellow dog with one ear bitten half off and one leg built on an entirely different plan from its fellow legs," and she concedes.

Filled with devotion and love for Hero, Stubby is devastated when his father tells him that Hero will be shot come August, since they can't afford to pay the $2.50 dog tax. Desperate to save his dog, Stubby commits all of his waking hours to earning the money he needs to pay the tax. To his family, who barely has enough to eat, his plot seems foolhardy.

One night, Stubby overhears his parents' conversation about anarchists and declares himself one, not really understanding its meaning or its implications. He decides he will shoot a policeman, because, "I don't think the government had ought to take things you like," he says. He writes this in a letter to the police station, concluding with his home address.

When the police and the press arrive at his house, Stubby thinks they've come to shoot Hero, mistakes the "black box" (a camera) for a gun, and jumps in front of Hero, shielding him from the nonexistent bullets. Awarded for his devotion and bravery, Stubby is allowed to keep Hero, and even his father recognizes "something remarkable about his son."

MARIO—FROM DEAD PILE TO GRAND PASTURE

Dead piles are commonplace on dairy farms. Because it would cost the operation to have a rendering company pick up an animal every time one of them dies, they drag the bodies to an out-of-sight location on their property and pile them up until they pay for a rendering company to pick up the decomposing animals.

One day, at a dairy in California, a rendering truck driver was horrified and distraught to find a 45-pound (20.4 kg) newborn Jersey calf lying helplessly atop a stack of corpses, alive and healthy except for an injured leg. It was clear that he had been discarded not only due to the injury but also because, as a male calf, he is considered worthless by the dairy industry and undeserving of humane euthanasia.

The young calf, by now named Mario, was rushed to the vet, where it was confirmed that he had a fractured humerus and needed surgery right away. The veterinary hospital's orthopedic department delivered the expected news that repairing the leg would be very challenging,

would require lengthy recovery and rehabilitation, and would be extremely expensive.

Although there were only two surgeons assigned to the calf's procedure, five surgeons assisted during his four-hour surgery when complications arose because, according to his attending veterinarian, everyone was so touched by his ordeal.

After ten days in intensive care, Mario was stable enough to make the trip home; his recovery proceeded even better than predicted. Now fully grown, Mario can buck and run, and wander our green pastures just like all his friends. He spends his days with his best buddy Linus, roaming through the tall grass, napping in the sun, and carousing with the more playful members of our herd. Watching him galloping and snorting happily, you would never know how close his life came to ending in tragedy.

—*Farm Sanctuary, Orland, California (U.S.)*

Beautiful Mario enjoying life at Farm Sanctuary
Photo courtesy of Farm Sanctuary

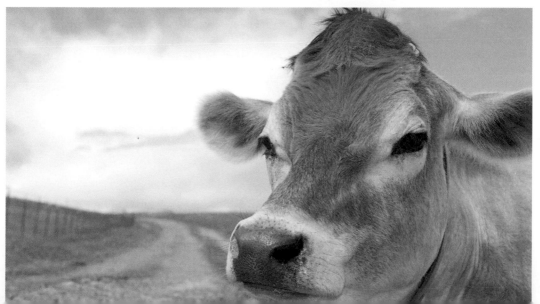

BLUEBERRY-LEMON MUFFINS

Enjoy these muffins for breakfast or as a quick snack.

> **2 cups (250 g) unbleached, all-purpose flour**
> **1½ teaspoons baking soda**
> **½ teaspoon salt**
> **Zest of 2 lemons**
> **¾ to 1 cup (150 to 200 g) granulated sugar**
> **1 cup (235 ml) nondairy milk (soy, rice, almond, hazelnut, hemp, or oat)**
> **⅓ cup (78 ml) canola oil**
> **1 teaspoon lemon extract**
> **1 tablespoon (15 ml) white distilled vinegar**
> **1½ cups (218 g) fresh blueberries, picked over to remove stems**

Preheat the oven to 400°F (200°C, or gas mark 6). Lightly grease your muffin tins.

In a medium-size bowl, combine the flour, baking soda, salt, and lemon zest. (Use a lemon zester or a Microplane, which is available in any kitchen supply store.)

In a large bowl, combine the sugar, milk, oil, lemon extract, and vinegar. Mix well. Add the flour mixture, stirring until the ingredients are just blended. Gently fold in the berries using a rubber spatula.

Fill the greased or nonstick muffin tins about two-thirds full. Bake until the muffins are lightly browned and a wooden skewer inserted into the center comes out clean, about 20 minutes. While the muffins are baking, lick the bowl clean. No eggs means no salmonella!

Remove from the oven and let sit for 5 minutes. Remove the muffins from the tins and cool on a wire rack.

Yield: 12 muffins

Originally published in *The Joy of Vegan Baking*

Soy-free, if not using soy milk

QUINOA

Pronounced *KEEN-wa,* this beautiful little grain (which is technically a seed) hails from South America, where it grows in the Andes Mountains of Bolivia, Peru, and Ecuador and has been a staple food for more than 6,000 years. The ancient Incas called it the "mother of all grains," or *chisaya mama.*

For cooking, the ratio of grain to water is about 1:2, though I usually add a little extra water to account for evaporation. Keep in mind before you cook quinoa that it contains a substance called saponin, a phytochemical that acts as the plant's own defense against birds. Convenient though that is for the plant, it can taste rather bitter to humans. To curtail this, rinse the quinoa first in a fine strainer under running water for a minute or two before cooking it.

Once it's rinsed, simply add it to a saucepan with water or broth. Cover, and bring to a boil. Reduce the heat, and simmer for 10 to 15 minutes, until the quinoa has absorbed all the water. You can tell quinoa is done when it is soft to the bite and the seeds have turned translucent. If there is still a lot of water once the quinoa is cooked, just drain it. Fluff with a fork, remove from the heat, and cover for 5 minutes to prevent the quinoa from becoming sticky.

Once it's cooked, you can enjoy it in many ways.

* Eat it plain with a little salt or tamari (soy sauce), or for added sustenance and nutrition stir in some frozen or fresh corn kernels (quinoa and corn pair beautifully together) or steamed kale.

* It can be used in place of brown rice as the bed for any stir-fry or vegetable sauté.

* Quinoa makes a delicious gluten-free tabbouleh.

* Fantastic as a breakfast food, quinoa can be prepared just as you would oatmeal or cornmeal. Once it's cooked, stir in walnuts, almonds, berries, cinnamon, and a little brown sugar. Top with almond milk.

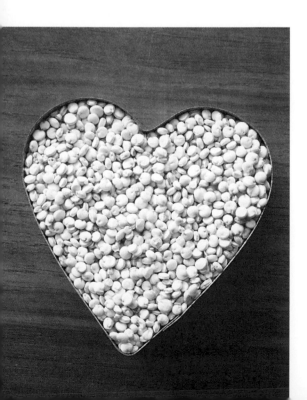

REMEMBERING YOUR STORY

When we go out into the world newly awakened, we become acutely aware of the vast consumption of animal products and we may become easily frustrated by those participating in it. We want to share what we've learned about animal cruelty, about the relationship between animal products and preventable diseases, and everything in between. We want to make others see what we see.

But we will neither make nor keep many friends if our approach is to force this awareness on everyone or judge them for not knowing. We will neither inspire many people nor do ourselves any good.

Remember that we, too, were once unaware. Once, we ate animals and their secretions in ignorant bliss. Perhaps we made stupid jokes, said silly things, defended our behavior. If we remember our story, we'll be less inclined to be

self-righteous, and our responses to non-vegans will become more about finding common ground—not acting superior.

When someone says, "I just love meat too much to give it up" or "I could never give up cheese," you can say: "I did, too. I loved meat. I never thought I'd be able to give up cheese, but I didn't stop eating meat and eggs and cheese because I stopped liking them; I stopped eating them because I just didn't want to cause any suffering." Or, "I thought the same thing—I know, I totally understand—I hear you—I can totally relate." All of these responses create a link between you and the non-vegan.

If people find ways to identify with you, they're more inclined to consider the changes they need to make themselves.

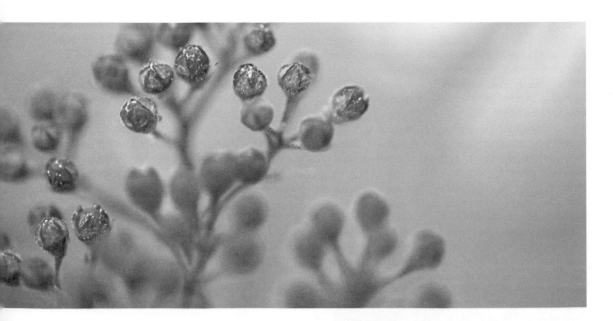

FINDING GRATITUDE

The expression of gratitude can be considered part of a spiritual practice or simply a psychological exercise. It can be a state of mind or a way of life. In its simplest form, it is a way of letting others know we appreciate them. For some people, gratitude comes easily; for others, it takes effort.

Being grateful is really just about being aware of what is already in front of us—and taking a moment to acknowledge it. When we are in a mental state of gratitude, we experience abundance rather than lack. When our consciousness is focused on what we have, there is no room for thoughts about what we don't have. By changing our thoughts, we have the power to change our mood.

This is not to say that we should deny our emotions if we're feeling down, but by making gratitude part of our daily lives, we become less inclined to stay down, and this is essential, particularly for activists who are painfully aware of and regularly exposed to abuses against animals.

Finding gratitude in the midst of despair can be challenging, but it is also vital. Choosing gratitude doesn't mean we deny reality or suffering; it means that we make a conscious decision to look in one direction over another.

And that's what gratitude is: a change in perception. We're continually making choices about how we perceive reality, about how to interpret the world around us. When we change our perception, situations don't change; we do. The way we choose to perceive events or circumstances determines our response to them.

Making a gratitude list each day is a good way to practice being grateful until it becomes natural. The list can be made in your head or written on a piece of paper, but the idea is to take a few moments each day to express gratitude.

The act of expressing gratitude aloud is very powerful, because when we say it out loud, it is so. This is especially true when we tell others how much we appreciate them. Simply uttering "thank you" can go a long way in making someone feel appreciated. In addition to writing our own gratitude list, perhaps we can choose one person each day to just say "I appreciate you" to. It goes a long, long way. Tell them via email, in a card, in person, or on the phone.

ANIMAL POEMS
BY WILLIAM COWPER

William Cowper (pronounced *COO-per)* was a popular English poet in his day, living from 1731 to 1800. A true lover and admirer of animals, he was given some pet hares to help him recover from one of his many plunges into depression, and it worked. He fell in love with these rabbits and named them Bess, Tiney [*sic*], and Puss, feminine names to be sure, but all three males.

Bess died in less than a year, but Tiney lived more than eight years, and Puss lived to nearly twelve, dying on March 9, 1786. The first poem is called "My Pet Hare," and the other, quite famous, is called "Epitaph to a Hare" written for Tiney and making mention of Puss.

Most remarkably, above Cowper's tomb, there is a beautiful stained-glass window, depicting Cowper reading to his pet hares.

My Pet Hare

> Yes—thou mayst eat thy bread, and lick the hand
> That feeds thee; thou mayst frolic on
>   the floor
> At evening, and at night retire secure
> To thy straw couch, and slumber unalarm'd;
> For I have gain'd thy confidence, have pledged
> All that is human in me, to protect
> Thine unsuspecting gratitude and love.
> If I survive thee, I will dig thy grave;
> And, when I place thee in it, sighing say,
> I knew at least one hare that had a friend.

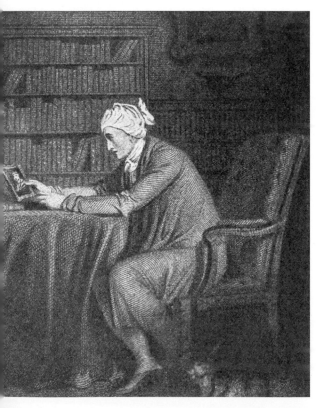

William Cowper (1731–1800)
© Lebrecht Music and Arts Photo Library / Alamy

ANIMAL "LOVER" BECOMES VEGETARIAN, THEN VEGAN

I have always loved animals. "Kitty" was my first word. I used to gently move insects off of walking paths so that my parents and friends would not step on them inadvertently. However, it took a while for me to make the connection between the animals and the food I liked to eat.

My paternal German grandmother, while not anywhere near vegetarian, rescued many animals and supported the Humane Society of the United States and People for the Ethical Treatment of Animals. I would read her PETA magazines when I was little. They turned my stomach and made me cry.

By the time I reached sixth grade, I became vegetarian. Thinking it was just a phase, my parents put meat on my plate for several weeks after I made the declaration that I would never eat meat again. They became very supportive once they realized that I was serious about my vegetarianism.

I soon stopped drinking [cow's] milk but would still eat products containing dairy; I stopped buying leather a few years after that, and I stopped buying wool a few years after that. I knew there was something wrong with eating egg and milk products, but I hid my head in the sand and chose not to read up on the topics. I didn't think it was possible for me to be vegan, mostly because I loved desserts, and I *loved* cheese.

I read *Fast Food Nation*, I watched *Super Size Me*, I felt guiltier and guiltier, and I noticed that my diet was becoming increasingly vegan. I'd grown passionate about animal rights over the years, and I'm embarrassed that it took me so long to finally switch to veganism. If only I had known how easy it would be!

I started listening to vegan podcasts and reading; I had always had vague concerns about nutrition and realized, once I started looking into what I'd need to do to stay healthy, that I would actually be much healthier after cutting out eggs and dairy. I feel so much better than I thought I would, both physically and mentally.

Knowing the reasons behind the importance of going vegan makes all the difference, and I am certain that I will never go back.

—*Lisa in Los Angeles, California (U.S.)*

APPLE COBBLER

Out of all the recipes I have tested, the cobblers were always the hardest to resist!

FILLING

- 5 cups (750 g) peeled and sliced tart apples
- ¾ cup (150 g) granulated sugar
- 2 tablespoons (16 g) unbleached all-purpose flour
- ½ teaspoon ground cinnamon
- ¼ teaspoon salt
- 1 teaspoon vanilla extract
- ¼ cup (60 ml) water

COBBLER BISCUIT DOUGH

- 1 ⅓ cups (165 g) unbleached all-purpose flour
- 3 tablespoons (40 g) granulated sugar, divided
- 1 ½ teaspoons baking powder
- ½ teaspoon salt
- 5 tablespoons (70 g) nondairy butter, melted
- ½ cup (120 ml) nondairy milk (soy, rice, almond, hazelnut, hemp, or oat)
- 1 to 2 tablespoons (15 to 30 ml) nondairy milk or 1 to 2 tablespoons (14 to 28 g) nondairy butter, melted, for brushing top of dough

Preheat the oven to 375°F (190°C, or gas mark 5). Have ready an ungreased 8- or 9-inch (20 or 23 cm) square baking pan at least 2 inches (5 cm) deep.

To make the filling, in a large bowl, combine the apples with the sugar, flour, cinnamon, salt, vanilla, and water. Spread evenly in the prepared baking dish, and set aside.

To make the biscuit dough, combine the flour, 2 tablespoons (26 g) of the granulated sugar, the baking powder, and salt. When completely combined, add the nondairy butter and milk. Stir just until it forms a sticky dough. Set aside.

Using a tablespoon, scoop the dough over the fruit. Either leave the dough in shapeless blobs on the fruit or spread it out. There will be just enough to cover the fruit. Brush the top of the dough with the 1 to 2 tablespoons (15 to 30 ml) milk or 1 to 2 tablespoons (14 to 28 g) butter and the remaining 1 tablespoon (14 g) sugar. Bake until the top is golden brown and the juices have thickened slightly, 35 to 40 minutes. Let cool for 15 minutes before serving.

Yield: 6 to 8 servings

*Soy-free, if not using soy milk

Originally published in *The Joy of Vegan Baking*

OATS

Oats have been touted as a health food for a long time, and they have withstood the pressure. They are indeed incredibly healthful little buggers, and they are one of my favorite foods. Who doesn't love oats?

Types of Oats

The many different oats we have to choose from has to do with how the oats are processed. First, you start off with the oat grain in the hull—nature's protection. When you remove that hull, you're left with the inner portion—the groat. The outer covering of the oat groat is the bran. So, once the hulls are removed, these groats are sized and separated based on the next step in the process, which is when they're sized again. Using a sharp, mechanical blade, the groats are "steel-cut" into, essentially, three different sizes: coarse, regular, and fine.

* Steel-cut oats are sold as is and aren't flattened or processed in any other way, and because they're just essentially coarse grains, they're nuttier, chewier, and more nutritious than rolled oats. They also take a little longer to cook.

* Rolled oats are these steel-cut oats that have been steamed, rolled, resteamed, and toasted.

* Quick-cooking oats are rolled oats that have been cut into several pieces before being steamed and rolled.

* Instant oats have been precooked and dried before being rolled.

* Oatmeal refers to a meal made from crushed, rolled, or cut oats.

* Porridge is a simple dish that can be made by boiling oats in water and nondairy milk. In Ireland and Scotland, it's traditional to use steel-cut oats. In England and the United States, rolled oats are used.

* Oat bran is intact in rolled and steel-cut oats; it's just the outer covering of that oat groat, but of course it can also be extracted and sold separately as oat bran.

Cooking Methods and Times

Different types of oats require slightly different cooking methods for making hot cereal or porridge.

* For all types, it's best to add the oats to a pot with cold water or nondairy milk and then cook at a simmer.

* The preparation of rolled oats and steel-cut oats require similar proportions of two parts water to one part oats.

* Rolled oats take approximately 15 minutes to cook, whereas the steel-cut variety takes about 30 minutes.

* The easiest way to prepare quick-cooking oats for oatmeal is to mix them with boiling water and let them sit for about 5 minutes.

* Prepackaged, flavored "instant oatmeal" offers fewer oats, less nutrition, and added sugar—for a lot more money. It's much better to just buy oats in bulk, and then add whatever you want to your porridge or oatmeal.

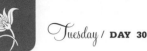
COMPASSIONATE ALTERNATIVE:
LIKE A CHICKEN WITH HIS HEAD CUT OFF

Although most people would say they "love" birds, our language certainly doesn't reflect that.

To "run around like a chicken with his head cut off" means, of course, to run around in a frenzied manner. The origin, as you can surmise, relates to birds who may sometimes run around frenziedly for several minutes after decapitation. This unpleasant phrase was known in the United States by the late nineteenth century, and it is recorded in print as being used as a simile from the 1880s. Preferring instead to let chickens keep their heads, I vote for less violent ways to make our point; something as simple as "He ran around in a frenzied state" is sufficient.

MAKING WHOLE FOODS THE FOUNDATION OF YOUR DIET

Bombarded with diet fads, biased information about nutrition, and sound bites from "experts," most people, including vegans, are utterly confused about what their guiding principle should be when it comes to making food choices.

I offer two words: *whole foods.*

Whole foods refers to food that is unprocessed and unrefined (or processed very little). Basically, it's food that is as close to its natural state as possible. For instance:

* Corn is a whole food. Corn flakes are not, because the corn has been processed.

* Brown rice is a whole food. White rice is not, because it's been stripped of its bran and fiber.

* Fruit is whole food. Fruit loops are not. Neither is fruit leather, fruit-flavored candy, or fruit roll-ups.

You get the idea.

Whole foods are fruits, vegetables, nuts, seeds, legumes, grains, and mushrooms. Whole foods don't have added ingredients; whole foods are colorful because of their phytochemical pigments—not because of additives, dyes, or packaging.

My recommendation is to make whole foods the foundation of our diet, which is a realistic and manageable goal. Notice that my recommendation is not to "eat only whole foods." Because it's not a realistic goal, it has the effect of making us feel bad about ourselves when we make other-than-whole choices.

Making the foundation of our diet whole foods means we can allow ourselves to have processed foods once in a while and still feel good about the majority of the food we put in our bodies.

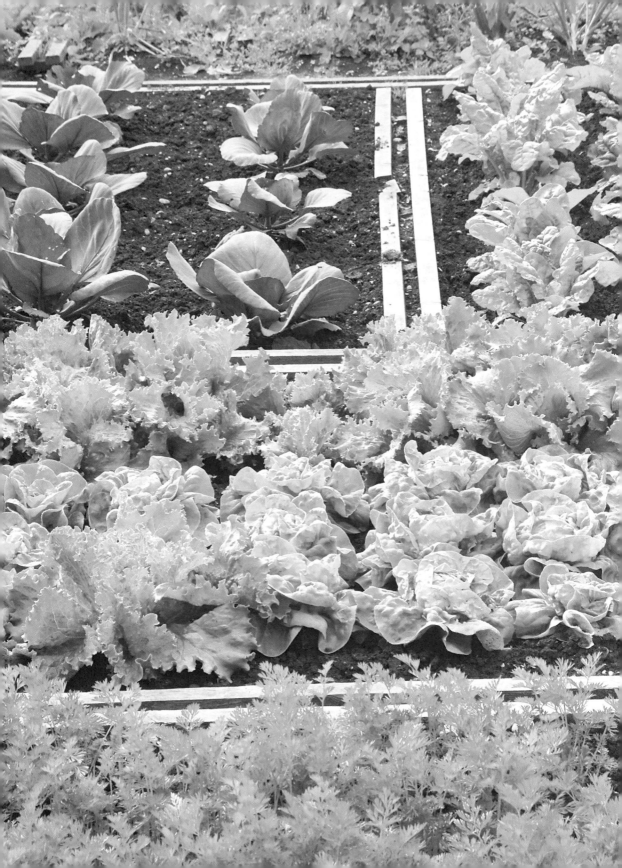

"THE LOTTERY"
BY SHIRLEY JACKSON

Although it's not an animal story, the short story "The Lottery" by Shirley Jackson sheds light on humanity's tendency to cling blindly to meaningless rituals and participate in pointless violence and speaks volumes about the tight grip our meat-eating habits have on us.

About the annual selection of a sacrificial victim in a small American town, the haunting story first appeared in *The New Yorker* magazine in 1948.

It opens on a warm summer day in a small New England town of about three hundred people, who gather to participate in an annual event, which is ostensibly a tradition among surrounding villages as well. Mr. Summers arrives with the black wooden box from which everyone is to draw a folded slip of paper. Whoever draws the slip of paper with the black dot on it "wins the lottery."

Despite the fact that no one in town remembers why or how the lottery began, everyone continues to observe it year after year solely because it is *tradition,* a tradition they are not willing to give up.

After each of the townspeople draws a slip of paper from the black box, Tessie Hutchinson is identified as the one with the black dot, and despite her protests, everyone, including her children, picks up rocks, closes in on her, and stones her to death.

By the end of the story, the reader is forced to confront our attachment to vacuous rituals that exist for their own sake. In my many years as an animal advocate, I've heard countless excuses for our use and abuse of animals, but I'm often taken aback by the one that concludes that certain practices are justifiable because they're embedded in the "culture" and sanctified by "tradition," as if that's all the reason we need to justify our behavior.

Nobody wants to see themselves as contributing to cruelty, but participating in cultural customs? Carrying out tradition? That doesn't sound so bad. To shroud our violence against animals in the sanctity of "tradition" is to romanticize our exploitation of them.

"Pack of crazy fools. Next thing you know, they'll be wanting to go back to living in caves," one of the townspeople declares when he hears about a neighboring village that has ceased holding the lottery. "There's always been a lottery," he says, justifying its continuation on its ritual past. We justify our use of animals in a similar way: "People have always eaten animals," we say.

But just because we always have done something doesn't mean we always have to. Just because we can doesn't mean we should. After all, one culture's traditions are another culture's taboos.

SEEING ANIMALS FOR THE FIRST TIME

I had been a meat-eater most of my life, but for the last ten years I had been really into fitness and a healthy lifestyle. This has made me look at vegetarian options and the benefits of being a vegetarian from a purely nutritional standpoint.

Recently, a vegan friend from college asked me why, if I believed "compassion" was so important, I ate "innocent animals." Something clicked. Just a few days earlier one of our dogs, Gidget, had passed away having been bitten by a black snake. I'm sure this, combined with my friend's question, somehow awakened my mind. Now I had both health and ethics to consider. That night, I typed "compassion" and "vegetarian" into Google and found the *Food for Thought* podcast, and I watched a video on slaughter. I literally "woke up."

I do not handle blood and gore very well, but I forced myself to watch the whole video. I had, and still have, that horrible feeling I think all vegans can identify with—where you just see the enormity of the problem and feel brainwashed by the media and the food lobbyists. I felt helpless but absolutely compelled to act.

The problem was telling my wife. She grew up with her family breeding "stud cattle." About six months ago, I told her I wanted to go vegetarian and was met with firm protests about how restrictive it would be. I did not follow through with it as a result, but this time I told her I was going vegetarian and that I was going to try and not have dairy. I then broke it to her the next day that I was adopting a vegan lifestyle. Because of my joy and conviction this time around, it went surprisingly well.

In addition to our remaining dogs and cats, we have horses, chickens, sheep, and a steer, whom we love as our companions. Wearing my new vegan cap, I feel like I am seeing these animals for the first time. The joy I now feel as a vegan is just amazing. It is easily the best decision I have ever made.

—*Ian in Dubbo, Australia*

CHOCOLATE MOUSSE

This quick and delicious dessert has been a favorite of mine for years, and it's a favorite of everyone who tries it. You won't miss the dairy in this rich and creamy mousse that's also perfect as a pie filling.

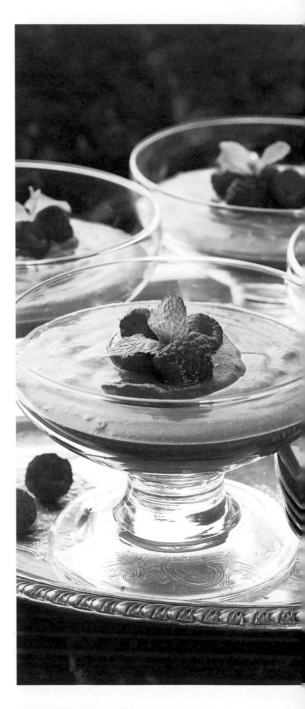

> 1 cup (175 g) nondairy semisweet chocolate chips
> 12 ounces (340 g) silken tofu (soft or firm)
> ½ cup (120 ml) nondairy milk (soy, rice, almond, hazelnut, hemp, or oat)
> ½ teaspoon vanilla extract
> Fresh berries for serving (optional)

Put the chocolate chips in a microwave-safe bowl, and set it in the microwave for 1 minute. Give the chips a stir, and heat for another minute. They should be melted at this point; just give it another quick stir. (You can also melt the chips by creating your own double boiler. Place the chips in a small saucepan. Set this pan in a larger pot that is filled with ¼ to ½ cup [60 to 120 ml] water. Heat over medium heat and stir the chips in the small pot until they are melted.)

Place the tofu in a blender or food processor. Add the melted chocolate, milk, and vanilla. Process until completely smooth, pausing the blender or food processor to scrape down the sides and under the blade, if necessary.

Chill the mixture in serving bowls—or in a low-fat graham cracker or cookie crust—for at least 1 hour before serving. Add fresh berries just before serving, if desired.

Yield: 6 servings

*Wheat-free, oil-free

Originally published in *The Joy of Vegan Baking*

CACAO NIBS

One of the most common misconceptions about being vegan is that you "can't eat chocolate." Aside from the fact that I *can* eat whatever I want (I just *choose not* to eat the flesh and secretions of animals), chocolate is indeed vegan! Chocolate comes from the cacao tree and more specifically from cacao seeds, which are contained in large pods. These seeds are essentially what we call the *cocoa bean*.

Cacao nibs are basically raw pieces of cocoa beans; they're sold in small pieces either raw or roasted.

With their smoky flavor, roasted cacao nibs taste similar to roasted coffee beans, and both the raw and the roasted nibs have a bittersweet flavor. Essentially, unsweetened cocoa powder is just finely ground cacao nibs. If you like very dark chocolate, you'll love nibs.

Often, nibs are eaten as part of other chocolate items, such as dark chocolate bars scattered with raw nibs, but you can also buy them separately to eat as a snack or to add to your own baked goods. Add them to cookies, brownies, and muffins in place of or in addition to chocolate chips; sprinkle them on chili or ice cream; or roll them into your favorite chocolate truffle.

It's true there are antioxidants in cacao nibs, but I'd rather see you look for these healthful phytochemicals in kale, carrots, or blueberries. If you want a dose of antioxidants from cacao nibs, be sure to buy them raw and unprocessed.

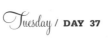

COMPASSIONATE ALTERNATIVES: **SKINNING A CAT**

Several idioms involve cats—many of which invoke violence against our feline friends.

One particularly horrific expression is, "There's more than one way to skin a cat." Apparently, the expression refers to a gymnastic move, whereby you hang by your hands from a bar, draw your legs up through your arms and over the bar, and pull yourself up into a sitting position. It did not appear in print until 1845, but it was most likely used verbally before it was written down.

Despite the fact that it refers to a gymnastic position, I'd rather use a less violent expression to communicate the fact that there's more than one way to do something. How about: "There's more than one way to peel a potato" or "There's more than one way to squeeze a lemon." They are even more colorful and evocative than the gruesome original.

GIVING YOURSELF PERMISSION TO CRY

Facilitating emotional healing and reducing stress, crying—like laughing—is good for our health. Though cultural norms are changing, men have traditionally been discouraged to cry, and evidence suggests this is why men tend to develop more stress-related diseases than women do.

For people exposed to images and stories of animal abuse, crying is essential for dealing with this trauma. On a smaller scale—but no less significant—vegans are often in scenarios that cause them added stress, such as the following.

* Dealing with insensitive remarks about being vegan.

* Coping with being a lone vegan without support from like-minded folks, continually confronted by meat and other products borne of violence.

* Enduring social pressure to conform and eat meat, dairy, and eggs.

Shedding a few tears can provide the relief and healing needed to feel empowered, strong, and refreshed.

"THE SLAUGHTERER"
BY ISAAC BASHEVIS SINGER

A prolific writer, Isaac Bashevis Singer, born in Poland, published at least eighteen novels, fourteen children's books, and a number of memoirs, essays, and articles, but he is best known for his short stories.

For the last thirty-five years of his life, Singer was a proud and vocal vegetarian, and he often included such themes in his works.

"The Slaughterer," a powerful and harrowing indictment against ritually sanctioned slaughter, describes the anguish that an appointed ritual slaughterer experiences as he tries to reconcile his compassion for animals with his job of slaughtering animals.

Although "he could not bear the sight of blood," Yoineh Meir is appointed the town's ritual

slaughterer. A pious and "soft-hearted" man, he is pressured by his wife and the town elders and begins a nightmare journey from which he does not return.

Constantly immersed in blood and violence, Yoineh Meir spirals into depression and eventually madness but begins to experience a profound love "for all that crawls and flies, breeds and swarms." He sees no way the Messiah can redeem the world as long as such injustice is perpetrated against animals. He concludes that "when you slaughter a creature, you slaughter God."

Finding no consolation even in his religion, Yoineh Meir, perceiving the whole world to be a slaughterhouse, flees to the river and drowns himself.

COMPASSION FOR DOGS AND CATS TURNS INTO COMPASSION FOR ALL ANIMALS

I have always considered myself an animal lover. We always had at least one cat while I was growing up and sometimes we had dogs, too. I thought of animal suffering in terms of dogs and cats being run over and left in the street, euthanized at the pound, or killed for no reason by cruel people.

In high school, I became aware of animals being used in laboratory testing for cosmetics and household products and requested information from People for the Ethical Treatment of Animals. I was shocked by the pictures showing the abuses suffered by rabbits, monkeys, and even dogs and cats. I began to buy only from companies that didn't perform tests on animals. Eventually, I became a member of PETA and started receiving their *Animal Times* magazine.

When I was twenty-two, I was working at Baskin-Robbins. I would read my *Animal Times* during my half-hour lunch break. I remember being so sad at the articles detailing animal testing, but not really reading much of the articles talking about farm animal suffering. I think I'd just look at the photos and say to myself, "Oh, that's so awful, those poor animals." I just thought it would be too hard to be vegetarian.

One day at work, I sat reading my latest issue of *Animal Times* while eating a 99-cent Whopper I'd just purchased from Burger King. I was reading an article about cattle, and how they're kept on feedlots. And it dawned on me . . . I'm eating a cow (well, several cows) who suffered terribly and who is an animal just like my beloved cats at home.

So I decided to go vegetarian. I checked books out of the library about how to eat, how to make sure I got enough of what I needed. I read all I could and vowed that "someday I'll be vegan." It took me nine years.

I feel that vegan is what I was meant to be—that there was simply no other way my life would end up. I love being vegan, and I'm just sorry it took me so long.

—*Kerrie in California (U.S.)*

PAN-GRILLED PORTOBELLO MUSHROOMS WITH HERB-INFUSED MARINADE

Portobello mushrooms are a wonderful "main dish" due to their heartiness, meatiness, and size.

8 to 12 large portobello mushrooms
½ cup (120 ml) balsamic vinegar
½ cup (120 ml) tamari soy sauce
½ cup (120 ml) water
2 or 3 sprigs fresh rosemary
  (or 1 teaspoon [1 g] dried)
2 or 3 sprigs fresh thyme
  (or 1 teaspoon [1 g] dried)
2 or 3 sprigs fresh marjoram or oregano
  (or 1 teaspoon [1 g] dried)
1 to 2 tablespoons (15 to 30 ml) olive oil,
  for sautéing
Freshly ground black pepper

Remove the stems from the underside of the mushrooms and lightly wipe the tops with a damp paper towel.

In a large bowl, combine the vinegar, tamari, water, rosemary, thyme, and marjoram. Stir to combine. Add the mushrooms and make sure each one is covered by the marinade. You may need to move them around to give the marinade a chance to coat the top mushrooms. Marinate the mushrooms for as little as 30 minutes or for as long as overnight in the refrigerator.

When ready to cook, add some of the oil to a large sauté pan over medium heat. Remove the mushrooms from the marinade, but do not discard the marinade. Put as many mushrooms as can fit in the pan, tops down. They will shrink as they cook. Cook for 3 to 5 minutes, until lightly browned. Turn and cook for 3 to 5 minutes longer.

Remove the fresh herb sprigs from the marinade, and pour the marinade into the pan, reserving some for additional batches of mushrooms. Cover and cook for 5 to 7 minutes. Flip the mushrooms, and cover and cook for 5 to 7 minutes longer. When fork-tender, remove from the pan, and repeat with the remaining mushrooms.

To serve the mushrooms hot, simply use multiple sauté pans on the stove at once. Serve 2 mushrooms per person.

Yield: 4 to 6 servings

*Wheat-free

Originally published in *The Vegan Table*

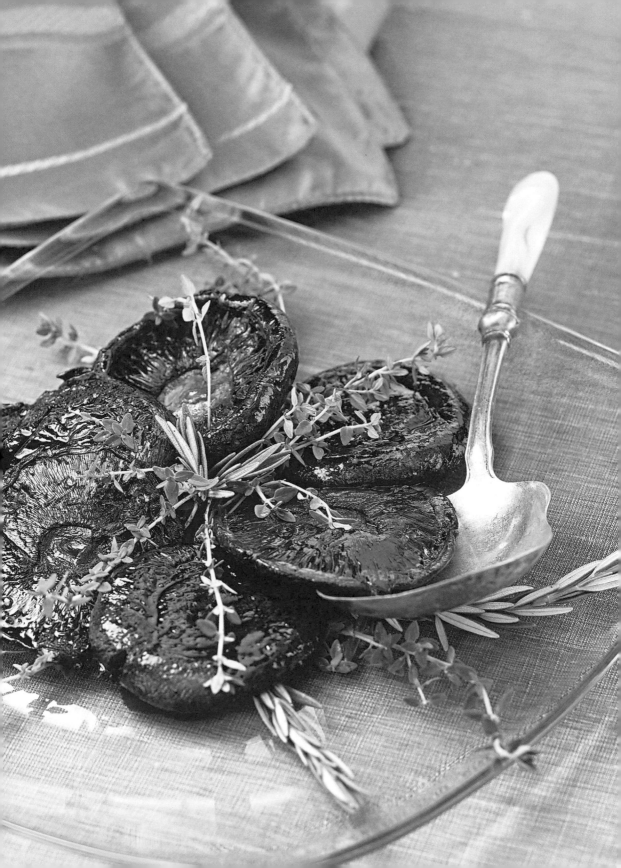

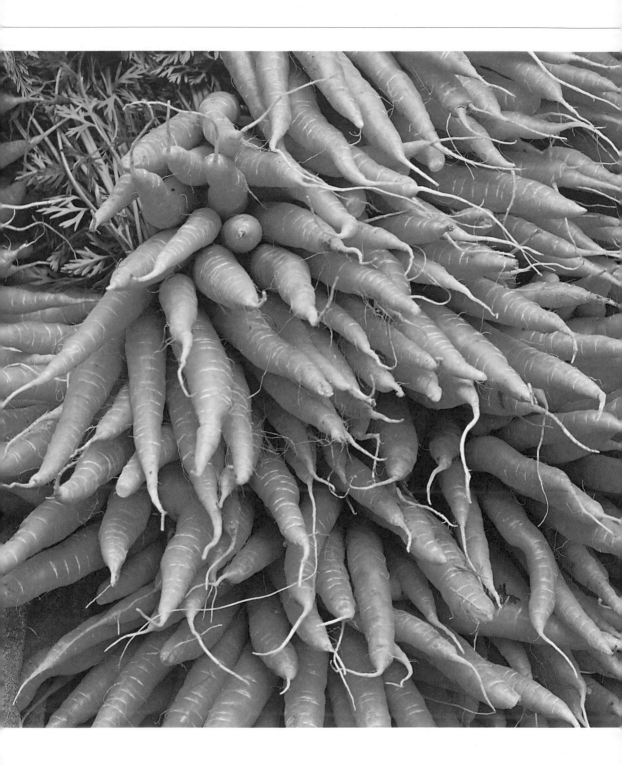

CARROTS

The bright orange color of the modern carrot is a clue to their healthfulness, though carrots were originally purple. The beta-carotene saturated in carrots—and other orange-yellow plant foods—has been found to provide protection against lung, bladder, breast, esophageal, and stomach cancers; heart disease; and the progression of arthritis.

These days, there is a lot of discussion about raw vegetables versus cooked vegetables, and carrots often come up in this context. Let me settle this once and for all: eat both! Technically, because the cell walls of raw carrots are incredibly strong, we tend to absorb less of the beta-carotene when we eat them raw. But that doesn't mean we should eat only cooked. Both have their advantages, and since raw and cooked carrots are equally delicious, eat both!

Some people talk about the "vegan glow" that many vegans emit, and I think most of it comes from the inside: the radiance that comes from living in alignment with your values and expressing that joyfully and compassionately in your behavior. But, it also comes from carrots!

Carrots, and other vegetables high in beta-carotene, quite literally do give you a glow—a bit of an orange glow. Increased consumption of carrots tends to tint your skin, which I think is a good sign that you're eating a healthful diet. Compare your skin to someone who's eating a typical American diet full of animal products and processed foods, and you may find a dull, pale, ashen hue versus the bright, sunny glow of someone consuming a diet rich in plant foods.

* Carrots are so easy to slice up and eat as a snack; they're portable; they're great with peanut butter; and I never eat a salad without them.

* Carrot juice is a regular staple in my diet. You can buy it already prepared or make it yourself. You do tend to sacrifice fiber when you juice carrots, because in juicing, you extract the pulp, and the pulp is where the fiber is. You can use the pulp to make carrot muffins or carrot cake.

* "Baby carrots" are bred to be small, not flavorful. Not only do they contain less beta-carotene than regular carrots, but also their flavor is artificial to me, lacking the earthiness of regular carrots.

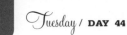

KNOWING YOUR INTENTIONS

Although this may come as a surprise, my intention in the work I do is not to make the world vegan. My intention is not to change someone else's mind. If those were my intentions, I would fail every time. It's not my role to make anyone do anything. All I can do is speak the truth and trust that it will inspire others to act on their own values. That's why I don't like the word *convert*. I prefer *inspire* or *empower*. I never set out to convert anyone.

Whenever I speak on behalf of animals, I make sure I'm clear about this intention. Before I speak to a group, record a podcast episode, or even answer someone's question one-on-one, I make sure—in my mind—I'm clear about my intention, and my intention is this:

* To raise awareness about the suffering of animals, to be their voice, and to speak my truth.

That's it.

Intention is everything, and people individually and collectively are smart enough to see right through you if you appear false to them—if you appear to have a hidden agenda, if you're saying one thing but you really mean another. Having a clear intention about your goal and making that goal about *truth* rather than *outcome* will make you a successful, effective advocate 100 percent of the time.

If someone asks me why I'm vegan, I tell *my* truth, *my* story, *my* reason for being vegan, which is—in short—to not contribute to suffering and violence where I have the power to do so.

Nobody can take away my story. No one can say, "That's wrong" or "That's not true."

So, if my intention is to raise awareness, be a voice for animals, and speak my truth, my intention will always be met. My goal will always be accomplished, because I didn't set out to do anything other than tell the truth, and I may have planted some seeds along the way.

DOING WHAT YOU LOVE

I hear from so many people who desperately want to work on behalf of animals or veganism but don't know what they're supposed to do or how they'll make money doing it.

The answer lies in two questions: What do you love? What are you good at?

I believe the work we're supposed to do in this world is an extension of our passion and our gifts. Each of us has a unique contribution to make, but many of us struggle with what it is, because we're asking the wrong questions. In our profit-driven culture, we're taught to ask, "What can I do that will bring me money?" As a result, millions of people are doing work that pays the bills but brings little joy and satisfaction.

That doesn't mean there's anything wrong with making money, but if that's all we're looking to gain, then that's all we'll get. If, however, our intention is to share our unique gifts with the world—and we are willing to work to make this happen—then we can be sure that we will be given what we need to support that.

I see so many people in unhappy jobs who admit they really want to be doing something else, but very few of them are doing anything about it. I believe that we create what we want, but it's not enough to just say, "What I really want to do is work with animals" or "I would love to work for a national park." We have to take the steps to make our dreams a reality. That might mean building our dream while we're working full time to earn a living.

When it comes to working on behalf of veganism and animal rights, in particular, I encourage you to be true to yourself. I don't believe that in order to do good work in this world, you have to be poor. On the flip side, I don't believe that if you make money, you're just a greedy mercenary. The animals don't need us to be martyrs; they need us to operate at our highest so that we can do the most effective work on their behalf and be joyful and supported while doing so.

With that as our goal, we can't help but succeed and find our calling.

"A MOTHER'S TALE"
BY JAMES AGEE

James Agee was an American novelist, screen-writer (he cowrote *The African Queen*), journalist, poet, and film critic. His autobiographical novel, *A Death in the Family*, published posthumously in 1957, won the Pulitzer Prize after he died, which was in 1955.

He wrote "A Mother's Tale" in 1952, and what a gem it is.

The story opens as a cow, her calf, and the other "spring calves" watch a cattle drive off in the distance. The naive calves want to know where the cattle are going, but the cow reluctantly tells them they're going to the railroad and assures the curious calves that it will most likely take them to a "nice" place, at which point her own calf declares that he wants to go, too. Unable to convince them that it's better to stay safe at home and goaded by their insistence to know the final destination, she tells them a grisly story about "one who came back," a story passed down from her great-grandmother.

Having been to the slaughterhouse, one particular steer—half alive, partially butchered—escapes and makes a painful journey back home to warn the others. He tells of the arduous train journey with no food and water, packed in the train cars such that "their sides pressed tightly together and nobody could lie down."

He tells of having been hung upside down by the tendons of his heels, of having his hide torn from him, of knives that "would slice along both flanks." He tells of jerking himself free and charging at the "men with the knives."

When he returns to the range, he urgently gathers the cattle together and warns them: "Break down the fences! Tell everybody, everywhere. All who are put on the range are put onto trains. All who are put onto trains meet the Man With The Hammer. All who stay home are kept there to breed others to go onto the range, and so betray themselves and their kind and their children forever. We are brought into this life only to be victims; and there is no other way for us unless we save ourselves."

Upon finishing the story, the cow realizes she has scared the calves and tries to convince them that the tale is untrue. "It's just an old, old legend," she says. "We use it to frighten children." Unmoved, her young calf tacitly decides he will go to the railroad and find out for himself.

FROM NEGLECT TO SANCTUARY

On one of my recent visits to Cleveland Amory Black Beauty Ranch, the sanctuary was still reeling from a huge rescue of hundreds of horses from a Nebraska ranch. Rescue staff and volunteers worked around the clock for weeks caring for 222 horses who had endured gross neglect and cruelty.

Eighty-four of those neglected horses arrived safely at CABBR where they were further rehabilitated and eventually adopted. Having seen footage and photos of the shameful condition of the horses when they were first brought in, I was amazed to see how fully they had recovered. Virtually unrecognizable, these horses were no longer underweight or covered in lice; they were thriving, healthy, energetic, and free.

The Humane Society, Habitat for Horses, and Front Range Equine Rescue transformed these wild horses into confident individuals and worked to find appropriate permanent homes for them. Most of the horses were stallions and geldings and required special care and handling.

In response to the many rescue cases CABBR takes on, the Doris Day Animal Foundation recently agreed to sponsor construction of a new state-of-the-art horse rehabilitation and adoption facility at the sanctuary, which will be called the Doris Day Horse Rescue and Adoption Center.

—*CPG*

A horse and a donkey footloose and fancy-free at CBBR

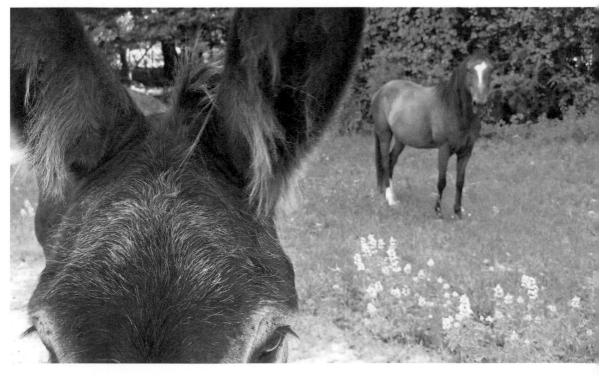

TOFU-CHARD BURGERS

A very easy recipe to throw together when you've got some chard and tofu begging to be used, these burgers can be made in advance and cooked the next day.

> 8 ounces (225 g) extra-firm tofu
> 2 tablespoons (30 ml) canola or olive oil, divided
> 1 bunch chard, finely chopped
> 3 tablespoons (45 ml) tamari soy sauce
> 2 teaspoons (14 g) agave nectar
> 2 teaspoons (10 ml) sesame oil
> 2 cloves garlic, minced
> 1 teaspoon (2.7 g) grated fresh ginger
> 3/4 cup (90 g) toasted bread crumbs
> 1/3 cup (27 g) finely ground walnuts

Cut the tofu into 1/2-inch (1.3 cm) slices and arrange them in a single layer on half of a dish towel. Fold the towel over, and place something heavy on top, such as a cutting board or a heavy sauté pan. This is to drain out some of the water in the tofu. Let stand for about 15 minutes. Once it's drained of excess water, crumble the tofu by hand, or pulse in a food processor until it's a coarse crumb.

Meanwhile, heat 1 tablespoon (15 ml) of the oil in a sauté pan over medium heat. Add the chard and cook until fully wilted, about 4 minutes. Transfer to a plate, and let cool. When cool enough, use your hands to squeeze out the excess water over the sink.

Using a paper towel, wipe out the sauté pan, and add the tamari, agave nectar, and sesame oil. Over medium heat, stir to combine the ingredients. After a minute or so, add the crumbled tofu, and toss until much of the liquid is absorbed, about 10 minutes.

Add the chopped chard, garlic, and ginger, and cook for another 5 minutes, until all the ingredients are thoroughly combined. Transfer to a bowl, and add the bread crumbs and ground walnuts. Mix until fully incorporated. Store in the refrigerator for up to 3 days if not using right away, or shape into 6 patties. (Even after you make the patties, you can put them in the fridge until you're ready to cook them.)

In a sauté pan over medium heat, add the remaining 1 tablespoon (15 ml) oil (or a little more, if needed), and cook the patties until browned on each side, about 10 minutes total.

Yield: 6 burgers

Serving Suggestions and Variations

* Substitute the bread crumbs for 1/3 cup (27 g) cooked oatmeal.

* Spinach is a good alternative if you don't have chard.

SWISS CHARD

Next to kale, Swiss chard is my favorite dark green leafy vegetable. The leaves themselves range from dark green to dark purple, with stems of white, yellow, pink, or red, depending on the cultivar. Often at farmers' markets, you'll also see "rainbow chard," which just refers to bunches of different-colored chard stems.

Packed with vitamins K, A, C, and E; fiber; folate; iron; and potassium, chard belongs to the same family as beets and spinach and is similar in taste to both: it has the bitterness of beet greens and the slightly salty flavor of spinach leaves. Both the leaves and the stems are edible, although the stems vary in texture, with the white ones being the most tender. Depending on how tough they are, the stems may take a little longer to cook if you add them to a dish at the same time as the leaves. One way to solve this is to slice the stems very thinly.

Reducing in size by half when it's cooked, chard—like spinach—becomes very soft and buttery when cooked.

* Add it to soups and stews.

* Use it in place of spinach.

* Add it to a vegetable sauté.

* Chop it finely to eat as a salad.

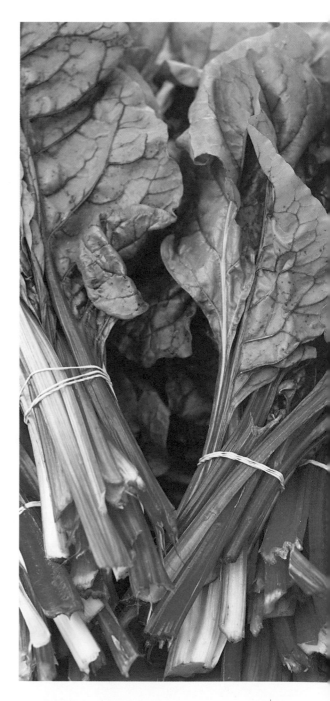

ASKING QUESTIONS INSTEAD OF HAVING ANSWERS

Because there are so many myths and misconceptions about being vegan, when people encounter a vegan, they often accost him or her with questions. They assume that you—the vegan—have all the answers; that you've thought it all through; that you have advanced degrees in nutrition, philosophy, anthropology, animal husbandry, ecology, and the culinary arts.

And because we feel that each encounter is our *one* opportunity to inspire people to think differently about the food they choose, we often feel that we have to have all the answers. It is important to be informed about related issues, but it is virtually impossible to be an expert in all these fields.

Sometimes, what's more important than having all the answers is *asking questions.*

Not only does this take some of the pressure off, but asking questions also engages other people in a way that makes them feel heard and gives you the information you need to respond to them personally—not in some generic, impersonal way. Asking questions invites dialogue, and that's what is sorely needed when it comes to this topic.

For instance,

* If someone says, "I could never be vegan," you could ask, "Why? What do you think would be so difficult for you?"

* If someone says, "I don't want to know what happens to the animals," you could ask, "What do you think would happen if you found out?"

* If someone says, "I tried being vegan, but I needed protein." Instead of spouting off the many protein-rich plant foods, you could ask, "How did that manifest itself? What happened to you physically that you realized it was protein you were missing?"

By asking questions, we explore with people where they're resistant. Most likely, no one has ever gently probed them to find out more about why they don't want to know. They may never have been encouraged to reflect on their own thoughts and feelings.

This doesn't mean you can never answer questions, but just don't be afraid to ask.

TOASTING BEFORE YOU DRINK

The practice of toasting began in ancient Greece, when the fear of being poisoned was a real concern. To alleviate his guests' concerns, the host would pour everyone's wine from a common decanter, take the first drink to demonstrate its safety, then raise his cup and invite his guests to drink in good health.

During Christmas celebrations in the United Kingdom, drinking wassail (a hot spiced punch) involves floating a piece of toasted bread in one's cup. The term *toast* may come from this practice.

Whether accompanied by a blessing or a wish for good tidings, the simple act of raising you glass to someone is all you need to constitute a toast. The Irish, with their gift for language, have made toasting an art form, though every culture partakes in this ritual in one way or another.

A ritual in its own right, a toast technically consists of three parts:

* The verbal toast, which could be as simple as "Cheers!" or as elaborate as an anecdote followed by a declaration of good wishes.

* The agreement, signified by the raising of glasses and often accompanied by words of concurrence, by either repeating the toast word ("Cheers!") or confirming the sentiment ("Hear! Hear!"). What follows next is the touching or clinking of glasses.

* The drinking of the beverage, which "seals" the blessing.

Many people panic at the idea of leading a spontaneous toast, but if you speak from the heart, you can't go wrong.

EXCERPT FROM "QUEEN MAB"
BY PERCY BYSSHE SHELLEY

This excerpt from Percy Bysshe Shelley's "Queen Mab," written in 1813, expresses his convictions about vegetarianism. For more about Percy Bysshe Shelley, see Day 326.

> How strange is human pride!
> I tell thee that those living things,
> . . .
> Is an unbounded world;
> I tell thee that those viewless beings,
> Whose mansion is the smallest particle
> Of the impassive atmosphere,
> Think, feel, and live like man;

> That their affections and antipathies,
> Like his, produce the Laws
> Ruling their moral state.
> . . .
> Immortal upon Earth: No longer now,
> He slays the lamb that looks him in the face,
> And horribly devours his mangled flesh,
> Which, still avenging nature's broken law,
> Kindled all putrid humours in his frame,
> All evil passions, and all vain belief,
> Hatred, despair, and loathing in his mind,
> The germs of misery, death, disease, and crime.

BONNIE, THE BURRO

Bonnie is a donkey (burro) who was brought to the Farm Sanctuary's California shelter in 1995. She was about five years young at the time. She's a little girl—not huge—with a beautiful brown coat. And she is an absolute sweetheart.

When she first arrived, she could barely stand or walk. The hooves on all four of her feet had overgrown by 11 inches (28 cm) or more and were curling underneath so far that they were hitting the backs of her legs. She struggled to simply remain upright, and with each step she took, she had to cautiously lift each foot high off the ground, set her mangled hoof down, and then try to regain balance all over again. She was covered in lice, and hair was missing in huge patches all along her body.

Rescued from a private home, she had been confined to a 10 by 15-foot (3 by 4.6 m) paddock—apparently her entire life. Each day for five years, she lived without proper shelter and without proper drainage, so when she was found, she was quite literally knee-deep in mud and manure.

The vet who looked at her right away determined that her hooves had never been trimmed. All four feet had severe and painful hoof rot, and as they trimmed away at the excess hoof material, Bonnie just endured it without complaint. Clearly, she knew who her saviors were.

X-rays showed that the bones in all four of her feet were rotated and severely deformed, and experts said she wouldn't live long. They also said that she would never be able to really walk or stand, and some suggested she be euthanized. Boy, did she prove them wrong.

With her incredible spirit, Bonnie continued to get stronger and healthier with each passing year, and she and her buddy, Waylon—a tall, handsome, gray and black burro—can be found in the far-off pastures of the sanctuary, eating, hanging out, and braying to one another. Bonnie has her hooves trimmed every six weeks and loves to be brushed and doted on by her caregivers.

—*Farm Sanctuary, Orland, California (U.S.)*

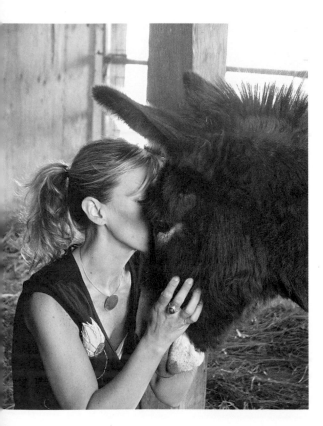

Colleen and Bonnie at Farm Santuary

PEANUT BUTTER–CHOCOLATE BARS

My good friend Tami Wall, who graced me with this delicious delight, recommends that the baking pan be very well buttered, so take heed!

2 cups (100 g) crispy rice cereal, crushed
1½ cups (390 g) natural peanut butter
2 cups (200 g) confectioners' sugar
½ cup plus 2 tablespoons (140 g) nondairy butter, melted, divided
1 teaspoon vanilla extract
½ cup (90 g) nondairy semisweet chocolate chips

Generously butter a 9 x 13-inch (23 x 33 cm) baking pan.

In a large bowl, combine the cereal, peanut butter, confectioners' sugar, ½ cup (112 g) of the butter, and vanilla. Press the mixture into the prepared baking pan.

In a small saucepan (or double boiler) melt together the chocolate chips and the remaining 2 tablespoons (28 g) butter, stirring constantly. Remove from the heat.

Spread the chocolate mixture over the top of the peanut butter mixture. Set aside for 1 to 2 hours to set.

Yield: 12 to 18 squares, depending on size

*Wheat-free, soy-free if using soy-free Earth Balance

Originally published in *The Joy of Vegan Baking*

COOKING GRAINS

Grains are one of the easiest things to cook, as long as you know how to boil water. Cooking times and grain: liquid ratios vary. Here is a helpful guide.

Grain Type	Grain: Liquid Ratio	Cooking Time
Brown Rice (short or long)*	1 cup (190 g): 2 or 2½ cups (470 or 588 ml)	45 minutes
Basmati Rice* (white)	1 cup (195 g): 1¾ cups (411 ml)	20 minutes
Basmati Rice* (brown)	1 cup (190 g): 2 cups (470 ml)	40 to 45 minutes
Bulgur Wheat	1 cup (140 g): 2½ cups (588 ml)	Simmer for 25 minutes, fluff, let sit for 10 minutes; or boil the water, pour over bulgur, cover, and let sit for 1 hour.
Quinoa* (pronounced KEEN-wah)	1 cup (173 g): 2 to 3 cups (470 to 705 ml)	15 to 20 minutes
Couscous (pronounced <KOOS-koos)	1 cup (175 g): 1½ cups (353 ml)	Bring water to a boil. Add couscous, 1 tablespoon (14 g) Earth Balance or olive oil, and ½ teaspoon salt. Remove from heat, stir, cover, and let stand for 10 minutes. Fluff with fork.
Amaranth*	1 cup (193 g): 3 cups (705 ml)	Mix with corn, scallions, and cooked beans. Simmer for 25 to 30 minutes. Do not salt until thoroughly cooked.
Pearled Barley	1 cup (200 g): 4 cups (940 ml)	Simmer for 60 to 70 minutes.
Millet*	1 cup (200 g): 2½ cups (588 ml)	Simmer for 15 minutes, remove from heat, fluff, and let sit uncovered for 20 minutes.
Wild and Brown Rice Mix*	1 cup (160 g): 3 cups (705 ml)	Simmer for 35 minutes.
Polenta* (cornmeal)	1 cup (140 g): 4 cups (940 ml)	Bring water to a boil, add 1 teaspoon (6 g) salt, and slowly add polenta, stirring constantly. Reduce heat to gentle simmer, stirring for 2 minutes more. Cover and cook for 40 to 45 minutes, stirring every 10 minutes.

*Gluten-free

NODDING: A FORM OF BOWING

When dogs pass one another (led on a lead by their person or leash-free in a park), they always greet or at least acknowledge each other. It isn't always possible for us to do the same to each other, but I still think there's something to learn from their behavior.

Smiling at strangers may seem natural, but it may come out looking more like a smirk than a sincere teeth-baring grin. It may be met with either a similar facial expression or no smile at all. This all changed dramatically when I started nodding to passersby.

When someone is walking toward me, I make a point to look into his eyes and give a nod; without fail, he nods back—and often adds a smile—which involuntarily forces me to produce a genuine grin, in return. This interaction all happens within a couple of seconds, and it is incredibly satisfying. A connection is made each time, and I think it makes people feel important.

The head nod is a mini version of a bow. Most prevalent in Asian cultures, bowing is a gesture of respect and denotes deference and humility. It is used to express gratitude, to apologize, to make a request, to greet someone, or to show reverence to an elder or someone of higher standing.

Demonstrating respect for others connects us to rather than separates us from our fellow humans. Though the etiquette surrounding bowing is extremely complex, just a simple nod of the head is all it takes to make people feel honored and respected, whether they're strangers we pass on the street, people we know and love, or people whose opinions differ from ours.

> The spoken or written version of this gesture of respect is *namaste*. This beautiful, simple Sanskrit word literally means "I bow to you." Derived from the words *namas* ("to bow in reverence") and *te* ("to you"), it can be used as a simple albeit respectful greeting or as a deeper, more spiritually minded salutation, such as "The highest in me salutes the highest in you."

Namaste.

GETTING YOUR VITAMIN D

Being healthy doesn't only mean taking in the proper nutrients; it also means making sure our bodies absorb these nutrients. One example of this is the relationship between calcium and vitamin D. As Jack Norris at Vegan Outreach says, "Calcium is important for bones because it is a major component of bones, which are constantly being broken down and built back up. Vitamin D regulates calcium absorption and excretion, especially when calcium intake is low."

The best source of vitamin D is the sun. When we expose our skin to ultraviolet light, our bodies respond by manufacturing vitamin D. This may seem to go against conventional wisdom of avoiding the sun to prevent skin cancer, but it's a matter of finding balance. Though sun exposure is essential, we can avoid going out when the sun is strongest, and 15 minutes is all that is necessary to derive the full benefit from the sun (in terms of vitamin D).

However, not everyone lives in a sunny California climate, and even those who do are spending inordinate amounts of time indoors. In the winter months or when you're unable to find 15 minutes a day to take in the sunshine, it is recommended that you ingest vitamin D through fortified food or supplements.

Most multivitamins include vitamin D, though people who are deficient or dark-skinned may want an additional supplement. Because dark-skinned people would have to spend significantly more time in the sun than light-skinned people, ensuring vitamin D intake through supplements is recommended. However, warm sun exposure (at least 15 minutes a day) is still recommended for all skin types.

"THE BOY WHO TALKED WITH ANIMALS"
BY ROALD DAHL

This story is further evidence that Roald Dahl was a writer who was sympathetic to animals and the people who care about them.

The narrator tells the story of his holiday in Jamaica and the mysterious—and moving—things he witnessed. Roused from his balcony repose by a loud commotion on the beach, he joins the gathering crowd gawking at the latest catch brought in by a group of fishermen: a huge turtle lying upside down on his back.

The beach patrons—some poking at him with a plank—begin debating about what to do with the turtle. One offers to buy him so his wife can take the "shell home and have it polished up by an expert" to be placed "smack in the center of our living room." The rest are excited to hear that the animal has already been sold to the beach hotel cook, who will most certainly make turtle soup and turtle steak.

Sympathetic to the defenseless animal, the narrator is in awe of the turtle's dignity and age.

Just as a number of the people start trying to drag the enormous animal up to the hotel using a rope, their plans are foiled. Running toward them, screaming, "Don't do it! Please let him go!" is an eight-year-old boy named David, whose parents are trying to hold him back. Admonishing them for being "horrible" and "cruel," the boy insists they let the turtle go.

Embarrassed, his father explains that his son is "crazy about animals. He talks with them." "He loves them," his mother explains. After some arguing, David's father convinces the fishermen to let the turtle go and pays them more than they would have received from the hotel manager. While haggling over money, David kneels down beside the turtle, puts his arm around his neck, and whispers to him. When he's finally turned over onto his legs and free to return to the water, David calls out, "Go, turtle, go! Go back to the sea!"

But the story doesn't end there. During the night the boy disappears, and the next day two local fishermen return insisting that they've seen David riding on the back of the turtle in the middle of the ocean.

MEAT-EATER ON BLOOD PRESSURE MEDS TO MEDICATION-FREE VEGAN

I am forty-three years old. For forty-two years of my life, I was a full-fledged omnivore eating whatever meat and dairy I could get my hands on.

A few years ago, I was diagnosed with high blood pressure and put on blood pressure medication and told to change my diet. I did for a while, but soon fell back into the junk food lifestyle. I had a pill that made things better and so eating what I considered "normal" again was okay in my mind. I started running and developed a passion for the sport, which resulted in my first marathon. But my nutrition and weight remained not where they should have been.

Six months after my marathon, I decided to get things under control and lose weight and eat properly. At first, this meant restricting the amount of meat and dairy I consumed and counting calories. By the end of the year, I had stopped consuming dairy products, and my meat consumption was very low, and eventually I became completely vegan.

I love my new life, and what I am doing for myself, the planet, and for animals. I've lost fifty-seven pounds (25.9 kg), my cholesterol is around 100, and recently my doctor took me off the blood pressure medication. I had been told that I would be on those meds for the rest of my life, and that people just didn't go off of those important medications. *I* did, and I now embrace a vegan lifestyle. Eating a plant-based diet and following that lifestyle has made me healthier and happier than at any time in my life!

—*Gordon in Alabama (U.S.)*

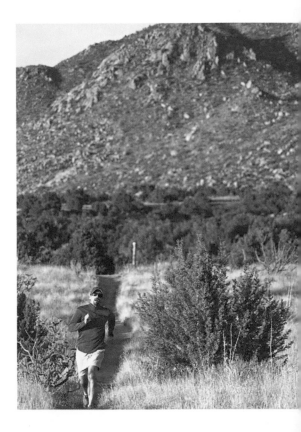

YELLOW SPLIT PEA DAL

This recipe is great served with brown or basmati rice—or even quinoa—and can also be made into a soup by just adding more water.

   3 cups (705 ml) plus 2 to 3 tablespoons
      (30 to 45 ml) water, for sautéing, divided
   1 medium-size yellow onion, finely chopped
   3 cloves garlic, pressed or minced
   1 teaspoon (2 g) finely minced fresh ginger
   1 teaspoon (2 g) curry powder
   1 teaspoon (2 g) ground cumin
   ½ teaspoon ground turmeric
   ¼ teaspoon chili powder
   2 tablespoons (32 g) tomato paste
   1 cup (225 g) yellow split peas, uncooked
   ¼ teaspoon salt (or to taste)
   Fresh cilantro or parsley, for garnish
      (optional)

Heat 2 to 3 tablespoons (30 to 45 ml) of the water in a 3-quart (3.5 L) saucepan. Sauté the onion, garlic, and ginger until they start to soften, about 5 minutes. To prevent sticking, use more water.

Add the curry powder, cumin, turmeric, and chili powder, and cook for 3 minutes, stirring frequently. Add more water, as necessary. Add the tomato paste and cook, stirring, for a minute or so, thoroughly mixing the paste with the other ingredients.

Add the remaining 3 cups (705 ml) water and the split peas, and stir to combine. Bring to a boil, then cover and simmer for 35 to 40 minutes, until the split peas are soft and broken down. Add more water, if necessary. Simmer, stirring frequently, until the mixture is thick. Add the salt.

Top each bowl with the fresh cilantro, if desired, and serve.

Yield: 6 servings

*Oil-free, wheat-free, soy-free

Originally published in *The Vegan Table*

LENTILS

Lentils are part of the vast legume family, which also includes beans. Essentially, if it's in the legume family, it is considered a seed that grows within a pod. You can easily differentiate lentils from beans, because the former live up to their name: they're *lens* shaped.

Lentils come in a variety of colors: brown, green, blue/green, red/pink, black, and yellow.

* Brown (also labeled "green") lentils are standard lentils found in most grocery stores. Flat and earthy-tasting, brown lentils become soft when cooked and are great for making patties, loaves, and dals.

* French green or Puy (pronounced *pwee*) lentils are smaller than your standard brown lentil and boast an absolutely beautiful slate-green color with blue marbling (see photo). Puy lentils hold their shape even when they're cooked, which makes them ideal for lentil salads; they're also great for soups and dals.

* Red lentils are flat and actually more pinkish. Typically the same size as brown lentils though different in flavor, they're also available on the small side. Red lentils become quite mushy when cooked, which makes them ideal for patties, loaves, soups, stews, dals, and pâtés.

* Black or beluga lentils are jet black and named such because they resemble the eggs of beluga whales. They also hold their shape when cooked and are great as the base of a lentil salad.

* Occupying the legume family along with lentils, yellow and green split peas are quite literally the dried, peeled, and split seeds of the pea plant. Picture round peas in a pod. That's how they start out; they're then dried, their skin is removed, and they're separated into two. One of the reasons they're split is to encourage faster cooking. The most popular (and delicious and easy) method of cooking split peas is to make split pea soup.

Cooking with Lentils

* Before adding lentils to the cooking pot, first place them in a strainer, and pick through them to remove any pebbles or stones. Finally, rinse them in running water to wash away any debris. *Note*: Don't ever rinse lentils before you store them—only once you're about to use them.

* When cooking lentils, hold off on adding the salt until the very end, because it could slow the cooking time.

* The ratio for most lentils is about 1 cup (192 g) lentils to 2 ½ cups (570 ml) water. Check the pot every 10 or 15 minutes to make sure the water hasn't evaporated, and keep the heat on medium-low.

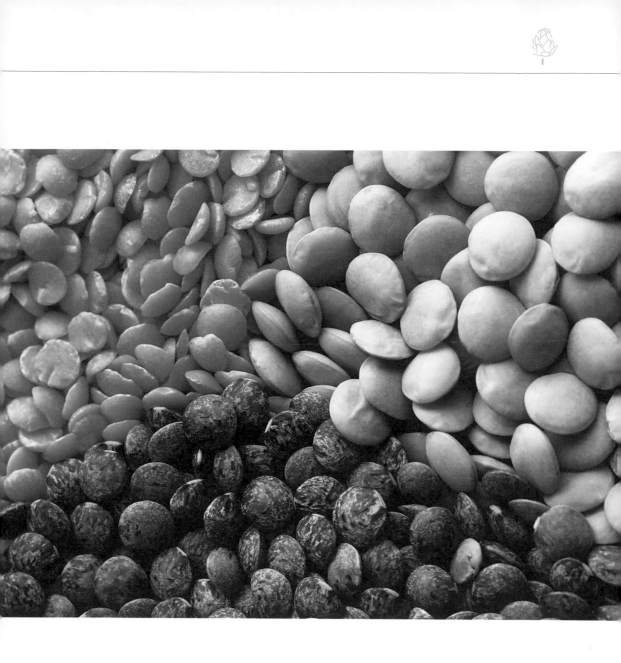

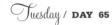
COMPASSIONATE ALTERNATIVE: **BEATING A DEAD HORSE**

Several idioms involve horses, including one that evokes a particularly unpleasant image: "It's no use beating a dead horse."

The original expression was most likely "It's no use flogging a dead horse," and though the origin is based in British politics (the British politician and orator John Bright used it in a speech in 1867 in Parliament), it's a pretty morbid expression. Bright was trying to rouse Parliament from its apathy on a particular issue,

and he said it was like trying to "flog a dead horse" to make it pull a load.

Clearly, the expression itself is trying to convey the idea of "trying to revive interest in a seemingly hopeless issue," and there are more compassionate ways to make the point. Perhaps we can try: "It's no use watering a dead flower" or "It's no use washing a clean shirt" instead.

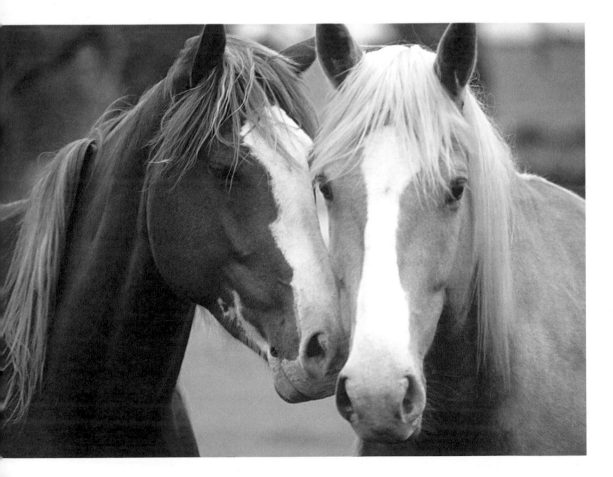

GETTING YOUR VITAMIN B$_{12}$

B$_{12}$ protects the nervous system and keeps the digestive system healthy; without it, permanent damage can manifest itself in blindness, deafness, or dementia. Symptoms of B$_{12}$ deficiency include unusual fatigue, tingling or numbness in the hands or feet, no appetite, nausea, and loss of menstruation.

Mild B$_{12}$ deficiency is less detectable, though no less significant. Because B$_{12}$ lowers homocysteine levels, it reduces the risk of heart disease and stroke. Vegans and near-vegans who don't supplement with vitamin B$_{12}$ have consistently shown elevated homocysteine levels, so even though you don't have any measurable side effects, it doesn't mean your body isn't affected in ways you can't see or feel.

Taking a supplement regularly prevents all of this. Our bodies require such a small amount that it's counted in micrograms. Research has shown that optimal intakes of vitamin B$_{12}$ are higher than the Recommended Dietary Allowance of 2.4 mcg; an optimum range is more like 5 to 10 mcg per day. Therefore, to ensure not only adequate but optimal intake of vitamin B$_{12}$, people should strive for 10 mcg per day from supplements. Some foods are fortified with B$_{12}$, but because we may not eat the same fortified foods every day, I think it's just easier to take a daily supplement. Plus, not all of these fortified foods contain reliable amounts.

B$_{12}$ deficiency doesn't occur only in vegans; these recommendations apply to nonvegans as well. People over fifty tend to lack proper B$_{12}$ absorption, and the Institute of Medicine recommends that infants of vegan mothers be supplemented with B$_{12}$ from birth, and the mother should be supplementing as well.

Some foods such as tempeh, nori seaweed, and spirulina have been touted as natural sources of B$_{12}$, but not enough research supports this. Although they do tend to contain B$_{12}$, they're not providing reliable or consistent amounts.

A daily multivitamin is a habit I highly recommend, but you also want to consider taking a separate B$_{12}$ supplement twice a week for maximum absorption and added insurance.

Being healthy is just a matter of creating new habits.

THE PLAGUE DOGS
BY RICHARD ADAMS

Often overshadowed by his more famous novel, *Watership Down*, Richard Adams's epic novel *The Plague Dogs* follows Rowf and Snitter, two damaged and scared dogs who escape from an animal research lab and fight to survive in the harsh hills of England's Lake District and in a human-centric world, whose cruelty they don't understand.

Written in 1977, *The Plague Dogs* is written from the viewpoint of the dogs—and other animals—who are given speech and language, just as the rabbits had in *Watership Down*. Adams's sympathy with the dogs and other victims of animal research is transparent not only through the narrative itself but also in several passages that—though they tend to slow the story down—belie his objection to animal research in general.

Not surprisingly, Richard Adams was active in animal welfare, serving as president of the Royal Society for the Prevention of Cruelty to Animals from 1980 to 1982 and explicitly stating that he "deliberately set up to satirize animal experimentation, government, and the press."

One of the reasons the book is so incredible—and painful—is its descriptions of actual experiments that continue to take place in labs all around the globe, including water-immersion experiments, brain experiments, and cancer and radiation research.

For public relations reasons, the laboratory decides to pursue the recapture of the dogs, and the media sensationalizes the escape itself, falsely stating that the dogs may be carriers of bubonic plague and depicting the dogs as vicious killers.

The cruelty they encounter reaffirms Rowf's dislike and distrust of humans, but Snitter only remembers the kindness of his former "master." Aided by the help of a fox, the trio take the reader on a journey that is at once exciting and heartbreaking. Only one or two compassionate humans appear in the story, including a research assistant who has a change of mind and heart about his work and releases a tormented monkey from a horrific experiment.

Adams brazenly depicts the cruelty and absurdity of animal research and the insensitivity of a government that allows it to happen merely for political and financial benefit. I confess to shedding several tears at each description of the useless torture the animals are subjected to, and I was in great distress through Rowf and Snitter's entire ordeal.

Although the narrative periodically becomes weighed down by some unnecessary exposition, and some dialect may be difficult for modern readers who don't live in the Lake District of England, the story is unforgettable. I still can't look at a fox terrier without thinking of Snitter.

FROM IGNORANCE TO AWARENESS

My parents own 150 acres (60.7 ha) of Texas farmland, upon which graze fifty beautiful bovines and a horse or two at any given time. One day when I was five years old, many of the old girls were bellowing their hearts out, making my little empathetic self squirm in my seat. What on Earth could be the matter?

My parents explained, "Their bodies made milk for their babies to drink, and now that their babies are gone, they're just a little sore. That's all."

"But, where did their babies *go*?"

"You see your hamburger here, sweetheart? Well, it's made from the cows. We take animals, and we make them into meat so we can eat them, so we can live."

To my fragile mind, this was devastating. My parents tried to fight the flames of my furious realization and soothe my troubled mind, but it was too late. From that day on I scrutinized my meals diligently, refusing to put anything in my mouth that my parents reluctantly admitted was, in fact, dead animal flesh.

They had hoped that this phase would end soon enough, that my mind would eventually separate the hunks of muscle that everyone around me continued to consume from the love and respect I felt for all the other living creatures— animals I felt were my equals.

I'm now vegan, and I'm so grateful to experience the bliss of total compassion and to live in such a way that celebrates all living beings.

—Jane in Milwaukee, Wisconsin (U.S.)

SESAME SALAD DRESSING

This delicious dressing comes from my friend Laurie Judd, who also uses it as a marinade.

> 5 tablespoons (75 ml) *ume* plum vinegar
> 6 tablespoons (90 ml) toasted sesame oil
> 3 tablespoons (60 g) agave nectar
> 2 tablespoons (30 ml) water

Combine all the ingredients in a blender or food processor, and blend until emulsified. Use right away, or store in a glass container in the refrigerator. Shake before using.

Yield: ½ cup (120 ml)

SERVING SUGGESTIONS AND VARIATIONS

* If you can't find *ume* plum vinegar, substitute rice vinegar. One tester even added 1 teaspoon (6.3 g) plum sauce to her rice vinegar, which worked beautifully.

* Great on any mixed salad, it also makes a wonderful dressing for shredded cabbage and carrots, tossed with peanuts.

* It also pairs well with avocado, bell pepper, cranberries, and almonds.

* Wheat-free, soy-free

BRUSSELS SPROUTS

Brussels spouts get a bad rap, and many parents will insist their kids won't eat them—or many other vegetables.

Kids don't dislike vegetables; kids dislike vegetables that don't taste good! When vegetables are overcooked or boiled to death, they don't taste good. When vegetables are covered in cream and butter sauces, their own natural flavors are not allowed to shine. When parents "sneak" and "hide" vegetables to get their children to eat them, they never learn to appreciate the value, flavor, and various textures of plant-based foods.

Brussels sprouts can be steamed, shredded and stir-fried, or roasted.

* To roast them, cut off the base of each Brussels sprout, along with any remaining stem, and peel away any outside leaves that are yellowing, browning, or just unappealing.

* Depending on the size, cut them in half or add them whole to a bowl and drizzle them with a little olive oil—just enough to coat. Sprinkle in some salt and press a few garlic cloves into the bowl. Then, just mix it all up by hand, and transfer them to a baking sheet in a single layer and roast them in a preheated 425°F (220°C, or gas mark 7) oven. Depending on the size, this may take 30 to 40 minutes; it's up to you how brown and crispy you like them. You want to make sure they are soft (but still chewy) on the inside and brown and crispy on the outside.

Packed with tons of vitamin A, vitamin C, folic acid, and fiber, Brussels sprouts get their name from the fact that they were grown as early as the 1200s in what is now Belgium; before then, it is likely they were cultivated in ancient Rome.

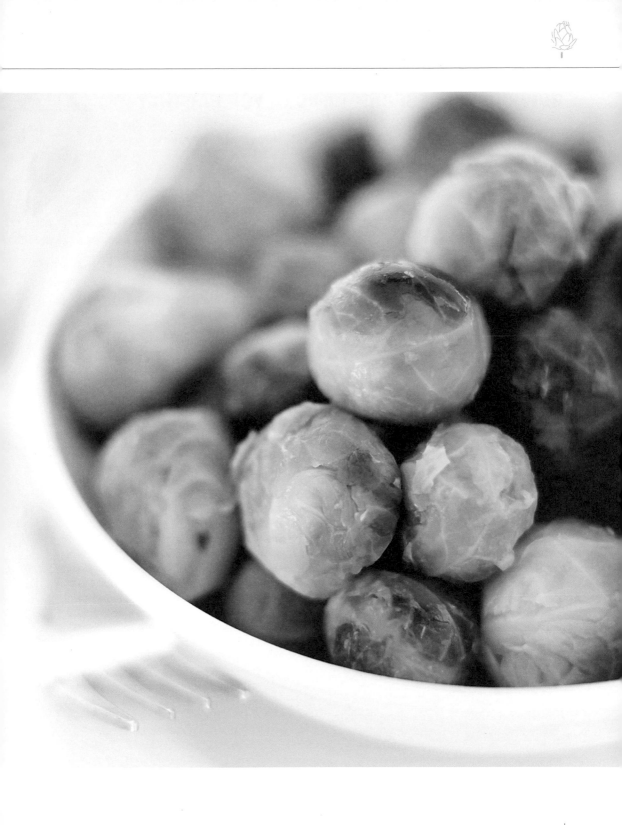

HOW DO YOU RESPOND TO, "CAN YOU EAT THAT?"

A few times in my life, I've been in a situation where people start talking about one of their favorite dishes or a delicious meal they just had at a restaurant. They realize *I'm* there—the *vegan*—and they say, with their head cocked and a sad expression on their face, "Oh, I'm so sorry. You can't eat that."

Here's the thing—I *can* eat whatever I want. There's nothing I *can't have*. But there are some things I *don't want*. Not consuming animals or animal secretions is a *choice*. I don't follow a set of dietary laws, and I am quite capable of physically putting food into my mouth.

It's not a matter of can and cannot. It's a matter of not *wanting* to.

The people asking if I "can" eat something are not trying to be malicious; if anything, they are being considerate, and I always let them know that I appreciate they've remembered I'm vegan.

But also, I don't want to miss an opportunity to offer them a different perspective about what it means to be vegan—that it is indeed about choice and not deprivation or willpower.

In these situations, I often just smile and find a friendly way to say, "It's not illegal. Of course I can have it. I just don't *want* it—thank you very much."

CONNECTING WITH LIKE-MINDED PEOPLE

Having a circle of people in your community—people you can dine with, people you can cry with, people you can laugh with, people who simply speak your own language—is so important. Connecting with like-minded people is easier than ever with all the social networking options available online.

* Find vegan meetups in your area or start one of your own (meetup.com).

* Attend vegetarian and animal rights conferences. Many vegetarian organizations host annual conferences and "veg fests," which are ideal places to meet fellow vegans, as are the larger national and international events.

* Join Facebook to connect with other activists through the numerous vegan and animal rights groups.

* Host a potluck or cooking party.

* Volunteer with your local vegetarian or animal rights group.

* Set up a table at farmers' markets and local fairs. By showing up, you'll attract like-minded people who didn't know you even existed.

* Attend veg social events in your area, such as Vegan Drinks.

* Make a love connection through vegconnect .com, veggieconnection.com, or veggiedate.org.

FROM "SONG OF MYSELF" IN *LEAVES OF GRASS*
BY WALT WHITMAN

Walt Whitman, an American poet and essayist, lived from 1819 to 1892. Controversial in his day, particularly due to the overt sexuality in his poetry, his work falls in between transcendentalism and Romanticism—and includes elements of realism. The celebration of nature plays a significant role, either as a backdrop or as a living character.

This particular section from his most well-known collection of poems, *Leaves of Grass*, has always been a favorite of mine. I think you'll see why.

> I think I could turn and live with animals, they are
> so placid and self-contain'd,
> I stand and look at them long and long.
>
> They do not sweat and whine about their
> condition,
> They do not lie awake in the dark and weep for
> their sins,
> They do not make me sick discussing their duty
> to God,
> Not one is dissatisfied, not one is demented with
> the mania of owning things,
> Not one kneels to another, nor to his kind that
> lived thousands of years ago,
> Not one is respectable or unhappy over the whole
> earth.
>
> So they show their relations to me, and I accept
> them;
> They bring me tokens of myself—they evince
> them plainly in their possession.

> I wonder where they get those tokens:
> Did I pass that way huge times ago, and
> negligently drop them?
> Myself moving forward then and now and
> forever,
> Gathering and showing more always and with
> velocity,
> Infinite and omnigenous, and the like of these
> among them;
> Not too exclusive toward the reachers of my
> remembrancers;
> Picking out here one that I love, and now go with
> him on brotherly terms.
>
> A gigantic beauty of a stallion, fresh and
> responsive to my caresses,
> Head high in the forehead, wide between the
> ears,
> Limbs glossy and supple, tail dusting the ground,
> Eyes full of sparkling wickedness—ears finely cut,
> flexibly moving.
>
> His nostrils dilate, as my heels embrace him;
> His well-built limbs tremble with pleasure, as we
> race around and return.
>
> I but use you a moment, then I resign you,
> stallion;
> Why do I need your paces, when I myself out-
> gallop them?
> Even, as I stand or sit, passing faster than you.

HEALTHY AND THRIVING

I am a 48-year-old man who has been married to my wife for twenty-eight years. We both were raised on farms. Her family is in the beef industry and mine is in the hog industry.

Over the last decade we both suffered tragic diagnoses. In 2004 I was a victim of sudden cardiac death syndrome but was revived and have a defibrillator implanted in my chest. Still we made no changes. Just recently my wife was diagnosed with viral cardiomyopathy and given 24 months to live. This made my brain scream, "Look around you—this doesn't have to be so!"

I went full-on vegan and at last health check my heart was found to be healthy, and no damage from the past trauma was apparent. I now prepare my wife's food. Her health has improved and she now only has to wear oxygen at night. Soon she will have another heart function study. I know it will show improvement.

As I did more research, I became overwhelmed by grief for all the victims of the slaughterhouse industry. I didn't want to become a tree-hugging vegan; I only wanted to save my wife. But now I have had an awakening that I never expected.

—*Wayne in Texas (U.S.)*

SWEET GARLIC AND TOMATOES WITH FARFALLE

My star recipe tester, Barbara Lyons, graced me with this simple and delectable recipe.

   16 ounces (455 g) farfalle (bow tie) pasta
   2 large heads/bulbs garlic, peeled and
      minced
   ¼ cup (60 ml) olive oil
   3 cups (540 g) diced fresh plum tomatoes
      (about 10 tomatoes)
   1 cup (100 g) chopped scallions
   1 teaspoon (1.2 g) red pepper flakes
   1 teaspoon (4 g) organic cane sugar
   2 cups (470 ml) vegetable stock
   1 bunch cilantro or parsley, finely chopped
      (reserving some for garnish)
   Salt and freshly ground pepper

Cook the pasta as directed until almost, but not quite, al dente. Drain and set aside.

Meanwhile, place the garlic and oil in a large sauté pan over medium heat. Cook, stirring frequently, until the garlic begins to turn a light brown.

Add the tomatoes, scallions, red pepper flakes, and sugar. Cook and stir for 10 minutes longer, or until the tomatoes begin to soften. Add the stock, and simmer to reduce slightly, about 5 minutes.

Add the pasta to the tomato mixture, allowing it to finish cooking completely for about a minute or two. Stir in the cilantro, and season with salt and pepper to taste.

Yield: 4 servings

*Soy-free

BLUEBERRIES

Although I love blueberries as a snack, my favorite way to eat them is in fruit smoothies. Any berry would work, but blueberries are my preference—not only because of how high they rank in nutritional superiority but also because they don't have annoying little seeds that get stuck in your teeth.

With a supply of frozen fruit, you can make fruit smoothies anytime—for a midafternoon snack or a healthful breakfast.

My go-to smoothie can be modified according to taste preference and what you have on hand. (Always be sure to keep banana chunks in the freezer, because bananas have a relatively short life outside the freezer. Simply peel ripe bananas, break them into chunks, and store them in a freezer bag. They keep for a few months in the freezer.)

* 1 banana

* 1 cup (145 g) blueberries

* ½ cup (70 to 90 g) other fruit (pineapple, strawberries, mango)

* 1 cup (235 ml) nondairy milk (almond, oat, soy, rice, hazelnut, hemp)

* 1 heaping tablespoon (16 g) nut butter (peanut and almond are my faves)

* 2 dates (optional)

* 1 tablespoon (7 g) ground flaxseed

Beyond smoothies, here are some other ways to enjoy blueberries:

* Mix them into your oatmeal.

* Top your cereal with them.

* Throw them in a bowl, and eat them plain or drizzled with a little agave nectar.

* Eat blueberry nondairy yogurt and top with more blueberries.

* Make blueberry pancakes, and top with blueberry sauce.

* Toss blueberries in a salad.

* Make a fruit salad with blueberries as the dominant fruit.

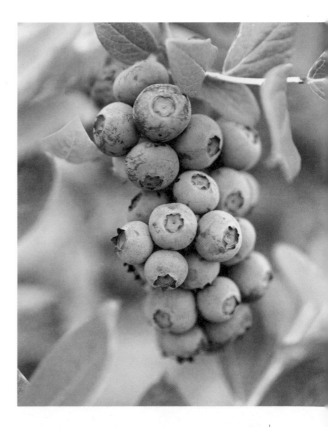

HOW DO YOU RESPOND TO, "EATING MEAT IS A PERSONAL PREFERENCE"?

This particular excuse has several variations but goes something like: "Eating meat is my personal preference, and since I respect your desire not to eat animals, I would appreciate your respecting my preference to dine on them."

The problem with this justification is that it assumes there is no victim, no *other*. It implies that the meat-eater's desires, traditions, culture, taste buds, or appetite are superior to anything—or anyone—else and that because of this, he or she is absolved from the harm eating meat causes, particularly to the one being eaten.

Whenever we hear people make such a declaration, we can gently remind them that as a society, we collectively decide that certain behaviors, certain actions, certain *personal preferences* are inappropriate or morally reprehensible, especially when they cause injury or harm to another. After all, when accused, abusive parents or spouses often justify their actions by protesting that it is nobody else's business how they treat their child/wife/husband, that people should not meddle in their affairs, and that they can do what they like in their own home. Although there was a time when the law protected such people and practices, this is no longer the case. We've created laws to make domestic abuse illegal and punishable.

When we take away the choice of another and then use that as license to hurt or kill, we're participating in an egregious act of cruelty, whether we do it ourselves or pay others to do it for us. We only tell ourselves that our personal choice is our own business—our own *preference*—so we can sleep soundly at night.

Remind them that a choice made from personal preference might be the color you paint your bathroom, the kind of car you buy, or the way you style your hair. But a personal choice to hurt someone else? That doesn't come out looking like a very pleasant credo to live by, but because millions of people do live by it, billions of animals unnecessarily die by it—year in and year out.

EATING BY COLOR

My message for eating healthfully can be narrowed down to three little words: eat by color. All of the nutrients we need are available in plants, and their color is a clue to their healthfulness.

We know we need to consume more plant foods; we know plant foods are good for us. But what is it about the color that makes them so healthful?

The answer is in the phytochemicals.

Phytochemicals (also called phytonutrients), from the Greek word for plant (*phyto*), are manufactured by plants to protect themselves from the damage caused by animals or insects, photosynthesis, and UV radiation. When we consume them, they provide the same protection for us that they do for the plant.

Phytochemicals are easy to identify because they are actually the pigments that give fruits, vegetables, flowers—all plants—their distinctive hues. We can detect the highest concentration of different phytochemicals just by looking at their color:

* blue anthocyanins in blueberries

* orange beta-carotene in carrots

* red betacyanins in beets

* green folate in kale

* yellow lutein in corn

And remember: there are no phytochemicals made by animals. (*Phyto*, after all, means "plant.") It's only when animals eat plants that they take in these and other nutrients. Cattle get calcium and protein from the plants they eat; salmon turn pink from the plants (and plant-eating animals) they eat; and egg yolks turn yellow from the lutein-rich plants the chickens eat (rather, today, yolks are a deep yellow because of the synthetic lutein added to chicken feed). The best thing we can do is skip the middle animal and go straight to the source for our nutrients: plants!

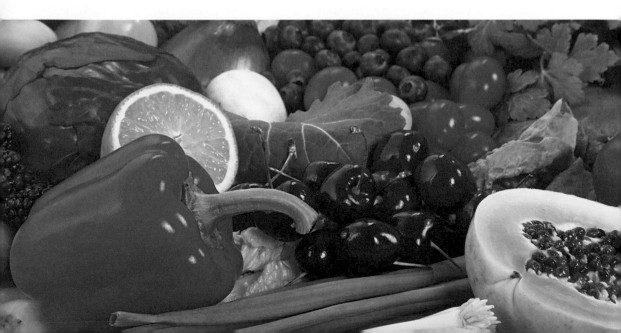

EXCERPT FROM *A VINDICATION OF THE RIGHTS OF WOMAN WITH STRICTURES ON POLITICAL AND MORAL SUBJECTS*
BY MARY WOLLSTONECRAFT GODWIN

British author-activist Mary Wollstonecraft Godwin, born in April 1759, is most famous for writing one of the earliest works on feminist philosophy. Although she wrote novels, travel narratives, and a history of the French Revolution, she is most known for the treatise *A Vindication of the Rights of Woman*, in which she argues that women are not inherently inferior to men but only appear to be because they have been denied the same education.

Wollstonecraft's life was tragically cut short when she died at the age of thirty-eight on September 10, 1797, due to complications during the birth of her second daughter, Mary. Mary became a well-known writer in her own right, subsequently writing *Frankenstein* as Mary Shelley, whose name she took when she married poet Percy Bysshe Shelley (see Day 326).

First published in 1792, *Vindication* advocates the education of women and offers one of the earliest arguments for the need for humane instruction in schools. With sensitivity and keen insight, Wollstonecraft makes the connection between cruelty to animals and violence toward human:

Humanity to animals should be particularly inculcated as a part of national education, for it is not at present one of our national virtues. Tenderness for their humble domestics, amongst the lower class, is oftener to be found in a savage than civilized state. For civilization prevents that intercourse which creates affection in the rude hut, or mud hovel, and leads uncultivated minds who are only depraved by the refinements which prevail in the society, where they are trodden under foot by the rich, to domineer over them to revenge the insults that they are obliged to bear from their superiors.

This habitual cruelty is first caught at school, where it is one of the rare sports of the boys to torment the miserable brutes that fall in their way. The transition, as they grow up, from barbarity to brutes to domestic tyranny over wives, children, and servants is very easy. Justice, or even benevolence, will not be a powerful spring of action unless it be extended to the whole creation; nay, I believe that it may be delivered as an axiom, that those who can see pain, unmoved, will soon learn to inflict it.

TIGER RESCUE

In November 2002, the California Department of Fish and Game seized ten tigers from a "pseudo-sanctuary" in Colton, California, called "Tiger Rescue," after finding them in filthy cages without water and suspecting the owner of illegal breeding. When officials executed a search warrant on the owner's residence, they discovered ninety dead tiger carcasses, including fifty-eight baby tigers dead in a freezer. Thirteen other cats were found barely alive. The state seized control of the facility, and the remaining animals were placed in sanctuaries, including the Performing Animal Welfare Society's new 10-acre (4 ha) tiger habitat in San Andreas, California.

Intensive medical intervention was provided for the tigers, because almost all of them had severe dental anomalies and several of the tigers arrived with premature arthritis.

One of the rescued tigers is Spanky, who arrived emaciated, sick with vomiting and diarrhea, and with a prognosis for recovery that was not very promising. After a comprehensive examination to determine why he was unable to digest his food, Spanky was diagnosed with pancreatic disease, a malady that creates an inability to digest food properly.

Chronic pancreatitis is often a result of inadequate diet. After careful research, Spanky was treated with the proper medication and enzymes to enable him to digest his food properly.

Happily, today Spanky is thriving, running, swimming, and playing with Artemis, his good friend and companion.

—CPG

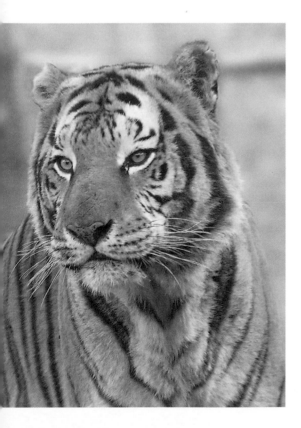

Spanky, healthy and safe at Performing Animal Welfare Society's tiger habitat

Photo courtesy of Performing Animal Welfare Society

NO-BAKE CHOCOLATE PEANUT BUTTER PIE

This is a rich and delicious no-bake pie that will have your guests clamoring for more!

- **2 cups (350 g) nondairy chocolate chips**
- **12 ounces (340 g) silken tofu (firm)**
- **1½ cups (390 g) natural peanut butter, crunchy or smooth**
- **½ cup (120 ml) nondairy milk (soy, rice, almond, hazelnut, hemp, or oat)**
- **1 store-bought or homemade graham cracker crust**
- **1 cup (175 g) nondairy chocolate chips (as an optional topping)**
- **1 cup (120 g) chopped nuts (as an optional topping)**

Melt the 2 cups (350 g) chocolate chips in the microwave or a double boiler. (To make a double boiler, place the chips in a small saucepan. Set this pan in a larger pot that is filled with ¼ to ½ cup [60 to 120 ml] water. Heat over medium heat on the stove and stir the chips in the small pot until they are melted.)

In a food processor or high-powered blender, combine the tofu, peanut butter, milk, and melted chocolate chips. Blend until very smooth, adding more milk, if desired. Pour the filling into the crust and refrigerate for 2 hours.

For a pie with a hard chocolate topping, after the pie has been chilled for 2 hours, melt the 1 cup (175 g) nondairy chocolate chips. Pour the melted chocolate over the top of the pie. If desired, sprinkle on the chopped nuts. Refrigerate for 2 hours longer.

Yield: 8 to 10 servings

Wheat-free if using wheat-free piecrust

Originally published in *The Joy of Vegan Baking*

ARUGULA (ROCKET)

Arugula, eaten in ancient Rome and Egypt (and considered an aphrodisiac), is also known as rocket arugula or rocket greens. It has a peppery (and some say bitter) taste and is rich in vitamins A, C, and calcium (½ cup [10 g] has 16 mg of calcium).

That's not all. It's a nutrition superstar. In just one 5-calorie cup (20 g) of arugula, you get almost half the recommended Daily Value of vitamin K (essential for blood clotting and for creating strong bones), an obscene amount of healthful carotenoids such as lutein and zeaxanthin, and a nice blend of anticancer properties.

* Arugula can be eaten raw in salads or added to stir-fries, soups, and pasta sauces.

* It's pretty powerful on its own, so it's often mixed with milder greens to produce a nicely balanced salad.

* It can also be sautéed in olive oil, like most greens, tossed into a pasta dish, or added as a pizza topping at the end of cooking time.

* Arugula can be substituted for basil in pesto.

Most any green can be substituted for it, but the closest matches are Belgian endive, escarole, watercress, and dandelion greens.

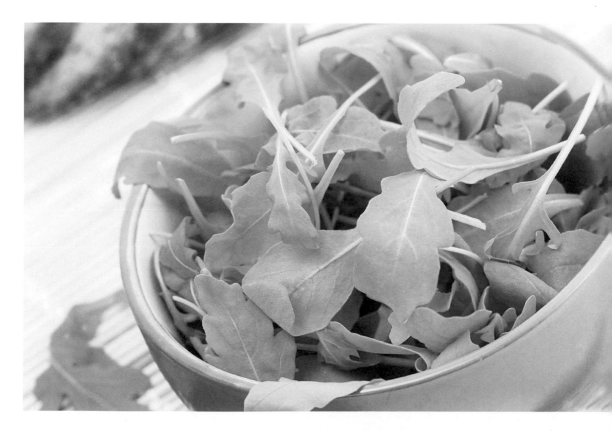

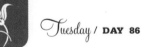
COMPASSIONATE ALTERNATIVES TO VIOLENT CATTLE IDIOMS

Like all nonhuman animals, cattle are also victims of our verbal assaults, generally calling them stupid, lazy, and fat. Common American idioms reflect our collective disdain for them—a necessity in a country that kills 45 million a year for consumption.

Some common idioms include: to be bull-headed, to shoot the bull, take the bull by the horns, kill the fatted calf, cash cow, big enough to choke a cow, why buy a cow when you can get the milk for free.

In addition to changing our language about cattle (cows, steers, bulls, oxen), we can encourage others to do the same. Whenever we hear someone making an insulting generalization about cattle, we can correct him by talking about all their wonderful, sensitive, maternal, sweet traits. Read some stories about amazing cattle in Friday: Stories of Rescue, Hope, and Transformation.

And practice using some compassionate alternatives to idioms that reflect violence or exploitation:

Shoot the bull—To refer to a social gathering where you hang around and talk, I've always preferred *shooting the breeze*.

Why buy a cow when you can have the milk for free? How about: Why pay for something that you can get for free otherwise?

CONSUMING OMEGA-3 FATTY ACIDS

We need omega-3 fatty acids, but we do not need to consume fish to ingest them. Apart from the damage fish and fish oil consumption is creating in the oceans and the unnecessary deaths of millions of sea animals, people are not necessarily healthier for eating fish. Fish is loaded with saturated fat, cholesterol, mercury and other heavy metals, and a variety of environmental contaminants (PCBs, DDT, dioxins, and so on). Farmed fish have the addition of antibiotics, pesticides, and more than 100 other pollutants.

Let's get this straight: Fish have high amounts of omega-3s in their flesh because they're eating the plant foods that contain these fats. Let's cut out the middle fish and go straight to the source by consuming plant foods rich in omega-3s.

Flaxseeds and hemp seeds are great sources of omega-3 fatty acids. Buy whole flaxseeds in the bulk section of any natural foods store, and use a coffee grinder to grind them. Store them in an airtight container in the freezer or refrigerator. (Whole seeds don't need to be refrigerated.) Add 1 tablespoon (7 g) ground flaxseed to your morning smoothie, oatmeal, cereal, salad, or soup.

Other omega-3-rich options include shelled hemp seeds (3 tablespoons [21 g]), walnuts (about 14 halves), and flax oil (1 teaspoon [5 ml]).

"MAN'S PLACE IN THE ANIMAL WORLD"
BY MARK TWAIN

Mark Twain was a forthright animal advocate, speaking out against bullfighting and vivisection, and animals factor into many of his stories. This important aspect of Twain's work is celebrated in a beautiful book edited by Shelly Fisher Fishkin and illustrated by Barry Moser. *Mark Twain's Book of Animals* is full of essays, excerpts, letters, and short stories that illustrate Twain's dedication to animal advocacy and his indignation about injustices and abuses committed against them.

One essay in the book that exemplifies Twain's criticism of our treatment of animals is "Man's Place in the Animal World." Full of Twain's wit and humor, it is written from one dog to another, as indicated by the full title: "Letters from a Dog to Another Dog Explaining and Accounting for Man by Author, Newfoundland Smith. Translated from the Original Doggerel by M.T."

Concerned by Darwin's theory of the "ascent of man from the lower animals," Newfoundland Smith argues that "that theory ought to be vacated in favor of a new and truer one, this new and truer one to be named the Descent of Man from the Higher Animals."

His reasoning is based on several observations and experiments; for instance, he presents the case where hunters organized a buffalo hunt for entertainment for an earl, killing "seventy-two of those great animals," eating only one and leaving "the seventy-one to rot." He decides to compare the difference between an anaconda and an earl, so he lures seven young calves into an anaconda's cage; "the grateful reptile immediately crushed one of them and swallowed it, then lay back satisfied. It showed no further interest in the calves and no disposition to harm them." He concludes: "The fact stood proven that the difference between an earl and an anaconda is that the earl is cruel and the anaconda isn't; the earl wantonly destroys what he has no use for, but the anaconda doesn't." He continues to catalog all the ways man is inferior to the "higher animals."

This anthology is a delightful book for animal people or Mark Twain fans.

FROM ATKINS TO VEGAN

When I was twenty-seven, I went on the Atkins Diet. I followed it perfectly, eating all the bacon and cheese I wanted. About two weeks into the diet, my left foot started swelling. Within days, the pain and swelling became so bad that I couldn't walk or even sleep. I spent most of my day in tears because of the excruciating pain. I went to the doctor, who was perplexed. He assumed it was an infection and gave me antibiotics. A few days later, nothing had changed.

I happened to be talking to a friend of mine— a podiatry student—who asked me if I had changed my diet recently. When I told him I was on a high-protein diet, he told me to get off the "stupid diet" and the pain and swelling would go away. He was right. Unfortunately, I now have gout.

After a few years of suffering, I decided to stop eating meat because meat has been shown in many studies to exacerbate gout. Nobody told me to; in fact, even my doctor merely said it "might" be a good idea. Eliminating meat from my diet has helped immensely, but I've continued to have attacks even with daily medication.

For all these years, my main protein sources had been eggs and cheese. I literally ate these foods almost three meals a day, every day. Once I met someone at a social event, and the topic of diet came up. He recommended I read *The China Study* and left me with just one final thought, which I couldn't shake: No other species on the planet except humans drinks lactation fluid after being weaned, and no other species drinks another species' milk. It blew my mind that it had never occurred to me before.

After listening to one episode of the *Food for Thought* podcast, I stopped eating dairy and eggs. Hearing the truth about the treatment of animals (even on supposedly "humane" farms) changed me forever. Few things in my life have felt this right.

My veganism is not a progression of affection for animals; it's a progression of belief in justice. Moreover, this has opened up a whole new appreciation for nonhuman animals.

Not eating animals is consistent with the way I already lived my life, is consistent with my beliefs about nonviolence and human rights, about compassion and reducing suffering in the world. I can't believe it took me this long, but I'm so grateful that I finally "got it."

—*Michael in San Francisco, California (U.S.)*

When Michael first wrote to me, he was still taking gout medications daily. Today, he is not.

LENTIL BOLOGNESE

Thanks to Barbara Lyons for contributing this recipe, which I can now share with you.

1 yellow onion, finely chopped
2 cloves garlic, crushed or minced
2 carrots, grated or finely chopped
2 stalks celery, finely chopped
1 tablespoon (15 ml) olive oil
1 cup (192 g) red lentils
2 large tomatoes, diced, or 1 (15-ounce, or 420 g) can diced tomatoes
2 tablespoons (32 g) tomato paste
2 cups (470 ml) vegetable stock
1 tablespoon (4 g) fresh marjoram or orega-no, minced, or 1 teaspoon (1 g) dried
3 tablespoons (19 g) finely diced black olives
Salt and freshly ground pepper
Finely minced fresh parsley or basil, for garnish

In a large saucepan, sauté the onion, garlic, carrots, and celery in the oil for about 5 minutes, or until they are soft.

Add the lentils, tomatoes, tomato paste, vegetable stock, marjoram, and olives. Bring the mixture to a boil over medium-low heat, then partially cover with a lid and simmer for 15 to 20 minutes, or until thick and soft. (Check halfway through the cooking time to make sure the water hasn't evaporated. Add a little more, if necessary.)

Add the salt and pepper to taste, and garnish with the parsley. Serve over pasta, if desired.

Yield: 4 servings

*Wheat-free, soy-free

NUTRITIONAL YEAST

Nutritional yeast is a nonlive, nonactive yeast fermented on molasses. It sometimes contains added vitamin B_{12}, which is why it is considered a supplemented food; it can also be thought of as a condiment or flavoring.

Nutritional yeast is different than brewer's yeast, which is also a nonlive, nonactive yeast, but it's fermented on hops rather than molasses, so it tends to have a bitter flavor.

Naturally low in fat and sodium, nutritional yeast boasts a cheesy flavor, so it's used to make sauces and gravies; sprinkled on popcorn, pasta, or baked potatoes; and added to tofu scrambles.

Cats and dogs seem to love it as much as humans do; a little sprinkle on their food is enough to spark their enthusiasm. (This is especially helpful if you need to hide medicine in their food.)

Nutritional yeast is available in powder or flake form, and I prefer the latter. It keeps indefinitely stored in a cool, dry place, though if you refrigerate it, it stays fresher.

COMPASSIONATE ALTERNATIVES: **VIOLENT PIG IDIOMS**

Pigs get a pretty bad rap in our society and are exploited and used by humans in a variety of ways, especially through language. The way we talk about pigs reflects the shame and discomfort we feel at treating intelligent, sentient beings with cruelty and disregard. At the same time, in order to continue treating them as mere production tools or research tools or tools for enjoyment or curiosity, the culture must shape our perception of them, so we view them as lowly, dirty, messy, sloppy, insignificant, and fat.

Here are a just a few expressions and words we use in our daily lives without thinking: self-righteous pig, capitalist pig, fascist pig, liberal pig, fill-in-the-blank pig, stupid pig, fat pig, filthy pig, greedy pig, sloppy pig, make a pig of myself, squeal like a pig, bleed like a stuck pig, male chauvinist pig, road hog, sweat like a pig, to pig out, the pig police, pig sty, go whole hog, hog-tie, hog the limelight, cast pearls before swine, drunken swine.

If we closely examine these insults that are normally associated with pigs, you'll find that the truth is quite the opposite.

Dirty, filthy, sloppy pig Pigs are actually the cleanest animals of all, and they refuse to excrete anywhere near their living or eating areas when given a choice. Pigs don't have functional sweat glands, so they cool themselves off using water or mud in hot weather. They also use mud as a form of sunscreen to protect their skin from sunburn; the mud also provides protection against flies and parasites.

Stupid pig Despite the insinuation, pigs are very curious and insightful animals; they are said to have intelligence beyond that of an average three-year-old human child and beyond that of our beloved domestic dogs. Pigs are incredibly friendly and loyal, and they form complex social units. Pigs have excellent memories, newborn piglets learn to run to their mothers' voices, and mother pigs sing to their young while nursing. When given the chance to live outside of animal factories, pigs spend hours playing, lying in the sun, and exploring their surroundings with their powerful sense of smell.

Lassen at Farm Sanctuary

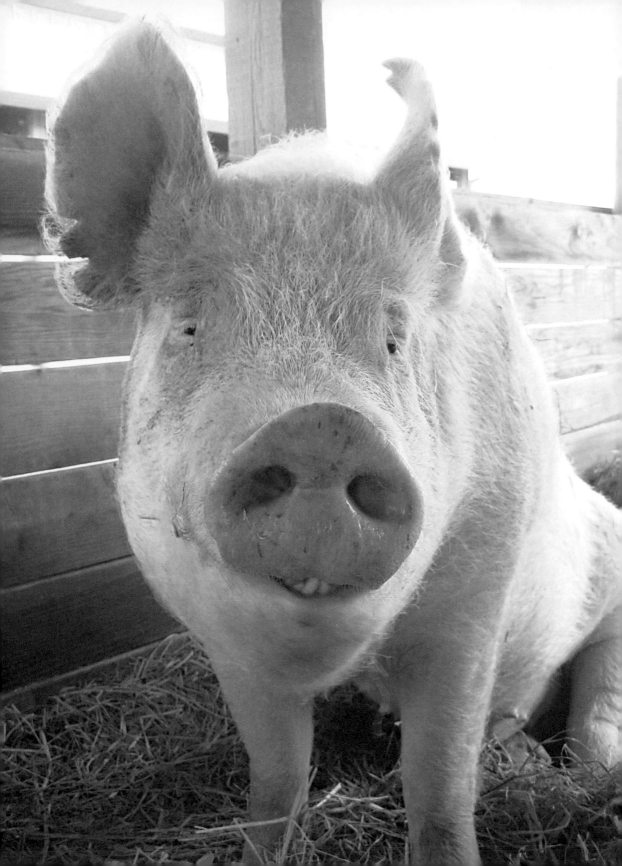

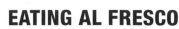
EATING AL FRESCO

There are so many ways to enjoy eating al fresco, whether you have a yard or not.

Splendor in the Grass

Nothing says summer like a picnic—whether it's in your yard, at a park, or on your balcony. The food options are endless, especially because you don't have to worry about everything spoiling as quickly as when you use egg- and dairy-based products. Emphasize what's in season, and don't forget the compostable plates, cups, and utensils. Keep the menu simple and fresh with salads and one-dish meals.

Moonstruck

Shut off the TV, turn off the lights, and get outside. Throw a blanket down on your balcony, patio, or lawn, and snuggle up with your honey by the light of the moon. Open a bottle of wine or sparkling juice, and enjoy organic strawberries dipped in melted chocolate, which you can keep warm with a portable butane stove.

Make a Request

When there's an outdoor seating option at a restaurant, take it. The air you're breathing will be fresher, and if you bring your pooch, he will most likely be able to hang with you while you dine.

Host a Barbecue

Portable grills are widely available, so barbecues don't have to be confined to your backyard. Fire it up, and add polenta squares, presteamed potatoes, marinated tempeh and portobello mushrooms, corn on the cob, seasoned eggplant slices, and skewers of peppers, red onions, and summer squash.

YES, PLAY BALL!
The food at sports venues is a-changin', too, believe it or not. If you don't want to bring your food anymore, many stadiums, parks, and arenas offer lots of veggie fare—from soy dogs and burritos to french fries and pretzels. Check out soyhappy.org for a veg guide to ballparks.

THE COCKPIT
BY WILLIAM HOGARTH AND DIARY ENTRY BY SAMUEL PEPYS

Just as in his series *The Four Stages of Cruelty* (see Day 284), Hogarth uses his art to take a stand against brutality. Cockfighting, a popular and legal activity when Hogarth made his engraving in 1759, attracted every sort of person, as depicted in the work. Banned outright in England, Wales, and the British Territories in 1835, cockfighting was banned in Scotland sixty years later in 1895.

In *The Cockpit,* Hogarth emphasizes the other effects of these bloody games—the gambling, the corruption, and the vulgarity of those who participate.

Even from Samuel Pepys's diary, we get a sense of the scene Hogarth was trying to convey. After attending a cockfight with Lord Sandwich in London, Pepys registers his reaction in his diary entry on December 21, 1663:

> [It is] strange to observe the nature of these poor creatures, how they will fight till they drop down dead upon the table, and strike after they are ready to give up the ghost, not offering to run away when they are weary or wounded past doing further, whereas where a dunghill brood comes he will, after a sharp stroke that pricks him, run off the stage, and then they wring off his neck without more ado, whereas the other they preserve, though their eyes be both out, for breed only of a true cock of the game. Sometimes a cock that has had ten to one against him will by chance give an unlucky blow, will strike the other starke dead in a moment, that he never stirs more.

Although he says it was worth attending if only for the sheer spectacle of it, he "soon had enough of it" and left—most likely never to attend again.

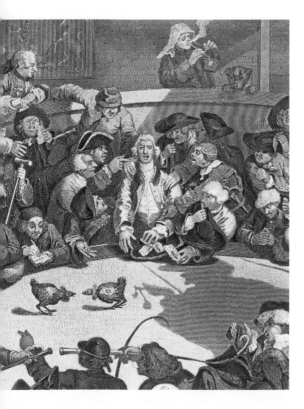

The Cockpit by William Hogarth, 1759
© Mary Evans Picture Library / Alamy

FROM AN UNCONSCIOUS VEGETARIAN TO A CONSCIOUS VEGAN

After emigrating to Miami from India, finding community we felt a part of was difficult enough, but being (lacto) vegetarian made us feel more alienated still. The norms of the American culture confused and bothered us. We didn't understand how people who kept petted and pampered animals (dogs and cats) could turn around and senselessly, viciously slaughter other beautiful, intelligent animals, like cows, pigs, and chickens.

Eventually, my mother found a vegan "meetup." Because most of the food of South India is vegan already, she had a very easy time throwing together delicious dishes that would get raves from all the vegans. For whatever reason, their truth didn't penetrate my dense skull at the time. They were vegan, and I was vegetarian.

No matter how clear the message, if you're not ready for it, you will not hear it. I thoughtlessly (literally) continued to consume dairy and eggs.

Finally, I stumbled upon the *Vegan Freaks* podcast. The hosts urged their listeners to try to go vegan for three weeks to see how they like it. I was willing to step up to the plate, so I "tried" it for three weeks.

Boom. I was vegan.

It wasn't that I hadn't heard the message before; it was that I wasn't ready to hear it or that the messenger wasn't speaking in terms that I understood. Once I got it, there was no turning back.

—*Dino in New York (U.S.)*

PURPLE CAULIFLOWER SOUP

Use any color cauliflower if you can't find purple.

- **1 tablespoon (15 ml) water, for sautéing**
- **1 large yellow onion, diced**
- **2 cloves garlic, minced**
- **1 large head purple, orange, or white cauliflower, cut into medium-size chunks**
- **1 large or 2 medium-size yellow potatoes, peeled and diced**
- **5½ cups (1,295 ml) vegetable stock**
- **½ teaspoon truffle or chile oil**
- **Salt and freshly ground pepper**
- **Chopped scallions or parsley, for garnish**

Heat the water in a sauté pan and sauté the onion until translucent, about 5 minutes. Add the garlic, and cook for 1 to 2 minutes longer. Add the cauliflower, potatoes, and vegetable stock.

Cook the soup over medium heat until the potatoes are fork-tender, about 25 minutes. Add the truffle oil, and stir to combine.

Transfer to a blender and blend until smooth. Add salt and pepper to taste, and garnish with the green scallions for a contrasting color.

Yield: 4 servings

*Soy-free, wheat-free

Originally published in *Color Me Vegan*

COOKING BEANS FROM SCRATCH

Unlike lentils, beans must be soaked before cooking, and this step trips people up. Accustomed to premade, fast, frozen, convenience foods, many people find the idea of planning in advance intimidating. It's this aversion that keeps people stuck in unhealthful eating habits. Planning meals in advance is the key to eating healthful, whole-food meals.

Soaking the beans softens them, returns moisture to them, reduces the cooking time, and helps release their sugar. The sugar in beans is what causes the digestive discomfort (bloating, gas, cramps) that some people have when eating them. When you soak the beans, you release the sugar from the beans into the water. This is why you should also always discard the soaking water—to get rid of all those hard-to-digest sugars.

Dried beans should soak for at least 6 hours and up to 10. (For 2 cups [500 g] dried beans, add 10 cups [2,350 ml] cold water.) However, you can also soak your beans in much less time by doing a "hot soak" or a "blanch soak." Add 2 cups (500 g) dried beans to 10 cups (2,350 ml) water, and bring to a rapid boil. Let boil for 2 to 3 minutes. Remove from the heat, cover, and set aside for at least 1 hour or up to 4 hours.

Once they're soaked, drain the soaking water, and rinse the beans. Cook the beans in fresh water. In general, beans take 1 to 2 ½ hours to cook depending on the variety, and you can also cook them in a slow cooker. (After 90 minutes, I usually check the beans every 20 minutes or so to make sure the water hasn't evaporated.)

Here are some general tips for the cooking stage:

* Flavor the beans while they cook. Add minced garlic and/or chopped onions, or spices and herbs such as cumin, chili powder, oregano, parsley, or thyme.

* Add salt and acidic ingredients, such as tomatoes, vinegar, wine, or citrus juices, only at the end of cooking, when the beans are tender. (Otherwise, they might hinder the cooking of the beans.)

ACTIVE LISTENING

With so many distractions, we listen to each other with divided attention, often more interested in hearing our own voice and ready to respond with a defensive answer or a witty quip. Instead of thoughtful exchanges of ideas, we've become accustomed to sound bites, we interrupt each other, we talk over cell phones ringing, or we talk while someone texts someone else. The anonymity of the Internet and email has dulled our discourse and dehumanized our dialogue.

We need a new approach. We need to make listening an active—rather than a passive—sport.

When we listen attentively, not only do we deepen our relationships with everyone around us, but we also become better voices for those who have no voice. Being a good communicator doesn't just mean that you can speak well; it also means that you listen well.

Listening takes energy—a lot of it. When we're actively listening, we're fully attentive, fully engaged. Active listening takes practice.

One of my favorite encounters with people occurs when they talk long enough that they wind up answering their own questions. Often when people are talking about their views on veganism or animal rights, I'm really just a sounding board for them. Many people already have the answers inside of them; they're often just looking for validation. Once they start talking, they discover things they may not have had I not been there in a listening role.

We need to relearn how to talk to one another, for our own relationships and for the sake of the animals.

KITCHEN SAFETY: **CHOOSING THE RIGHT CUTTING BOARD**

Next to using an improper knife (see Day 129), using an improper cutting board is the second leading cause of both kitchen accidents and cooking apathy.

Some of the worst culprits are glass cutting boards and flexible cutting "boards," both of which are dangerously slippery. Small cutting boards are also dangerous, because they make chopping difficult and awkward. The best size cutting board is at least 18 inches (45.7 cm) long and 12 inches (30.5 cm) high.

In terms of material, my favorite cutting board is made from bamboo, though any wood is good, too. They're both hard and solid and great to cut on (though bamboo is even harder and typically from a sustainable source). I recommend buying a cutting board made from a solid piece of wood or bamboo; I've seen too many cutting boards crack where two pieces are joined.

Properly cleaning and storing your wood/bamboo cutting boards ensures they have a longer life.

Don't leave veggie scraps and water sitting on your cutting board; they warp the wood. The same applies when you wash it: dry it right away, and never immerse it and let it soak in a sinkful of water. The wetter it remains, the higher the chances it will become warped.

If the board does become a little warped or it doesn't sit flat on your counter or if you find it tends to slide, then place a dish towel underneath it. If it becomes so warped that it wobbles every time you use it, then either return it to the manufacturer or chuck it.

Avoid placing hot pots and pans on the boards right off the stove or right from the oven. It might not happen right away, but over time, it the heat can dry out your board and cause cracking.

With these techniques, you'll keep your board—and fingers—for years to come.

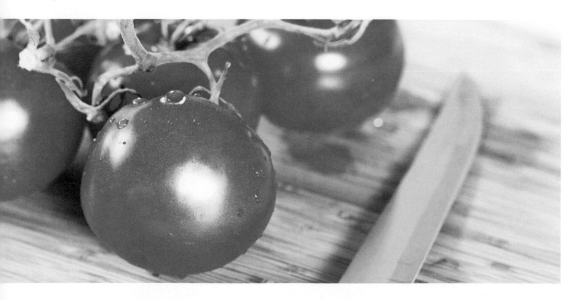

"LITTLE BOY PIG: A GENETICALLY MODIFIED TALE"
BY SHAD CLARK

"Little Boy Pig" is the tale of a mutant in search of his mother's heart. Born to an industrialized supply line of universal organ donors, young Ziggy is supposed to look like an ordinary pig, even if his eyes, lungs, liver, pancreas, kidneys, intestines, and heart are, more or less, human. But unlike all the other cloned pigs, Ziggy's human parts aren't confined to his insides; he's born with human hands and feet. Although this alarms the geneticist in charge of Animal Pharm, his concern is outweighed by intrigue.

Ziggy's value as a unique specimen saves him from imminent destruction, and the little boy pig becomes the unknowing subject of a new experiment. The geneticist orders that Ziggy be raised as a "normal" child in a house with no mirrors, and there in the care of his doting nanny, the little boy pig begins walking on two legs.

Developing like a human child but at the growth rate of a modern, industrialized pig, he's soon talking and reading. Before long, he asks the nanny if she's his mother. She confesses she's not and is then forced to lie, saying his parents passed peacefully away, and though it's not what he hoped to hear, Ziggy manages to carry on. The world is a bit bleaker now but still full of exhilarating discovery—until he sees his reflection in a pond: his true nature staring back at him.

Convinced that only one person could love such a misfit creature, Ziggy asks again about his mother. How did she die? His nanny doesn't know for sure and can only assume the worst, and so she encourages the little boy pig to confront the geneticist.

What's revealed rattles Ziggy's world and his perception of his place in it. Ultimately, and with the nanny's undying support, Ziggy seeks out—and finds—his mother's heart.

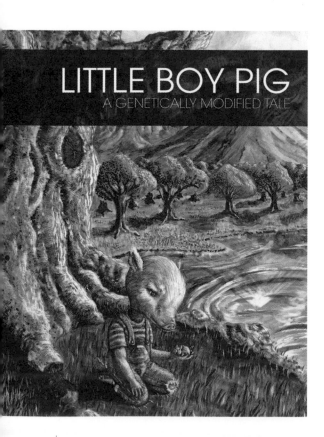

Cover Art of "Little Boy Pig"

MOTHERHOOD MADE ME VEGAN

I had dabbled in veganism and vegetarianism both after reading *Skinny Bitch* and then during my first pregnancy when the smell of cooking flesh made me sick. Although I supported the principles veganism stands for, I went back to eating meat.

Recently, I found the *Vegetarian Food for Thought* podcast and was listening to all of the back episodes; I watched *Food, Inc.* and read *The Face on Your Plate* and began to ask, "Is there such a thing as humane dairy?" As so many other people say, cheese was the hardest thing to let go of, but the more I researched, the more convinced I was that there wasn't a humane dairy option. How could there be?

When I listened to the podcast episodes on the dairy industry about the mother cows having their babies taken away, I broke. I had the information I needed to hear. As a new mother, I was crushed by the torment that dairy animals endured, and at that moment I wished I could recoil from myself for contributing to that pain by eating dairy. I would die inside if someone tried to take away my son.

I knew this was the right choice: Ironically, I knew it was the right choice even before I could make the choice for myself; when my son began eating solid foods, before my moment of clarity, I made him vegan meals. It was I who followed in his tiny footsteps.

Abby in Decatur, Illinois (U.S.)

WHITE BEAN DIP

Here is a nutritious and delicious last-minute dip for fresh veggies or crackers.

> **2 (15-ounce, or 420 g) cans cannellini beans, rinsed and drained**
> **⅓ cup (5 g) chopped fresh cilantro**
> **3 cloves garlic, peeled**
> **⅓ cup (80 ml) olive oil**
> **Juice from 1 large lemon**
> **Salt and freshly ground pepper**

In a food processor, combine the cannellini beans, cilantro, garlic, olive oil, and lemon juice. Process until smooth, or to your desired consistency. Taste, and season with salt and pepper.

Yield: 4 cups (960 g)

*Wheat-free, soy-free

TEMPEH

A soybean-based food, tempeh (pronounced *TEM-pay)* has been a staple in Indonesia for hundreds—possibly thousands—of years and is still building its reputation in the West. Less familiar than its more popular cousin, tofu, tempeh most likely originated on the island of Java in present-day Indonesia, unlike tofu, which came from China and Japan.

Whereas tofu starts with soybeans boiled and made into a milk, tempeh is simply whole soybeans that have been fermented with a grain, usually rice. Less processed than tofu and making use of the *whole bean*, tempeh tends to be easier to digest, is higher in protein, and is higher in fiber than tofu.

The flavor of tempeh is very different from that of tofu. It is nutty, earthy, and somewhat sweet, whereas tofu is more neutral. Tempeh is firm and chewy in texture, contrasted with the spongy, fluffier texture of tofu. The fermentation process causes it to have somewhat of a bitter edge to it, but that's not necessarily a bad thing. It is simply part of its flavor profile.

However, to reduce the bitter flavor, steam it first. Whether you're ultimately going to sauté, grill, stir-fry, or deep-fry it; crumble it into chili; or marinate and bake it, steam it first for just 10 minutes. Once you smell its nutty aroma and notice the color lighten a bit (from tan to a whiter color), it's sufficiently steamed.

Once it is steamed, you can do whatever you like to it.

* Cube it and fry it up in a little oil. Add to a vegetable stir-fry.

* Combine steamed, cooled cubes with your favorite eggless mayonnaise and finely chopped peppers and carrots for a tempeh "better-than-chicken" salad.

* Crumble steamed tempeh into pasta sauce or chili for a "meaty" texture.

* Grate steamed tempeh and mix with taco seasonings for a Mexican feast.

* Marinate steamed tempeh in barbecue sauce, and grill or bake in a glass baking dish for 30 minutes.

* Add cubed to soups and stews. (*Note:* Because the tempeh will spend a long time in a soup/stew, there's less of a need to steam it first.)

Tempeh also freezes well. Just thaw it completely before using in a recipe.

AVOIDING ARGUMENTS ONLINE

It's one thing if a friend, family member, or co-worker has a question sent via email that stems from a place of genuine curiosity, but it's quite another to get into a debate with someone via email, on a social networking site, or on a message board. This applies to whether you know the other person or not.

The Internet as a means of deep communication is simply inappropriate. There is no way to detect tone, inflection, irony, humor, or sarcasm, and innocent remarks are too easily misinterpreted. I can think of a million better ways to spend our time than explaining a misinterpreted email or blog comment.

The Internet creates the illusion that there's not another human on the other side of that computer. It's simply too impersonal and leaves open too many opportunities for anonymous attacks.

Unless someone is genuinely asking you for resources or advice or tips or recipes, just keep animal rights and vegan-related discussions and debates face-to-face and respectful.

KITCHEN SAFETY: USING THE PROPER KNIFE

Truth be told, you really need only one good knife: a chef's knife—and perhaps a serrated knife for cutting bread. Visit a cutlery or kitchen supply store to hold different knives in your hand to see which one you like the best. Chef's knives come in 6-, 7-, 8-, and 9-inch (15.2, 17.8, 20.3, and 23 cm) blades, the latter two being my personal favorites.

I'm convinced that one of the reasons people don't cook often enough is because they're using improper tools and not caring for the ones they have. Once you have a good knife, there are many things you can do to prolong its life.

Sharpening Knives

There are a lot of fancy sharpeners out there these days, but the simple "steel" sharpener is the most reliable. About 9 inches (23 cm) long,

it has a sturdy handle and blunt tip. In addition, consider getting your knives professionally sharpened every 6 months or so.

Cleaning Knives

Never put your knives in the dishwasher. The very high temperatures can damage the blades. Wash them by hand each time you use them, so food residues don't damage the blade. As soon as you wash them, dry them with a soft cloth.

Storing Knives

Don't store knives in a drawer. Aside from the fact that this is dangerous, the blades can also become dull when rubbing against one another. Buy a proper knife block or magnetic strip to hang.

DISCOURSE ON THE ORIGIN AND FOUNDATION OF THE INEQUALITY AMONG MEN
BY JEAN-JACQUES ROUSSEAU

Living at a time when traditional customs and institutions were critically dissected, philosopher Jean-Jacques Rousseau (1712–1778) wrote about everything from the nature of humans to the manner in which they should be educated.

In *Discourse on the Origin and Foundation of the Inequality Among Men,* written in 1754, Rousseau responds to the question, "What is the origin of inequality among men; and is it authorized by the natural law?" In order to understand the nature of humans, it is necessary that Rousseau study their treatment of and compassion toward nonhuman animals.

In proceeding thus, we shall not be obliged to make man a philosopher before he is a man. His duties toward others are not dictated to him only by the later lessons of wisdom; and, so long as he does not resist the internal impulse of compassion, he will never hurt any other man, nor even any sentient being, except on those lawful occasions on which his own preservation is concerned and he is obliged to give himself the preference. By this method also we put an end to the time-honoured disputes concerning the participation of animals in natural law: for it is clear that, being destitute of intelligence and liberty, they cannot recognise that law; as they partake, however, in some measure of our nature, in consequence of the sensibility with which they are endowed, they ought to partake of natural right; so that mankind is subjected to a kind of obligation even toward the brutes. It appears, in fact, that if I am bound to do no injury to my fellow-creatures, this is less because they are rational than because they are sentient beings: and this quality, being common both to men and beasts, ought to entitle the latter at least to the privilege of not being wantonly ill-treated by the former.

Every animal has ideas, since it has senses; it even combines those ideas in a certain degree; and it is only in degree that man differs, in this respect, from the brute. Some philosophers have even maintained that there is a greater difference between one man and another than between some men and some beasts.

Compassion, which is a disposition suitable to creatures so weak and subject to so many evils as we certainly are: by so much the more universal and useful to mankind, as it comes before any kind of reflection; and at the same time so natural, that the very brutes themselves sometimes give evident proofs of it. Not to mention the tenderness of mothers for their offspring and the perils they encounter to save them from danger, it is well known that horses show a reluctance to trample on living bodies. One animal never passes by the dead body of another of its species: there are even some which give their fellows a sort of burial; while the mournful lowings of the cattle when they enter the slaughter-house show the impressions made on them by the horrible spectacle which meets them.

PHOENIX, THE RABBIT WHO ROSE FROM THE ASHES

In shelters across the United States, rabbits— neglected by people who are no longer willing or able to care for them—are the third most commonly euthanized animals. Given all this, it's a wonder how a dismembered rabbit foot could possibly represent "good luck."

Unfortunately, it is not only the obvious dangers that threaten them, but also humans committing acts of violence against them.

In 2005, police in the San Francisco Bay Area responded to a call from a person who found a horribly injured rabbit, along with cigarettes, lighter fluid, and a lighter. A teenage boy had doused him with lighter fluid, lit a match, and forcibly restrained him while he burned. The rabbit was taken to the local humane society, where he began to get treatment—and survived against great odds.

Phoenix was appropriately named after the mythical bird that dies in flames and is reborn from the ashes. He endured second- and third-degree burns over much of his body, eventually lost his ears, and had extensive ear canal surgery because of infections that had developed from the attack.

Phoenix required months and months of care but amazed his caregivers with his resiliency, strong will to live, and ability to heal—both physically and emotionally.

Although it took months, the fur on his back fur grew back completely—even over the deepest of the wounds—and his coat is a very soft, thick white and gray. Phoenix is thriving at his lifelong home at SaveABunny in Mill Valley, California, where he will always be loved and protected.

—CPG

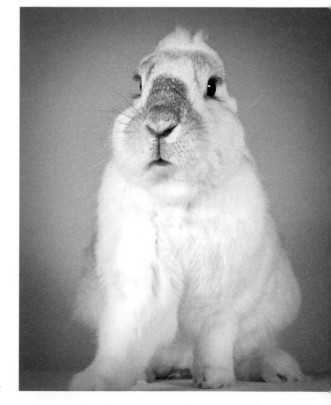

Phoenix, beautiful and safe
Photo courtesy of Save A Bunny

ASPARAGUS AND CARROTS WITH WALNUT DRESSING

This recipe is modified from one in *The Enlightened Kitchen* by Mari Fujii.

- 20 asparagus spears, thick ends removed
- 6 carrots, peeled and finely sliced into 1-inch (2.5 cm) matchsticks
- 1 cup (100 g) walnuts
- 4 teaspoons (20 g) white or "light" miso paste, or 2 teaspoons (10 g) red miso paste
- ¼ cup (60 ml) mirin
- 4 teaspoons (20 ml) tamari soy sauce
- ¼ cup (60 ml) white wine
- ¼ cup (60 ml) rice vinegar or any other white vinegar

Steam the asparagus and carrots for 5 to 7 minutes, until tender but not completely soft. Set aside. (You also can roast the vegetables.)

Meanwhile, using a food processor, blend together the walnuts, miso, mirin, tamari, white wine, and rice vinegar.

In a large-size bowl, combine the carrots and asparagus with the dressing, and arrange on a serving plate. Although you can serve this at room temperature, it is best served warm.

Yield: 6 servings

WHAT IS MIRIN?

Mirin is a kind of rice wine similar to sake, but with a lower alcohol content. It has a slightly sweet taste and is a common ingredient in teriyaki sauce.

*Oil-free, wheat-free

Originally published in *The Vegan Table*

WHITE BEANS

This general category contains such beans as cannellini, Great Northern, and navy. The small, white navy bean might also be called a pea bean or haricot, and it's used in such popular dishes as Boston baked beans. My favorite way of preparing white beans is either in a simple red sauce or just cooked slowly in garlic, sage, and olive oil.

- Because of their mild taste and texture, white beans complement Mediterranean dishes very well.

- On that same note, white beans and tomatoes (fresh or sun-dried) were made for each other.

- They pair well with stronger herbs such as sage and rosemary.

- I love the texture contrast between white beans and soft greens, such as spinach and chard, which cling to the beans when they're cooked.

- White beans can be added to any soup, stew, or chili.

ARE YOU SERIOUS?

Our desire to cling to familiar habits can be so strong that sometimes we reach for the most absurd argument for fear we may be forced to rethink our position. I, like many a vegan, have been on the receiving end of some pretty silly arguments.

When questions are at their most absurd, I first gauge the authenticity of the person asking the questions. Vegans known too well how exhausting and frustrating—not to mention ineffective—it can be to respond to someone whose intention is not to have a productive dialogue. The truth is sometimes:

* People are just goading you on.

* They're trying to trivialize your genuine concern for animals.

* They just want to hear themselves talk.

So, in the spirit of creating dialogue, I may ask them one of several questions:

* Are you serious?

* Do you really want me to answer that?

* Are you kidding?

* What do *you* think?

The secret to all of these questions is using the right tone and looking them right in the eye.

If asked in the right way and often with a smile, these questions (or variations thereof) accomplish one of several things.

* It disarms people, as they realize the absurdity of their question. Often, they chuckle and say, "I'm just teasing," which diffuses the situation.

* It highlights their snarkiness, at which point they may not want to bother pursuing it and choose to walk away.

* They confirm that they are serious and want you to answer, but now you've at least created some breathing room and established a connection.

And keep in mind that some questions may not even deserve an answer. If someone is just being obnoxious, it's better to just laugh and walk away rather than get sucked into a pointless argument.

SPENDING TIME WITH ANIMALS

A growing body of research suggests that interacting with animals may have health benefits, from decreasing blood pressure, cholesterol, and triglyceride levels to alleviating feelings of loneliness. Those of us fortunate to live with furred, feathered, or finned animals are already aware of the many intangible benefits we derive from this special bond. After all, we humans have been doing it for a long time.

Although new studies are being conducted all the time, many have found that dog guardians—who walk their four-legged friends—get more exercise and are less likely to be obese than people without dogs. There is evidence that there are social benefits as well, because people who walk dogs tend to have more interactions and conversations with strangers. There is a lot of clinical and epidemiological evidence suggesting that animal guardianship fosters healing—hence the rise in animal-assisted therapies in hospitals and nursing homes. Animals also play a critical role in child development, encouraging empathy, providing comfort, improving mood, and reducing anxiety.

You don't necessarily have to live with a dog or cat (or rabbit or other animal with whom you bond); there are many opportunities to interact with animals, many of which benefit the animals as much as—if not more than—they benefit you.

* Volunteer with your local SPCA or rescue organization.

* Foster an animal. Most people or organizations who do direct, hands-on animal rescue are in desperate need of volunteers to foster animals in their home.

* Visit a farmed animal sanctuary and spend time with cattle, pigs, goats, sheep, chickens, burros, rabbits, and turkeys.

* If you don't have your own animals, offer to walk your neighbor's dog or sit for a friend's cat when she's away.

* Volunteer at a local wildlife sanctuary.

* If you're looking for a career change, consider becoming an animal groomer, dog walker, or cat sitter.

* Spend quality time with your own animals—or encourage your children to do so—by brushing, petting, playing, or just sitting with your companions.

* Sit in nature to revel in the complex behaviors and interactions of wild animals.

* Pass the benefits on to others: enroll your own dog in a class to become a therapy dog.

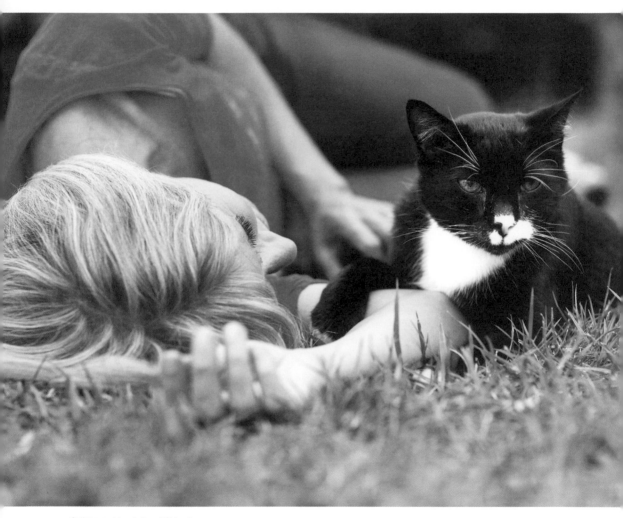

Colleen and her beloved Schuster
Photo by Sara Remington

UMBERTO D.
DIRECTED BY VITTORIO DE SICA

Directed by the great Italian neorealist Vittorio De Sica, *Umberto D.* is the story of an old man's struggle to keep his dignity—and his dog—as he falls further into poverty. With no family of his own, save his faithful terrier companion Flike (Italian for "flag"), Umberto struggles to afford the small ant-infested room he rents by selling his prized possessions, skipping meals, and, in one of the most heartbreaking moments on film, reminiscent of Charlie Chaplin, begging in the streets—almost.

While the story—always sympathetic but never sentimental—is certainly a larger commentary on society's forsaking of people as they age (Umberto is a former civil servant who can barely survive on his state pension), it is—at its heart—the story of a man and his dog.

Tired and battered, Umberto arranges to go to the hospital—not because he is incurably ill, but because he needs a few days of good food and restful sleep. Always mindful of his dog, Umberto trusts the building's maid, Maria, to care for Flike while he's gone.

When he returns, he discovers that Flike has run away—most likely to look for Umberto—and what follows is a long search and a painful visit to a dog pound. Here he sees how abandoned, neglected, and lost dogs are put to death, as he desperately tries to identify Flike among the terrified dogs arriving in trucks and barking in cages. They are reunited in an emotional albeit unsentimental scene.

Facing eviction and hopelessness, Umberto coolly and logically decides that he has exhausted his options and that the only path before him is suicide. He cannot, however, kill himself before he finds a good home for his beloved Flike. And his standards are high. He will not leave Flike to just anyone.

In the end, it is Flike who saves Umberto. Though the film concludes on a question mark, one thing that's certain is that Umberto will do what is necessary to survive, precisely because of his love for his dog. Just as Flike refuses to leave Umberto, Umberto will not abandon Flike.

"HUMANE MEAT-EATER" TURNED VEGAN

I've eaten a loose vegetarian diet off and on for fifteen years. Last year, I stopped eating land animals for good. Before going vegetarian, I had sought out meat from locally raised, authentically grazing animals—what the industry calls "humane."

Explaining why *some* meat is okay became fuzzy and felt hollow. If most meat comes from tortured animals, why eat it at all when there are so many other options?

For a year, I ate no meat but continued to consume milk, eggs, and cheese. I avoided thinking about the conditions under which the animals who produce these products lived. The animals producing milk, cheese, and eggs were still suffering, living in unbearable conditions as they produced the organic milk and cheese I consumed each day.

And so, I finally *went there*. I finally let myself think about the conditions the animals lived in and that my life was being sustained by their suffering. There are so many other ways to sustain my life than animal products—so many wonderful ways—and so I became vegan.

Since then, I've gained so much more knowledge not only about the raising and killing of animals but also about nutrition and health and about the importance of being joyful about embracing veganism. It's a relief to no longer open the refrigerator to see eggs and cheese and feel my mind close to their origins. Bringing plant-based foods to the center of my life and to meals that I share with family and friends is nourishing physically and spiritually.

—*Victoria in Colorado (U.S.)*

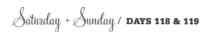

CARROT-GINGER-TAHINI SOUP

If you've never added tahini (sesame paste) to a creamy soup, you're in for a real treat. With its nutty flavor and smooth texture, it adds dimension and pairs particularly well with carrots.

- **7 or 8 large carrots, peeled and cut into rounds**
- **1 yellow onion, diced**
- **2 teaspoons (5.4 g) grated ginger**
- **4 cups (940 ml) vegetable stock or water**
- **2 tablespoons (30 g) tahini**
- **¼ cup (60 ml) nondairy milk (soy, rice, almond, hazelnut, hemp, or oat)**
- **Salt and freshly ground pepper**

To a 4-quart (3.6 L) saucepan, add the carrots, onion, ginger, and vegetable stock. Cook over medium heat for 40 minutes, or until the carrots are soft.

Transfer to a blender, add the tahini and milk, and blend until smooth. Season with salt and pepper.

Return the soup to the pot to heat and serve, or transfer to a container and store in the refrigerator until ready to heat and serve. Garnish with freshly ground pepper.

Yield: 4 servings

*Oil-free, wheat-free, soy-free if not using soy milk

LEEKS

A member of the onion family and resembling overgrown scallions (green onions), the leek is found in abundance in Welsh, British, Scottish, and Irish recipes. A delicious vegetable in its own right, leeks are often used as the base for soup stock—not only for its flavor but also because, when cooked, it thickens the liquid.

Slightly sweeter than onions, leeks can be used in stir-fries, sautés, tofu scrambles, quiches, and stews. Because the dark green top is fibrous and tough, you'll want to use only the light green and white portions of this cylindrical vegetable.

The main issue with leeks is making sure you clean them thoroughly. Because of the way they grow (they are a root vegetable, after all), they amass dirt and sand within their overlapping layers. To prepare for cleaning and cooking, first remove the root base, some of the tough green tops, and the outermost layer. Make a lengthwise incision down the center, fold it open, and run the leek under cool water, separating the layers and rinsing each one as you go. Once thoroughly washed (or soaked), slice and chop as needed for your recipe.

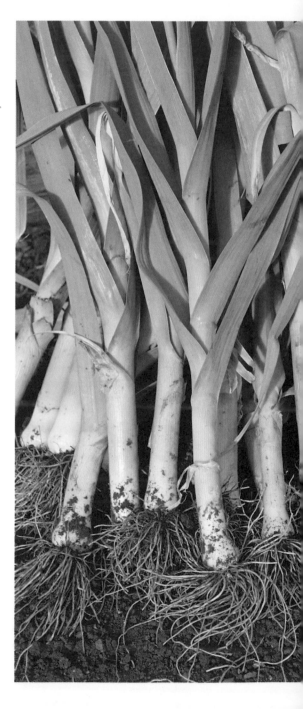

HAVING A SENSE OF HUMOR

Keeping a sense of humor is vital to developing an authentic rapport with people. Both vegans and non-vegans get uptight around such a personal and sensitive subject, and humor has a way of diffusing tension.

In all of our interactions, we act as mirrors to one another. We reflect back to each other what we might need to see about ourselves, and food issues in particular bring up a lot of emotions.

Just by declaring you're vegan, some people take it as an attack and may retaliate with passive-aggressive—and sometimes aggressive—behavior or comments, such as, "If animals aren't supposed to be eaten, then why are they made out of meat?" or "Don't you care about plants?"

Some may be passive, snarkier, or even more aggressive. Maybe they don't understand what "vegan" really means. Maybe they feel guilty. Maybe they tried being vegan but didn't continue. For whatever reason, they're uncomfortable and need to say or do something to make themselves feel bigger. They do this by making you feel small, by making a joke at your expense.

If you respond with a cranky quip or you walk away or you insult them in return, you're giving them the power they want. *What they don't expect you to do is laugh or smile.*

By laughing at their joke or at yourself and by not taking them (and yourself) so seriously, it shows that you're approachable. It smashes the cliché that vegans don't have a sense of humor, and it shows them that you're someone they can come to with questions. Just like the little boy who pulls the braids of the girl he has a crush on, they *really are* curious. They just don't want *you* to know that they are.

By responding with levity, they relax a little, too, and it opens up the possibility of a fruitful and enjoyable dialogue.

SHOPPING AT YOUR LOCAL FARMERS' MARKET

Farmers' markets and farm stands are popping up all around, making it easier for us to choose locally grown fruits and vegetables. The benefits are numerous for everyone.

Benefit to Farmers

* Selling directly to the consumer and cutting out the middleman allows farmers to control prices, enabling them to yield a higher return.

* Because transport and packaging requirements are reduced, so are the costs.

* Markets provide a secure and regular outlet, which is especially valuable for smaller or newer farmers who can't compete in large grocery stores.

Benefit to Consumers

* Consumers can communicate directly with the farmers and find out exactly how their vegetables are grown.

* Eating produce picked at their peak ensures fresher, better-tasting food, but it also ensures higher quantities of phytochemicals (see Day 80).

* Many vendors are a wonderful source of information about how to prepare and cook their fruits and vegetables.

* Market prices are often lower than at grocery stores.

* Shopping at farmers' markets incline people toward eating in season.

Benefit to the Environment

* Transporting produce only a few miles—rather than a few thousand—from local farms means reduced vehicle pollution, noise, and fossil fuel use.

* Transported in boxes and reusable crates, produce at farmers' markets requires little packaging.

* Most farmers' markets encourage environmentally friendly growing practices, such as organic or pesticide-free. Some farmers' markets sell only 100 percent organic produce.

* Farmers' markets encourage farm diversification and hence biodiversity.

The Local Economy and Communities

Encouraging interaction between rural and urban communities, many farmers open their farms up to visitors in addition to bringing their produce to the cities.

Farmers' markets stimulate local economic development by increasing employment and encouraging consumers to support local business, thus keeping the money within the local community. Business retailers in the vicinity of the farmers' markets also benefit.

Many people don't even know where to begin when they visit their first farmers' market. Ask the farmers for their advice. They'll be more than happy to help!

"TO SERVE MAN"
BY DAMON KNIGHT

More people know the TV adaptation "To Serve Man" than the short story itself, written by Damon Knight and published in 1950. Adapted into a *Twilight Zone* episode and airing in 1962, it's an unforgettable story (and a delightfully campy but classic episode).

Set in 1950 during the cold war, the story is a flashback told in the first-person narrative by a United Nations translator named Gregori. During a special session of the UN, members listen to testimony given by three Kanamit representatives, a race of aliens who resemble both pigs and humans.

Having learned the means of producing free unlimited energy, doubling agricultural yields, and creating "taller, stronger, healthier" humans, they simply want to share these discoveries with the human race—no strings attached. And the Kanamit do just that.

Meanwhile, Gregori and a friend, suspicious of the aliens, steal and partially translate a Kanamit book that appears to be a guide of sorts. After several weeks, they decipher the title to be *To Serve Man* and almost leave it at that. But Gregori persists and translates the first chapter of the book, leaving him distraught at what he discovers.

"It's a cookbook!" he declares, and the story ends.

GRATEFUL

I had been a vegetarian since I was fourteen, but I was someone who swore I could never give up cheese. I had already given up milk and eggs; cheese was my sticking point.

My grandparents ran a dairy farm, and I remember being a very young child playing in an old veal crate. I asked my father what the box was for. He said that calves were put in there, and I remember thinking that they must have misbehaved and were being punished. Even with this childhood memory I never really made the connection or at least denied the connection between the dairy industry and the veal industry.

Once I made the decision to become vegan, my life changed completely. I taste so many more flavors in my meals now that they're not smothered in what was once my favorite food. I feel like I've eaten so many more things since losing the cheese, and I'm so grateful for these changes. I also lost 10 pounds (4.5 kg), which is a wonderful bonus.

I was always somewhat apologetic to people about my vegetarianism, never wanting to be the center of attention, but that has changed, too. Now, when people wrinkle their nose at me and say in that wonderfully condescending tone, "Oh, you're vegan?" I give them a huge guilt-free smile and say, "Yes, isn't it great?"

—*Shana in Madison, Wisconsin (U.S.)*

THAI SALAD

Peanut butter sauces are my favorite for noodle dishes or cabbage salads—warm or cold. This recipe is from star tester Barbara Lyons.

1 cup (260 g) salsa (smooth, not chunky)
¼ cup (260 g) smooth peanut butter
2 tablespoons (40 g) agave nectar
3 tablespoons (45 ml) orange juice
2 tablespoons (30 ml) water, or more as needed
1 teaspoon (5 ml) tamari soy sauce
1 teaspoon (2 g) grated or finely minced fresh ginger
½ head green cabbage, shredded
½ cup (8 g) chopped cilantro
¼ cup (75 g) coarsely chopped peanuts
½ cup (75 g) red pepper strips
Salt and freshly ground pepper

Combine the salsa, peanut butter, agave nectar, orange juice, water, tamari, and ginger in a small saucepan. Cook and stir over low heat until the mixture is smooth and blended.

Toss the cabbage with the peanut sauce (warm or cooled) until thoroughly combined. Arrange the cabbage on a platter, and sprinkle the cilantro, peanuts, and pepper strips over the top. Season with salt and pepper. Serve immediately.

Yield: 4 to 6 servings

*Oil-free, wheat-free

KIDNEY BEANS

A type of red bean, the kidney bean was named for its visual resemblance to an actual kidney. Loaded with antioxidants, kidney beans (as well as smaller "red beans") were named by the USDA as one of the top-scoring foods in terms of nutrient density.

Kidney beans are a large part of the cuisine of northern India as well in the popular red beans and rice dish of Louisiana Creole cuisine. I love the heartiness of kidney beans and find they work with most cuisines. I add them to green salads, bean chili, pasta sauce, and bean salads and even make bean dip with them.

In a food processor or blender, combine 1 can of cooked kidney beans with garlic, cumin, and chile peppers for a delicious spread that can be used as a crudité dip or sandwich filling.

DID YOU KNOW?
Cannellini beans are simply white kidney beans.

SPEAKING YOUR TRUTH

In the many years I've been a vegan and an animal advocate, I've concluded that the *eating* aspects of being vegan are a breeze, but dealing with the social aspects can be a little challenging. Most of us have been brainwashed into believing we need to consume animal products, so the burden remains on the vegan to justify his or her eating habits. I think this is why many people retreat from it in the first place.

We often say that we value individuality in our culture, but I think we value conformity a lot more. "Nonconformity" is a dirty word in many people's vocabulary.

Many people shy away from being vegan because they're afraid to make anyone uncomfortable. When they go to dinner at friends' houses or out to lunch with non-vegan friends, they don't want to appear difficult. Where we stand on certain issues—namely, that animals are here for their own purpose and not here for our pleasure—is not something we have to apologize for.

Frankly, it would be pretty self-centered to try and control other people's reactions—being afraid of telling someone you don't eat animals because it might make them uncomfortable? How can we truly guess what someone's reaction is going to be? Who are we to protect people from the very thing that might open up their own suppressed feelings?

As long as we think we're "protecting" people from discomfort, we're not only denying our own ethics and perpetuating the socially sanctioned abuse of animals, but we're also—potentially—denying other people their own transformation. Because how else does this occur than through honest interaction and communication with others?

We need to learn to speak our truth without being attached to what that truth will do to other people. After all, if we don't stand up for what we believe in, we might as well have no opinions at all.

EXERCISING

We are creatures who are built to move. We aren't designed to lead the sedentary lives we currently live. Cardiovascular exercise—the kind that gets your heart pumping—has numerous physiological, psychological, emotional, and even social benefits, especially if we use it as an opportunity to connect with friends.

* Endorphins released during exercise ease depression and reduce stress.

* Our immune systems are boosted as a result of exercise, which results in fewer colds.

* The exercise glow makes us look healthier, which in turn boosts our self-esteem.

* Exercise increases energy and strength.

The American College of Sports Medicine recommends a combination of aerobic exercise (dancing, walking, jogging), strength-training (weight or resistance training), and stretching.

Modifying our habits even slightly will be an improvement:

* Take the stairs instead of the elevator (down and up).

* Go for a walk with a friend at lunch instead of sitting in a restaurant.

* Get up from your desk several times a day to take a brief walk.

* Walk or bicycle to work.

* When you send your kids outside to play, take 15 minutes to run around with them.

* Walk your dog twice a day instead of once.

* Do jumping jacks during TV commercials.

There are so many wonderful ways to move: running, hiking, walking, cycling, swimming, yoga, jumping rope, dancing, lifting weights, joining a sports team, playing tennis, bowling, skating, rollerblading, skiing, golfing, or doing aerobics.

The key to adding exercise to your everyday routine is doing something you love.

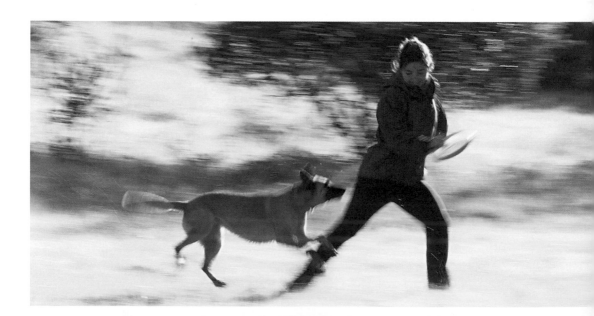

AU HASARD BALTHAZAR
DIRECTED BY ROBERT BRESSON

Au Hasard Balthazar (1966) is an exquisitely beautiful and heartbreaking film directed by Robert Bresson (1901–1999), whose titular main character, a donkey, is as much a victim of human cruelty as his human counterpart, Marie, is.

Depending on whose hands he falls into, Balthazar is used as a pack animal, forced to perform in the circus, and used to generate power for a mill by being tied up and forced to walk in endless circles. Finally, he's used to smuggle contraband for the same thugs who take advantage of Marie.

The film can be easily read as a religious parable of sin and suffering, especially when viewed through Bresson's deep Catholic sensibilities. In this story of purity and transcendence, Balthazar endures a Christlike journey, during which he is beaten, whipped, slapped, burned, mocked, and ultimately killed on a hillside. He's even called "a saint" for having abided so much suffering.

Balthazar—and the martyred Marie—are both victims in a fallen paradise. Here, idyllic beauty belies a world of cruelty and moral depravity, from which neither Marie nor Balthazar can escape. To great effect, Bresson depicts human brutality with little emotion, until the final scene, which is—accompanied by Schubert's exquisite Piano Sonata No. 20—one of the most sublime moments in cinematic history.

Balthazar is a beautiful and tragic story that illuminates the common roots of cruelty and violence, whether they're aimed at humans or animals.

NEWBORN CALF AND HIS MOTHER REUNITE FOR LIFE

Days old and barely breathing, Harrison was lying alone in an open field and only hours away from death when he was discovered by a compassionate humane officer in Santa Cruz, California. The newborn—the son of a cow bred to replenish a herd of beef cattle—was nonresponsive, bellowing only briefly in pain when the officer checked his vitals and determined that he was in desperate need of medical attention.

Harrison was rushed to a nearby veterinary hospital, where medical personnel determined that he was suffering from a severe navel infection, which had begun to spread throughout his body. He was administered antibiotics and fluids, but these measures would not be enough to see him safely through his ordeal.

Learning from veterinarians that Harrison's chances of survival would increase with access to his mother's milk, Santa Cruz Animal Services swiftly retrieved the mother, Loretta, from the ranch and reunited her with her son. The pair immediately picked up where they left off— Loretta taking over the care of her son and Harrison basking in the attention only a mother can provide.

When Animal Services asked the rancher why he left the calf for dead, he merely replied, "The calf is only worth $5, so why would I pay to treat it? If it lives, it lives. If it dies, it dies."

After convalescing under the care of veterinarians, a healthier and happier mother-son duo traveled to Farm Sanctuary's California shelter, where they remain inseparable. Having the opportunity to shelter Loretta and Harrison from an industry that inevitably tears farm animal families apart has been a true gift, one that goes unmatched for everyone involved.

—*Farm Sanctuary, Orland, California (U.S.)*

Loretta nursing Harrison, the only offspring she ever got to keep and nurture
Photo courtesy of Connie Pugh

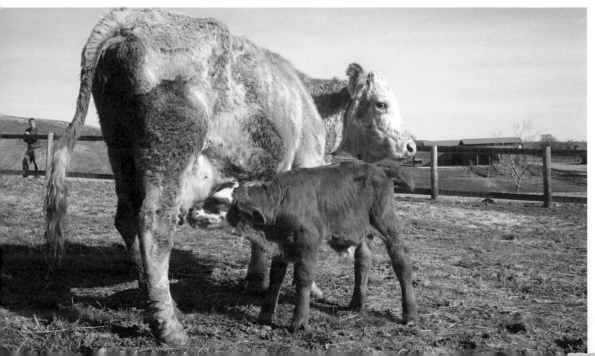

BORSCHT (BEET SOUP)

Warning: This soup will make a beet lover out of you!

3 medium-size beets, plus greens
6 cups (1,410 ml) water
1 ½ teaspoons (9 g) salt
½ cup (65 g) finely chopped carrots
5 yellow potatoes such as Yukon gold
    (3 peeled and quartered, 2 diced;
    peeling optional)
2 tablespoons (28 g) nondairy butter
1 yellow onion, finely chopped
1½ cups (270 g) chopped fresh tomatoes or
    1 can (15 ounces, or 420 g) diced tomatoes
¼ cup (60 ml) nondairy milk (soy, rice,
    almond, hazelnut, hemp, or oat)
    or soy creamer
1½ cups (105) finely shredded red
    or green cabbage
1 tablespoon (4 g) fresh dill
Salt and freshly ground black pepper
1 large bunch fresh dill, snipped
    with scissors

Using a sharp knife, carefully cut off the skin of the beets, without taking too much beet flesh. Cut the peeled beets into quarters. Wash the beet greens to remove any soil and roughly chop. Set aside.

Place the water, salt, carrots, the 3 quartered potatoes, beets, and beet greens in a large soup pot over high heat. Bring to a boil.

Meanwhile, in a separate sauté pan over medium heat, melt the nondairy butter. Sauté the onion until tender, approximately 5 minutes. Stir in the tomatoes, reduce the heat to medium-low, and simmer for 10 minutes. Set aside.

When the beets are tender, about 30 minutes later, use a slotted spoon or tongs to remove them from the pot, along with the potatoes. Chop up half of these beets into bite-size pieces, and place the other half in a blender or food processor, along with the potatoes. Add the milk, and blend until smooth. (You can also mash them by hand.) Return the bite-size beets and mashed beets/potatoes to the soup pot.

At the same time, add the remaining 2 diced potatoes, shredded cabbage, dill, and tomato/onion mixture. Simmer the soup until the potatoes are just tender but still firm, 10 to 15 minutes. Season with salt and pepper to taste.

Spoon into individual serving bowls, and top with a generous amount of dill. Fresh dill is key to this dish, so don't be stingy with it!

Yield: 8 servings

Oil-free, wheat-free, soy-free if not using soy milk

Originally published in *The Vegan Table*

SEEDS

An excellent source of fiber, protein, selenium, and vitamin E, seeds should be a regular part of a healthful diet. It's true they're high in fat, but most of it is monounsaturated fat, and that's a good thing. Whole fats are a necessary component of our diets, and seeds are a wonderful source.

* Flaxseeds—A superior source of omega-3 fatty acids, these gorgeous little seeds must be ground before you eat them so that your body can utilize the nutrients.

* Hemp Seeds—Also a wonderful source of omega-3 fats, which strengthen brain cells and improve memory, hemp seeds have a delicious, nutty flavor. No need to grind them as you do flaxseeds; hemp seed butter is also available.

* Pumpkin Seeds—Packing a nutritional wallop, pumpkin seeds are a rich source of minerals, as well as protein, zinc, and fiber. Sprinkle raw pumpkin seeds on oatmeal or any type of salad—pasta, noodle, green, tofu—or eat as a snack. For a treat, toss pumpkin seeds with a little olive oil and cayenne pepper and bake them until crisp.

* Sesame Seeds—Truly an ancient seed, sesame is the oldest known plant cultivated for its seeds and oil. They add crunch to any dish and pair beautifully with Asian and Middle Eastern flavors. Try the Japanese condiment *gomasio,* which is a delicious blend of toasted whole sesame seeds mixed with sea salt. Sprinkle it on soups or any favorite dish.

* Sunflower Seeds—Harvested from the huge head of the sunflower and containing a rich quantity of vitamin E and selenium, sunflower seeds make tasty additions to trail mix, granola, stuffing, and baked goods. Avoid sunflower oil, however. It is too high in omega-6 fatty acids.

* Chia Seeds—The newest seed on the block to be touted for its high omega-3 content, chia seeds are a member of the mint family and are grown abundantly in southern Mexico. Unlike with flaxseeds, chia seeds don't need to be ground up to make their nutrients available. Add them to oatmeal, nondairy yogurt, breads, muffins, or biscuits.

COMPASSIONATE ALTERNATIVES: LET THE CAT OUT OF THE BAG

When you "let the cat out of the bag," you disclose a secret. What is the cat doing in the bag in the first place? On that point alone, we should try to use a different expression, such as "Keep it under wraps." Or "Keep it under your hat." Or just "Keep it secret." You could even say, "The secret's out of the bag." Or "The secret's been revealed."

The origin of the idiom itself is not certain, but there are two speculations. One relates to the supposed fraud of substituting a cat for a pig at markets where they're sold for slaughter. So, if you let the cat out of the bag, you disclose the trick. The other theory is that the "cat" refers to the cat-o'-nine-tails, a leather whip that was supposedly stored in a bag when it wasn't being used to flog sailors. Let's just do away with the cat in the bag altogether, and make letting said cat out of the bag obsolete.

GETTING CALCIUM

Calcium is a mineral found in the ground. Although it's true that cow's milk contains a lot of calcium, this is only true because cows eat grass. Grass—like all green leafy plants—contains high amounts of calcium. However, because most dairy cows are raised on dry lots and not given grass to graze on, their feed is supplemented with calcium to make up for the calcium they're not consuming naturally.

Humans have absolutely no nutritional requirement to drink the milk of another animal—whether that animal be hoofed or clawed; in fact, the link between cow's milk and many preventable Western diseases, including diabetes and certain types of cancer, is indisputable, such that we are actually harming ourselves with this seemingly innocuous secretion.

Humans do, however, have a nutritional requirement for calcium. The best way to consume calcium is to go straight to the source, just like the cows do: to dark green leafy vegetables—kale, collard greens, chard, beet greens, mustard greens—as well as broccoli, beans, nuts, and seeds.

Adults should aim for 1,000 to 1,200 mg of calcium per day. Also, keep in mind:

* Many nondairy milks are fortified with calcium, vitamin D, and/or vitamin B_{12}. Many orange juices are also fortified with calcium.

* Because the calcium can settle to the bottom of the container, shake calcium-fortified nondairy milks before drinking.

* Calcium supplements can inhibit iron absorption if eaten at the same time.

See Day 59 for more on increasing the absorption of calcium.

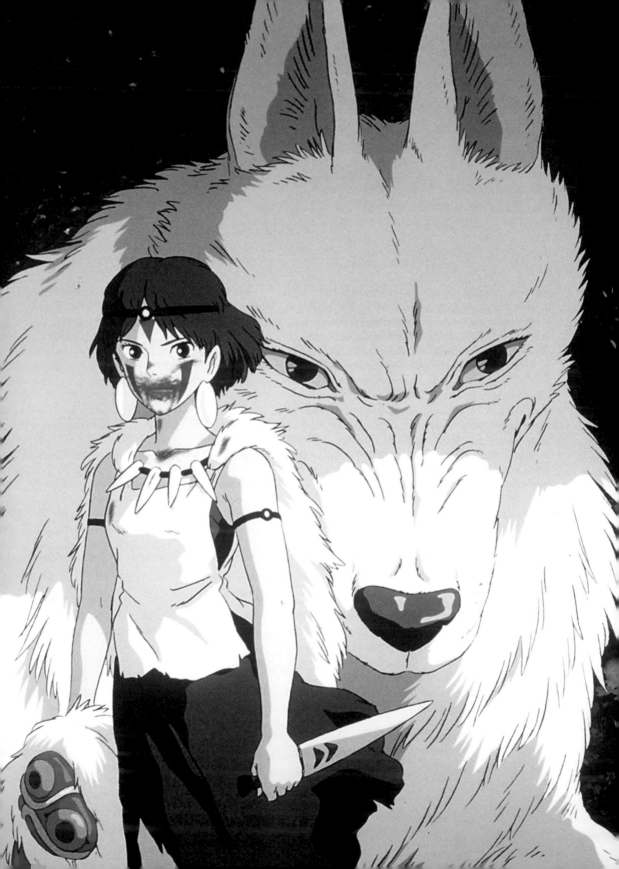

PRINCESS MONONOKE
DIRECTED BY HAYAO MIYAZAKI

A relevant film in these days of environmental awareness, *Princess Mononoke* is a 1997 Japanese animated drama about the struggle between the supernatural guardians of the forest and the human beings who destroy nature in favor of industry.

Both mythic—the film contains some of the most fantastical figures on screen—and historic—set in Japan in the sixteenth century—*Princess Mononoke* opens with a boar god being shot with a bullet made of iron, a material so anathema to his nature that it turns him into a demon. He attacks a local village but is killed by its young prince, Ashitaka. In the fight, Ashitaka's arm is cursed by some of the evil that possessed the boar god and he is told it will spread and overtake him if he does not have the curse lifted by the Forest Spirit who lives deep in the woods. Heeding the advice, he travels to the forest on his red elk and encounters Iron Town, whose inhabitants have destroyed the surrounding forest to make charcoal, iron, and firearms.

In defense of their home, the animal spirits of the diminishing forest attack the town, led by Princess Mononoke, named San, a mysterious human girl who was raised by three wolves, including the wolf god Moro. (*Mononoke* is a Japanese word for "spirit.") Ashitaka joins San and fights to protect the forest against the leader of Iron Town, Lady Eboshi, who is determined to destroy the Forest Spirit so she can expand her ironworks.

After a few bloody battles, Ashitaka and San save the Forest Spirit, the land turns green once more, and Ashitaka's curse is lifted. In a renewed Iron Town where even Lady Eboshi is reformed, Ashitaka settles down to help transform it into a peaceful village.

In an early scene in the film, Ashitaka asks Moro, "Can't humans and nature live together in peace?" In the beautiful images of rejuvenation that end the film, director Hayao Miyazaki seems to suggest that we *can*. But if we are to survive, we must find a sustainable balance between our technological advancements and the needs of the natural world.

Princess Mononoke after saving one of her wolves by sucking the poison out of his wound.

ONCE-BLIND CHARLIE

When Charlie arrived as a blind beagle, we noticed his pupils reacted to the camera flash when we took his photo, which meant his retinas were detecting light. Maybe he could see behind his thick cataracts?

Our vet also found the same pupillary light reflex, and the electroretinogram confirmed that his retinas were really working. This meant Charlie could have surgery to restore his vision!

Normally the surgery takes about 75 minutes; Charlie's cataracts were so old and dense it took 165 minutes. But when he awoke from anesthesia, it was clear Charlie could see. During his post-op evaluation, he saw the exam room door was open and walked out.

Back at the hotel, we took Charlie for a walk and watched as he looked in awe at everything around him. Vehicles moving, birds flying, people strolling—Charlie soaked it all in. In the hotel room, Charlie kept going over to the mirror to stare at himself. It's as if he was thinking, "I'm as handsome as I thought I was!"

But nothing compared to his excitement the next day when he saw Alayne for the first time. Charlie kept jumping up and down, trying to get closer to her face. His tail wagged so fast we thought it might come loose. He could barely contain himself.

Just when we thought it couldn't get any better, it did. A wonderful couple adopted Charlie as a companion for their other beagle, Hugo.

—Rolling Dog Ranch Animal Sanctuary, Lancaster, New Hampshire (U.S.)

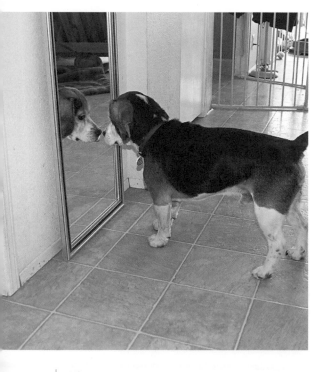

Charlie admiring himself in the mirror after the successful surgery through which he regained his sight

Photo courtesy of Rolling Dog Ranch Animal Sanctuary

NIÇOISE-STYLE SALAD

As suggested by the name, this colorful salad hails from the city of Nice in the Côte d'Azur region of France. My version is much healthier and compassionate, replacing the tuna with artichoke hearts (which were in the original recipe anyway) and eliminating the eggs.

3 yellow potatoes, peeled and cubed
1 large garnet or jewel yam, peeled
    and cubed
8 ounces (225 g) green beans, ends trimmed
1 cup (55 g) shredded salad greens
1 roasted red bell pepper, cut into strips
1 (6-ounce, or 170 g) jar marinated artichoke
    hearts, roughly chopped
2 plum (Roma) tomatoes, quartered
    or chopped
½ cup (75 g) halved yellow pear tomatoes
2 tablespoons (12.5 g) pitted and halved
    Niçoise or kalamata olives
1 (15-ounce, or 420 g) can red kidney beans,
    rinsed and drained
¼ cup (60 ml) olive oil
¼ cup (60 ml) white wine vinegar or
    apple cider vinegar
2 teaspoons (8 g) Dijon mustard
2 cloves garlic, minced
2 tablespoons (8 g) minced fresh parsley
2 tablespoons (5 g) minced fresh basil
2 tablespoons (8 g) minced fresh tarragon
Salt and freshly ground pepper

Steam the potatoes and yam until tender enough to be pierced with a fork.

Steam the green beans until they are cooked but still firm, about 7 minutes. Remove from the heat immediately, and submerge in ice water to stop the cooking and keep them crisp. Drain, and set aside.

At this stage, you can either arrange everything on a plate traditional style or combine as a mixed salad. If you opt for the former, place a layer of the salad greens on 4 dinner plates. Arrange a portion of the potatoes, yam, green beans, roasted pepper, artichoke hearts, plum and pear tomatoes, olives, and kidney beans decoratively on each plate. If you opt for the latter, simply toss the ingredients together in a large bowl and divide among 4 plates or bowls.

In a small bowl, combine the oil, vinegar, mustard, garlic, parsley, basil, tarragon, and salt and pepper to taste. Whisk until blended, then drizzle some of the dressing over each salad (or if combining all the ingredients together, drizzle on enough dressing to coat and toss gently).

Yield: 4 servings

*Soy-free, wheat-free

TEA

Never having had a cup of coffee in my life, I'm a self-proclaimed tea junkie and drink several pots of tea a day.

All tea comes from the same plant, the *Camellia sinensis*, an evergreen shrub or small tree indigenous to China but also grown in other parts of the world. Most premium teas come from the mountainous regions of China, Taiwan, Japan, Korea, India, and Sri Lanka.

The difference in teas has to do with how the leaves are processed.

White tea: White teas represent the most natural form of tea. Steamed instead of air-dried to stop the oxidation process (which naturally begins occurring once the leaves are picked), "white teas" are plucked from the downy premature leaves of the White Tea varietal and also include some buds because they're picked just before the buds have opened. Based on Western medical findings, white teas are reputed to be higher in antioxidants than green teas, and they're extremely low in caffeine.

Green tea: The next grade is green teas, which have been pan-fired or steamed to retain their color and nutrients, and indeed, green teas have been found to be rich in antioxidants and vitamins and nutrients. Green tea flavors can be sweet, nutty, buttery, smoky, marshy, or floral depending on the location and time of year the tea was picked.

Oolong tea: Next, you've got your oolong teas, which have been semioxidized and roasted, containing medium levels of caffeine. Clay *yixing* (pronounced *ee-SHING*) teapots and the numerous accoutrements used for oolong teas were developed by the Chinese and Tawainese.

Black tea: Finally, black teas are fully oxidized through an intense rolling or tearing process. They're higher in caffeine content than greens and whites but are still moderate compared to coffee.

Pu-erh tea: Pu-erh (pronounced *poo-AIR*) teas have a strong, earthy aroma and a full-bodied flavor, which increase as they age. Pu-erhs come in many forms, are compressed into any number of sizes, and may be aged in baskets, bamboo stalks, or citrus rinds.

Tisanes: If it doesn't come from the *Camellia sinensis* plant, it's not tea. Anything made from flowers, herbs, twigs, or spices is a *tisane*, an herbal infusion—not tea.

COMPASSIONATE ALTERNATIVES TO VIOLENT BIRD IDIOMS

A chicken in every pot—During the 1928 presidential campaign, a circular published by the Republican Party claimed that if Herbert Hoover won the presidency, there would be "a chicken in every pot and a car in every garage," referring to the prosperity they promised. However, the public lost their confidence in Hoover when the stock market crashed in 1929, plunging the United States into the Great Depression. Reportedly, in the seventeenth century, Henry IV wished that each of his peasants would enjoy "a chicken in his pot every Sunday." Rather than wish dead chickens for the poor, we could wish for:

* Abundance for all

* Beans in every pot

* Rice in every cupboard

Ducks in a row/ducks in order—Referring to the act of being well organized and having everything in place before you start a project, this idiom most likely alludes to a mother duck who leads her ducklings in an orderly single file. The image alone is one that makes me smile, and it is one of those animal idioms we can keep.

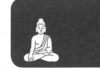
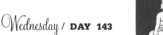

TAKING SUPPLEMENTS

A multivitamin that contains B$_{12}$ is what many experts recommend—not as a substitute for good nutrition but as insurance—even if you are eating the healthiest diet possible based on whole foods.

* Based on recent evidence that antioxidant supplements actually cause more harm than good (or no good at all), experts recommend choosing a supplement that contains no or low doses of vitamin A, isolated beta-carotene, and vitamin E.

* Some recommend choosing an iron-free multivitamin and only taking iron supplements when there is a true deficiency or when you need additional quantities (such as when you're pregnant).

* Keep vitamins in a place where you'll see them and be reminded to take them, such as by your toothbrush.

"ON SEEING A WOUNDED HARE LIMP BY ME WHICH A FELLOW HAD JUST SHOT AT"
BY ROBERT BURNS

Regarded as the national poet of Scotland, Robert Burns (1759–1796) was a poet and lyricist, most famous for his poem (and song) "Auld Lang Syne" (which loosely translates to "Long, Long Ago").

Influential on other Romantic poets—namely Coleridge, Shelly, and Wordsworth—Burns also inspired American writer John Steinbeck, who took the title for his novel *Of Mice and Men* from Burns's poem, "To A Mouse, on Turning Her Up in Her Nest, with the Plough"—a "murdering plough-staff," no less. In this tender poem in which the narrator apologizes to a mouse for upturning her home, the penultimate stanza contains the well-known lines:

> But little Mouse, you are not alone,
> In proving foresight may be vain:
> The best laid schemes of mice and men
> Go often askew.

Burns died too young at the age of thirty-seven and is regarded as one of Scotland's most beloved figures. Concerned with the social justice causes of poverty, gender and class inequalities, and Scottish cultural identity, he was also clearly attuned to the suffering of animals, as seen in his 1789 poem "On Seeing A Wounded Hare Limp By Me, Which A Fellow Had Just Shot At."

Inhuman man! curse on thy barb'rous art,
And blasted be thy murder-aiming eye!
May never pity soothe thee with a sigh,
Nor ever pleasure glad thy cruel heart!

Go live, poor wanderer of the wood and field,
The bitter little that of life remains!
No more the thickening brakes and verdant plains
To thee shall home, or food, or pastime yield.

Seek, mangled innocent, some wonted rest;
No more of rest, but now thy dying bed!
The sheltering rushes whistling o'er thy head,
The cold earth with thy bloody bosom prest.

Perhaps a mother's anguish adds its woe;
The playful pair crowd fondly by thy side;
Ah! helpless nurslings, who will now provide
That life a mother only can bestow?

Oft as by winding Nith I, musing, wait,
The sober ever, or hail the cheerful dawn,
I'll miss thee sporting o'er the dewy lawn,
And curse the ruffian's aim, and mourn thy hapless fate.

ETHEL, THE GREATEST TURKEY OF ALL TIME

Ethel arrived with six other turkeys, fortunate escapees from an industry that grows close to 300 million birds annually—and then kills them.

Fortunately, Ethel was to have a different fate.

From her first day, it was clear that Ethel was a standout, curious kinda gal. Turkeys are gentle; Ethel groomed our truly free-range chickens, sheep, and pigs. Turkeys are affectionate; Ethel became our first lap turkey.

Ethel craves connection. Whether you're turkey, sheep, horse, chicken, rabbit, pig, human, or other is irrelevant. Her criteria are simple: If you live and breathe, Ethel wants to know you.

Despite her love of animals, Ethel seems to find the greatest joy in connecting with humans. When I sit down and cross my legs, Ethel sidles up to me until her big bird body touches my side, trills her lovely turkey trill, and stares at me. When I pick her up and place her in my lap, her body relaxes and her eyes quickly grow heavy with sleep. For those moments, all is right in my world, and, it seems, in hers.

Every weekend throughout our visiting season, both tour guides and guests struggle not to step on Ethel. When we're in the barn, she settles into the middle of each group, moving with us as we move from animal to animal. She moves from one guest to the next, looking deeply into their eyes. In these moments, whatever's in that big turkey heart seems a lot like love.

—*Kathy Stevens, founder of Catskill Animal Sanctuary, Saugerties, New York (U.S.)*

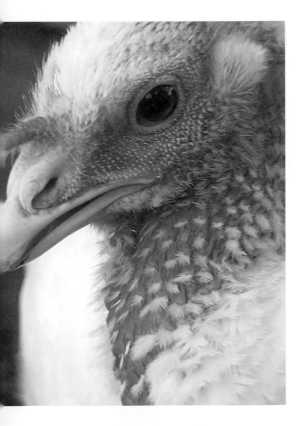

Ethel at Catskill Animal Sanctuary

FALL FRUIT CRISP

Any autumn fruit can be used for this delight-ful dessert that fills the home with an inviting fragrance.

FILLING

> **6 to 8 cups (900 to 1,200 g) cored and sliced or chopped pears and/or apples**
> **1 cup (145 g) blueberries, fresh or frozen (optional)**
> **1 cup (145 g) raisins (optional)**
> **Juice from 1 lemon**
> **¼ cup (85 g) pure maple syrup**
> **1 teaspoon (2.3 g) ground cinnamon**
> **½ teaspoon ground allspice**

TOPPING

> **1 cup (80 g) rolled oats (not quick-cooking)**
> **1 cup (150 g) chopped walnuts or pecans, toasted for 10 minutes**
> **½ cup (62 g) whole wheat flour**
> **½ cup (112 g) nondairy, nonhydrogenated butter such as Earth Balance**
> **¼ cup (55 g) firmly packed light or dark brown sugar**
> **1 teaspoon (2.3 g) ground cinnamon**
> **¼ teaspoon ground allspice**
> **¼ teaspoon ground nutmeg**
> **¼ teaspoon salt**
> **½ teaspoon anise seeds (optional)**

Preheat the oven to 350°F (180°C, or gas mark 4). Have ready an ungreased 8- or 9-inch (20 or 23 cm) square baking pan at least 2 inches (5 cm) deep.

To make the filling, in a medium-size bowl, combine the pears, blueberries (if using), raisins (if using), lemon juice, maple syrup, cinnamon, and allspice and pour into the baking pan.

To make the topping, in a separate bowl (or simply rinse out the one you just used), combine the oats, walnuts, flour, butter, brown sugar, cinnamon, allspice, nutmeg, salt, and anise seeds (if using). The topping should be crumbly (and chunky from the walnuts) and have the texture of wet sand. If it's too dry, add a little more butter or a couple teaspoons of water.

Sprinkle the topping over the fruit mixture, making sure it's evenly distributed. Bake for 35 to 45 minutes, or until the pears and apples are soft when pierced with a toothpick or fork. Remove from the oven and serve hot, warm, or at room temperature; you can also serve it plain or à la mode.

Yield: 6 to 8 servings

Soy-free if using soy-free Earth Balance

Originally published in *The Joy of Vegan Baking*

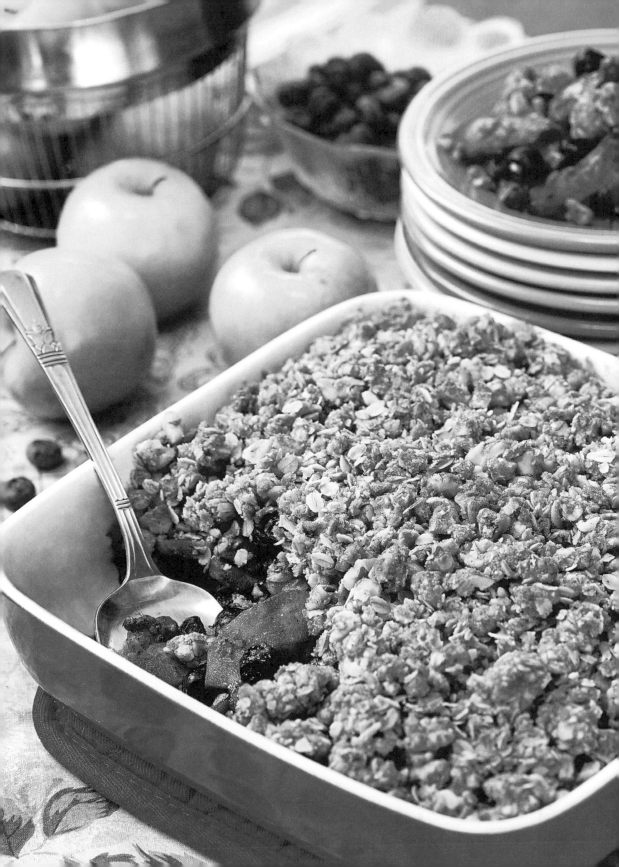

ARTICHOKES

I confess when I'm making a soup or salad that calls for artichoke hearts, I rely on the frozen or jarred variety for the sake of convenience. Nothing, however, beats sitting down to a whole artichoke and enjoying it petal by petal.

Artichokes are a perennial thistle, and the head we eat is actually the bud of the flower. If left to flower on the plant, the bud emerges into a gorgeous pink and purple blossom. Although I do harvest the buds from our own artichoke plants, I always leave one on the plant to allow it to flower.

The easiest way to prepare artichokes is to cut off the stem just at the base (so they can sit flush on a plate), snip away the pointy tip of each leaf, and steam them until tender—about 40 to 50 minutes, depending on the size of the artichoke. Then the fun begins!

Eating an Artichoke

Pull off the outer petals, one at a time. Dip the bottom of each leaf—the white fleshy end—into melted nondairy butter or eggless mayonnaise. Tightly grip the top end of the petal. Place the dipped end in your mouth, bite down, and pull the leaf through your teeth to remove the soft, delicious portion of the petal. Discard the remaining part of the petal. (It's too tough to eat.) Continue until all the leaves are removed and the heart and choke are revealed.

Some people become flummoxed at this point, but it's really very simple. You just need to remove the furry *choke* and get to the *heart*. Once you've eaten all the leaves and have reached the choke, scrape the top of the heart with a spoon to remove all the white feathery part. All that is furry is the choke. What you have left when you've cleared away the choke is the heart. Cut that into bite-size pieces, dip, and enjoy!

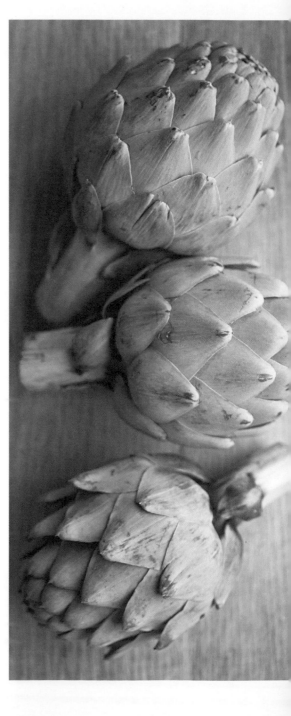

EQUIVOCATE

In a brilliantly written play called *Equivocation* by Bill Cain, the protagonist (one William Shakespeare—or "Shagspeare" as he's called in the play) is confronted with the challenge of telling the truth in what are dangerous times. He consults Father Henry Garnet, who wrote "A Treatise of Equivocation" to learn how to handle hostile and tricky questions with skill.

What Garnet teaches him is that you don't answer the question that is posed but rather the question that is really being asked, and this same technique can be used in our correspondence with people who are simply curious about or even hostile to veganism and animal rights.

For instance, when people ask, "Don't you care about plants; they have feelings, too" (see Day 324), they are not really that concerned about the emotional distress of vegetables. What they are really asking is "How extreme is this vegan thing? Is there a way to make ethical choices in this world with all its hypocrisies and contradictions?"

If you answer the literal question about plants, you'll make absolutely no headway in terms of guiding people to a more reasonable and compassionate understanding about animal rights. But if you look past the question they're asking on the surface, you'll find there is a more profound concern lurking about.

Try it with the more absurd questions you may encounter. Answer the question that's *really* being asked, and be prepared for a much more engaging conversation that is based on common ground rather than hostility.

AVOIDING BURNOUT AS AN ACTIVIST

Burnout is common among animal activists, mainly because the problem is a large one, there is much work to do, and compassionate people have huge hearts that compel them to work endlessly to make all the suffering disappear.

The challenge is finding balance between being an effective advocate and staying healthy and sane. We also need to make sure our relationships with our loved ones don't suffer.

I won't pretend I've mastered this thing called balance—I've recently admitted to being a workaholic—but balance is something I strive for every day. The problem is I feel best when I'm doing something to end the suffering of animals, to raise awareness of their suffering, and to empower people to live according to their own truth and compassion.

I'm an ACTivist through and through. I can't but ACT if I see a problem.

But I'll be honest. Some of my workaholism stems from the pangs of guilt I have felt when I'm not doing these things. I've thought, "Who am I to relax and enjoy life when there is so much suffering out there?" And though that might sound noble, I really do believe now that:

* It sounds too much like martyrdom, and I don't do this work to be a martyr.

* I will be no good to the animals or to other people if I don't take care of myself.

With that in mind—and it's something I have to remind myself of all the time—I make sure I:

* Set realistic goals

* Create reasonable expectations of myself

* Find time to relax and recharge

* Make my relationships a priority

* Make time to exercise

The healthier I am emotionally and physically, the better representative I am for the animals, and the better I am to myself and those around me. I'm also happier. I've seen too many activists become so uptight from stress that they're just not pleasant to be around.

Although my role as an animal advocate is central to who I am, it is not my only identity. I am also a daughter, a wife, a friend, and a neighbor. Finding balance means tending to these roles as well.

POETRY'S PLEA FOR ANIMALS: AN ANTHOLOGY
EDITED BY FRANCES E. CLARKE

We modern folk tend to forget that our contemporary ideas have roots in the past. Animal advocacy has a long history that stretches back centuries. Many people came before us with forward-thinking ideas, paving the way for those of us who work today to liberate animals from human exploitation and oppression.

Considering the prevalence of justice movements in the United States in the early part of the twentieth century, the collection of poems in *Poetry's Plea for Animals* (1927) is not really so remarkable—and yet it is. That so many poems were written on behalf of animals, that such a diverse collection was ever compiled at all, and that these poems are not just about how lovely animals are but also how cruelly they are treated is truly extraordinary.

The book is broken up into several sections, characterized by subject. Some poems are devoted to those who are less frequently thought of, and remarkably, there are poems dedicated to those who are victims of our appetites and vanity. One section is called "For Vanity," which encompasses poems about fur-bearing animals trapped for their fur; other such sections are called "Braves of the Hunt," "In Captivity," and "Performing Animals."

To be made the subject of poetry is the highest honor you can receive, and so in and through these poems, the status of nonhuman animals is elevated to a much higher degree than that which they experience in actual life. As subjects of these poems, they are exalted in ways they have yet to witness off the page.

Although *Poetry's Plea for Animals* is no longer in print, some rare copies can be found with a little investigating. The original publisher was Lothrop, Lee, and Shepard in Massachusetts, and the editor was Frances E. Clarke.

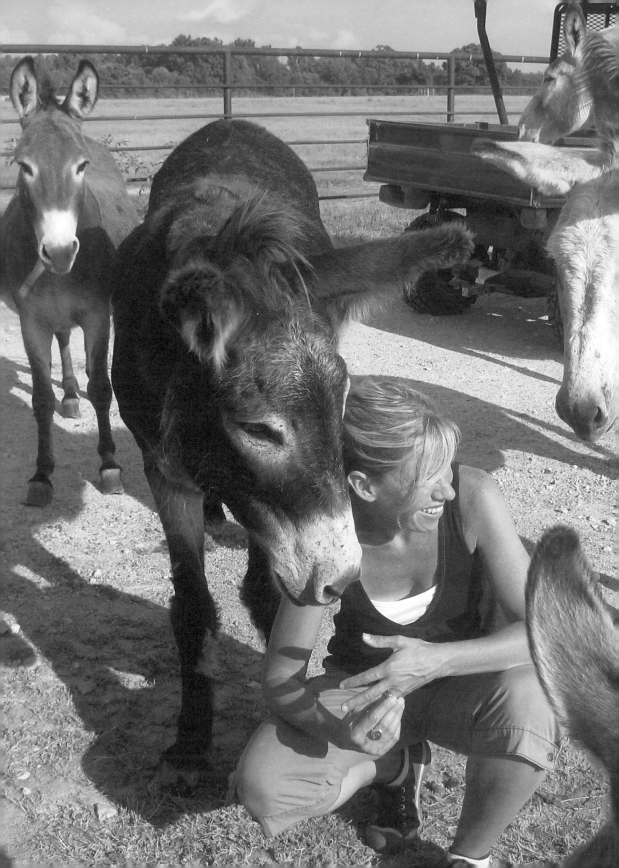

AN UNPRECEDENTED RESCUE

In 1979, the National Park Service planned to kill hundreds of burros then living in the Grand Canyon. The burros, whose ancestors were cast-offs from the gold rush era, grazed the canyon and lived as wild equines on public lands. Private cattle and sheep ranchers had long resented their presence, claiming the animals were eating food meant for their "livestock." Determined to exterminate them, the Park Service first tried to run the burros off the trails, but they were unsuccessful. Their next recourse was to shoot the animals from a small aircraft.

When Cleveland Amory, founder of the Fund for Animals and author of *The Cat Who Came for Christmas*, heard of the park's plans, he arranged for their rescue—an arduous endeavor that first entailed acquiring hundreds of acres of land in east Texas that would serve as a sanctuary for the burros. This would be Black Beauty Ranch.

The aerial shoot was stalled during a lawsuit that tried to prevent the killing of these animals, and when the lawsuit lost, Cleveland declared that he would organize the safe removal of hundreds of burros himself.

The rescue began on August 9, 1979, meeting with many obstacles but ultimately succeeding. The rescue ended up being a two-year operation, during which no animal or person was injured. In the end, all 577 burros were carefully airlifted out of the Grand Canyon and brought to safety at Cleveland Amory Black Beauty Ranch.

During the rescue itself, one burro Cleveland named Friendly didn't trot away from her rescuers but stood her ground and eventually even came closer. Cleveland explains in his book, *Ranch of Dreams*:

"Friendly had come up in a sling in the very first batch of burros, and I was in the corral when she was lifted up over the rim and delicately dropped to the ground. I was one of the crew who untied her. She must have thought . . . we all were [crazy]. But she also realized, I felt then and still feel, that no one had really hurt her, and therefore we were not all bad."

Well over thirty years old, Friendly most certainly lives up to her name. She is one of more than 1,200 domestic and "exotic" animals who live on the 1,300 acres (526 ha) of land.

Cleveland Amory passed away on October 15, 1998, at the age of eighty-one. He is buried at Cleveland Amory Black Beauty Ranch next to his beloved cat Polar Bear (the first resident of the sanctuary). When her time comes, Friendly will rest alongside them both.

—*CPG*

Colleen enjoying quality time with the many rescued burros at Cleveland Amory Black Beauty Ranch

NUT BUTTER DIP (A.K.A. CRACK DIP)

My friend Laurie Judd gave me this recipe, warning me to change the name from "Crack Dip" to something else. Her sister bestowed this moniker upon it, because she finds it so addictive. Though I modified the recipe only slightly, I can attest that its appeal remains the same.

> 6 tablespoons (96 g) almond or peanut butter
> 3 tablespoons (45 g) tahini (sesame butter)
> ¼ cup (60 ml) tamari soy sauce
> 2 tablespoons (40 g) agave nectar
> 1 tablespoon (15 ml) apple cider vinegar
> 1 tablespoon (6 g) minced ginger
> 2 cloves garlic, peeled
> ¼ teaspoon cayenne pepper
> ¼ cup (60 ml) water
> 1 tablespoon (15 ml) olive oil

Combine the almond butter, tahini, tamari, agave, vinegar, ginger, garlic, and cayenne in a food processor or blender. Slowly add the water and olive oil and continue blending to reach the desired consistency. The mixture should be smooth and thick.

Serve with a combination of raw fruits and vegetables: celery, cucumber, beets, turnips, radishes, apple slices, carrots, and bell peppers.

Yield: 1 cup (250 g)

SERVING SUGGESTIONS AND VARIATIONS
To prepare it as a salad dressing instead of a dip, replace the ¼ cup (60 ml) water and 1 tablespoon (15 ml) olive oil with ¼ to ⅓ cup (60 to 80 ml) olive oil and enough water to reach the desired consistency. It should be pourable.

*Wheat-free

CREMINI MUSHROOMS

Essentially a baby portobello, cremini mushrooms have an earthy flavor and firm texture, making them suitable for soups, stir-fries, topping for pizza, or stuffing for ravioli.

When choosing mushrooms, look for those that are firm, plump, and clean—not wrinkled or slimy. Store them in the refrigerator in a loosely closed paper bag, and use them within three days. Enjoy them in a variety of ways:

* Sauté sliced mushrooms and onions and serve as a side dish or topping for grilled tempeh.

* Add finely chopped mushrooms to tomato sauce. Pour on pasta.

* Remove the stems and stuff with vegetables.

* Add sliced mushrooms to a tofu scramble.

* Include sliced and sautéed mushrooms in your favorite vegan lasagna recipe.

* Mince cremini mushrooms, add binding ingredients and herbs, shape into patties, and you've got mushroom burgers.

COMPASSIONATE ALTERNATIVE:
NEVER LOOK A GIFT HORSE IN THE MOUTH

Horses make their way into a number of idioms (see Day 65). One expression we use a lot is "Never look a gift horse in the mouth," and there are variations of this proverb in French, Italian, Spanish, and other European languages. Apparently, this expression is so old that its origins cannot be determined. It has been traced to the writings of St. Jerome, one of the Latin Fathers of the fourth century, who then labeled it a common proverb.

The expression refers to the bad manners of one who receives a gift but examines it for defects. Its reference to a horse's mouth comes from the fact that up to a certain age, the age of a horse can be determined by looking at his teeth. And though it may seem like an innocent expression, the fact that you'd need to check the value of the horse based on his teeth, based on his age, implies that you intend to *use* the horse for some purpose. For me, an animal's *value* is determined not by what he can do for humans but simply that he is alive and thus worthy of consideration.

Charles Earle Funk, who was editor in chief of the *Funk & Wagnalls Standard Dictionary* series and who wrote a number of books on the origin of common expressions, wrote about this proverb: "Though it ["it" referring to the horse] may appear to be young and frisky, the number or condition of teeth may show it to be almost fit for nothing but the glue-works." That seals it.

One compassionate alternative is: "Don't look for bugs in a flower bouquet"—not that there's anything wrong with bugs, of course! But when you smell a flower, the last thing you want is a bee stinging your nose!

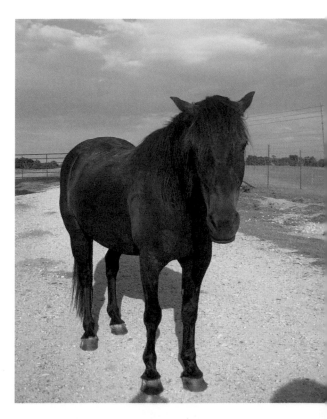

A rescued horse at Cleveland Amory Black Beauty Ranch

TAKING RESPONSIBILITY FOR SOCIETY'S ANIMALS

I admit to being one of those people who can't resist greeting every animal I encounter. My husband has accepted that our evening walks are often interrupted by my need to pet every dog being walked and every cat lounging on the sidewalk.

I've also been known to bring animals home with us—dogs who are clearly lost, cats who are clearly homeless.

I don't seek out wandering dogs or hungry-looking cats, but they seem to find me. And at that moment when I realize I have to intervene, my first thought is always, "Oh no, I'm in a rush. I don't have time. This isn't my problem," but that voice is never loud enough to make me turn away. It would be easier to do—certainly more convenient, especially for my own cats, who have to relinquish part of their living space for whatever refugee happens to come home with us.

But if it's not my problem, then whose is it? By virtue of being part of a larger community, I can't help but feel a responsibility to care for all its members, particularly those who are the most vulnerable.

Gandhi once said, "The greatness of a nation and its moral progress can be judged by the way its animals are treated"; by that definition, we have a long way to go. But there is so much we can do to make sure that no one suffers needlessly.

* Keep leashes, treats, and blankets in your car.

* Store the number for your local animal shelter in your cell phone.

* Keep your eyes open when driving and consider pulling over to move a lifeless body out of the street, calling when there's a telephone number on the tag, and creating a proper burial when there's not.

* Take home dogs and cats who are lost or sick. Find their people, bring them to the shelter (where you can follow up to make sure they are adopted), or find a home for them yourself.

* Or, simply return a dog—who has broken out of his backyard—to his home.

Basically, I've come to accept that whatever plans I have on any given day may be curtailed by an unexpected critter who happens to cross my path.

These small steps reap huge rewards, namely reuniting animals with their people and knowing that a few moments of inconvenience for us makes a world of difference in the lives of others.

AN EXCERPT FROM "A WINTER WALK AT NOON"
BY WILLIAM COWPER

An animal lover all his life, English poet William Cowper (pronounced *COO-per*) lived from 1731 to 1800 and wrote affectionately about the animals with whom he lived and whom he admired. (See Day 25 for more.)

In "A Winter Walk at Noon," published in 1785, Cowper celebrates the joy we feel in the company of animals and guarantees the consequences we experience when we choose cruelty over compassion.

> The heart is hard in nature, and unfit
> For human fellowship, as being void
> Of sympathy, and therefore dead alike
> To love and friendship both, that is not pleased
> With sight of animals enjoying life,
> Nor feels their happiness augment his own.
>
> The seeds of cruelty, that since have swell'd
> To such gigantic and enormous growth,
> Were sown in human nature's fruitful soil.
> Hence date the persecution and the pain,
> That man inflicts on all inferior kinds,
> Regardless of their plaints. To make him sport,
> To gratify the frenzy of his wrath,
> Or his base gluttony, are causes good,
> And just in his account, why bird and beast
> Should suffer torture, and the streams be dyed
> With blood of their inhabitants impaled
> Earth groans beneath the burthen of a war
> Waged with defenceless innocence.

> Witness, the patient ox, with stripes and yells,
> Driven to the slaughter, goaded as he runs
> To madness, while the savage, at his heals
> Laughs at the sufferer's fury spent
> Upon the guiltless passenger o'erthrown.
> He too is witness, noblest of the train,
> That wait on man, the flight-performing horse:
> With unsuspecting readiness he takes,
> His murderer on his back, and push'd all day,
> With bleeding sides and flanks that heave for life,
> To the far distant goal, arrives and dies.
> So little mercy shows, who needs so much!
> Does law, so jealous in the cause of man,
> Denounce no doom on the delinquent? None.
> He lives, and o'er his brimming beaker boasts,
> (As if barbarity were high desert)
> The inglorious feat, and clamorous in praise
> Of the poor brute, seems wisely to suppose,
> the honors of his matchless horse his own.
> But many a crime, deem'd innocent on earth,
> Is register'd in heaven; and there, no doubt,
> Have each their record, with a curse annex'd.
> Man may dismiss compassion from his heart,
> But God will never.

GUILT AS A MEAT-EATER, PEACE AS A VEGAN

I first became vegetarian in 1995 when my mother was diagnosed with stage-4 breast cancer and I began to read about ways to cure her. I learned about people who had cured themselves from cancer through their diets, particularly macrobiotic, and the growing research documenting the terrible effects of meat and dairy products on the body. I became vegetarian at that time but still ate eggs; I hadn't eaten milk products for years due to allergy.

My mother passed away a short time later, and I continued my vegetarian lifestyle as a health concern. I explained to people that the animals were raised in such horrible and unsanitary conditions that it could not be healthy to eat such products. I understood on some level the horrors that the animals suffered to feed us, but I allowed it into my heart and mind superficially.

Years later, I began to eat meat again. I was surrounded by people who ate meat, and my husband at the time, who had gone vegetarian with me, went back to eating meat, too. I had felt alone in my vegetarianism and an inconvenience to friends and family.

Once I saw the film *Peaceable Kingdom*, and the seemingly endless number of male chicks sliding down chutes and conveyor belts on the way to the dumpster—useless by-products of the egg industry—there was no turning back to eating meat.

Being vegan for ethical reasons is very different than giving up meat for health reasons. I've experienced rewards I never would have imagined. I feel peace within me, and I feel like I have learned to love again in the truest sense—a love that knows no boundaries. For most of my life, I felt disconnected from the world, as if there were some hole in my being, something holding me back.

Becoming vegan, I feel whole again. I feel as if a weight has been lifted, and my heart is free.

—*Janice in Lincoln Park, New Jersey (U.S.)*

DIANE'S FAMOUS MANICOTTI

My dear friend and mentor Diane Miller shared this recipe with me after I begged for it for years. Rich, satisfying, and familiar to anyone who grew up on manicotti (me!), it is a pleasure to share this crowd-pleasing recipe. It yields enough to serve a large group!

2 (8-ounce, or 225 g) packages manicotti shells (approximately 16 to 20 shells)

2 (32-ounce, or 905 g) cans fire-roasted diced tomatoes

2 (6-ounce, or 170 g) cans tomato paste

4 cups (280 g) chopped cremini or portobello mushrooms

6 to 8 cups (180 to 240 g) coarsely chopped fresh spinach, divided

12 cloves garlic, minced, divided

1 cup (160 g) diced yellow onion

2 tablespoons (8 g) Italian seasoning (or a combination of dried basil, oregano, and thyme)

2 teaspoons (12 g) salt

1 teaspoon (2 g) black pepper

¼ cup (60 ml) extra-virgin olive oil

16 ounces (455 g) firm or extra-firm tofu

16 ounces (455 g) nondairy cream cheese, such as Tofutti

8 ounces (225 g) favorite vegetarian meat crumbles

1 cup (160 g) diced purple onion

Preheat the oven to 400°F (200°C, or gas mark 6). Lightly oil a large casserole pan or two or more medium-size pans.

Prepare the manicotti shells by cooking them in boiling water until they are a very firm al dente; do not cook until tender or they will split and fall apart while being stuffed. Set them aside to cool in a single layer. Applying a very light coating of olive oil can help prevent the shells from sticking to one another.

Prepare the sauce by combining the diced tomatoes, tomato paste, mushrooms, 3 to 4 cups (90 to 120 g) of the spinach, half of the garlic, the yellow onion, Italian seasoning, salt, pepper, and olive oil in a large bowl. Set aside.

Prepare the filling by mashing together the tofu, cream cheese, and vegetarian meat crumbles. Fold in the red onion and the remaining half of the garlic and the remaining 3 to 4 cups (90 to 120 g) spinach. The mixture should be thick and lumpy but creamy at the same time.

Assemble your dish. Cover the bottom of the pan(s) with 1 inch (2.5 cm) of the sauce.

Carefully stuff the manicotti shells with the filling and line them up in the pan on top of the sauce. When the pan is filled with stuffed shells, generously cover them with the remaining sauce. Cover the pan with foil, sealing the edges. Bake on the top shelf for 50 to 60 minutes, or until the sauce is somewhat browned.

Yield: 16 to 20 manicotti shells

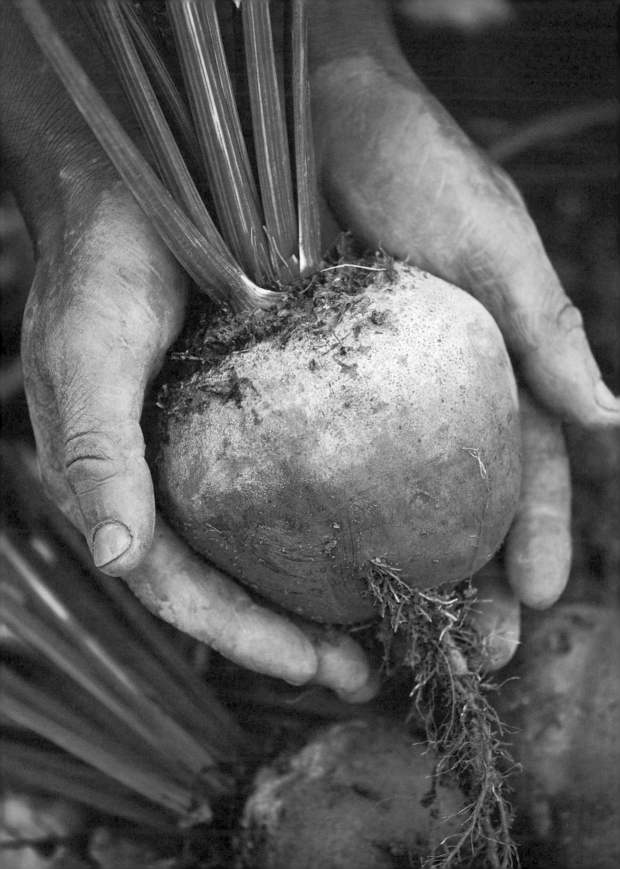

BEETS

Betacyanin, the pigment that gives beets their red-purple color, is a powerful cancer-fighting agent. Other plants that contain concentrated amounts of this protective phytochemical include red carrots, red grape skin, red chard, elderberry, and red cabbage. Aside from the popular red beets, there are many varieties, including those that are orange, yellow, and white.

Beets belong to the same family as chard and spinach, and their leaves can be prepared just as you would any other leafy green.

As with all vegetables, choose beets that are firm and unwrinkled. When a vegetable or fruit appears wrinkled, it means it is losing water and thus freshness. Plump and firm is what you want. If you're buying beets with their greens still attached, make sure the leaves are a nice, solid green—not yellowish.

Raw beets are a favorite addition in my salads; they can be shredded or julienned and added to mixed greens. They add such a striking color, and their crunch—like carrots—complement the softer lettuce leaves. Beet salads—consisting mostly of the beets themselves—are also delicious and nutritious, and raw shredded beets also make a beautiful garnish on soups.

Beets can be steamed, roasted, boiled, or baked, and they're wonderful simply tossed with your favorite vinaigrette. I confess to never having had a pickled beet, though this is a popular form of preparation.

You don't need to remove the skin before cooking beets; in fact, it's much easier if you don't. Because of their rough texture, peeling beets can be somewhat laborious. Use a good vegetable peeler, or cut away the thin skin with a good, sharp knife. If you are going to cook them, it's just as easy to cut off the tops, halve or quarter them if they're large, and steam or roast them. Periodically poke them with a fork to test for doneness, and remove from the heat when a fork easily penetrates the flesh. Give them a little time to cool, then slip off the peel, which will easily slide off.

At this point, you can chop them and toss them with oil, vinegar, mustard, and salt. Or make a citrus vinaigrette by leaving out the mustard and adding some orange juice and zest. Citrus and beets pair beautifully together.

HOW DO YOU RESPOND TO, "SO, YOU'RE VEGAN. DO YOU EAT FISH?"

Many a vegan has been asked this question, and though it might make you want to give the asker a little Laurel-and-Hardy smack on the head, I suggest you refrain.

Although it may be obvious to you that "vegan" food means only that which is derived from plants, some people have been misguided by others who call themselves vegan but who state explicitly that they eat fish or chicken—or any number of animals.

Although they clearly need a patient and kind explanation of what it means to be vegan, keep in mind that they clearly want to identify as a vegan. They know enough to think that the label is a positive one, and it's important to recognize and appreciate that.

At the same time, you must remind them that fish aren't plants. Sadly, some people think that because fish are so unlike *us*, they must be closer to the plant family than the animal family.

Fish are animals, and as animals, they feel pain. They are killed by being crushed in a net, by having their swim bladders explode when they are brought to the surface, or by being asphyxiated when they're denied oxygen through water.

So next time someone asks if you eat fish as a vegan, gently but definitively remind him that fish are not plants. With your wisdom and understanding, you can help him see otherwise.

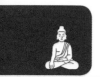

VOLUNTEERING

After a short time of going vegan, many people want to get involved in more direct ways by volunteering their time and energy to a cause they feel strongly about. They begin exploring what type of activism they should get involved in and often feel overwhelmed by how much there is to do—and how to go about doing it.

I highly recommend finding something you're passionate about and that reflects your skills and talents. You're going to be most effective at something that brings you pleasure and that comes naturally to you. For instance, if you are terrified of public speaking but are a good writer,

then you'd probably want to focus on the latter. If you love to talk to people but hate sitting in front of a computer writing, then it's an obvious choice which one is for you.

Once you've decided what you have to contribute, get in touch with organizations you admire and ask them how you can help. The main thing is to get involved. If you have just one hour a week to give, then give it. Two hours? All the better.

I highly encourage you to read Mark Hawthorne's *Striking at the Roots: A Practical Guide to Animal Activism* for many ideas.

"INSCRIPTION ON THE MONUMENT OF A NEWFOUNDLAND DOG"
BY LORD BYRON

George Gordon Byron, known to us as Lord Byron, was a prolific English poet and a leading figure in literary Romanticism along with William Wordsworth, Samuel Coleridge (see Day 214), Percy Shelley (see Day 326), Mary Shelley (see Day 186), and John Keats. Considered one of the greatest European poets, he was born in 1788 in London and died very young at the age of thirty-six in 1824.

In his 1808 poem "Inscription on the Monument of a Newfoundland Dog," Byron recognizes that by virtue of writing a poem about this dog, he is glorifying him in art. Lamenting the fact that so many dogs—and by implication *any nonhuman animal*—die "unhonored" and "unnoticed," he wrote this poem to *honor* and *notice* them.

> When some proud son of man returns to earth,
> Unknown to glory, but upheld by birth,
> The sculptor's art exhausts the pomp of woe,
> And storied urns record who rests below;
> When all is done, upon the tomb is seen,
> Not what he was, but what he should have been:
>
> But the poor dog, in life the firmest friend,
> The first to welcome, foremost to defend,
> Whose honest heart is still his master's own,
> Who labours, fights, lives, breathes for him alone,
>
> Unhonour'd falls, unnoticed all his worth,
> Denied in heaven the soul he held on earth:
> While man, vain insect! hopes to be forgiven,
> And claims himself a sole exclusive heaven.
> Oh man! thou feeble tenant of an hour,
> Debased by slavery, or corrupt by power,
> Who knows thee well must quit thee with disgust,

> Degraded mass of animated dust!
> Thy love is lust, thy friendship all a cheat,
> Thy smiles hypocrisy, thy words deceit!
> By nature vile, ennobled but by name,
> Each kindred brute might bid thee blush disgust, for shame.
>
> Ye! who perchance behold this simple urn,
> Pass on—it honours none you wish to mourn:
> To mark a friend's remains these stones arise,
> I never knew but one, and here he lies.

KITTY—FROM RESEARCH TO RESCUE

In 1997, Kitty became the companion for Nim Chimpsky, the first chimpanzee who arrived at Cleveland Amory Black Beauty Ranch in 1982. Famous for his ability to use sign language, Nim had recently lost his longtime companion and was displaying signs of depression, such as lethargy and loss of appetite.

An inquiry for a new companion was made to the Coulston Foundation Chimpanzee Project in New Mexico. This now-defunct facility bred chimpanzees for hepatitis research and was looking to find a new home for Kitty, a chimpanzee who had been there for more than twenty years.

Acquired in 1972—most likely wild-caught—from an animal dealer at the age of ten, Kitty had been used as a "breeder" chimp, producing offspring for Coulston's research projects. Ironically, due to her competent mothering skills, she was forced to give birth, and then, only briefly, allowed to care for her babies, repeatedly grieving for her young as she suffered the trauma of each one being taken from her.

After fourteen pregnancies, Kitty would have soon been unsuitable as a "breeder," and it was only a matter of time before she would have been taken for hepatitis studies.

Nim and Kitty were initially placed in separate quarters but in full sight of each other and indicated an immediate affinity for one another. After some time, they were joined, and they remained compatible until Nim died suddenly of heart problems on March 10, 2000, at the age of twenty-six. Kitty and two other rescued chimpanzees, Midge and Lulu, continue their lives together at the sanctuary, where they presently enjoy a large new outdoor enclosure.

Intelligent and inquisitive, Kitty loves to hang out in the suspended skywalk that connects to the indoor chimp house, where she enjoys a panoramic view of the busiest area of the sanctuary.

—*Cleveland Amory Black Beauty Ranch, Murchison, Texas (U.S.)*

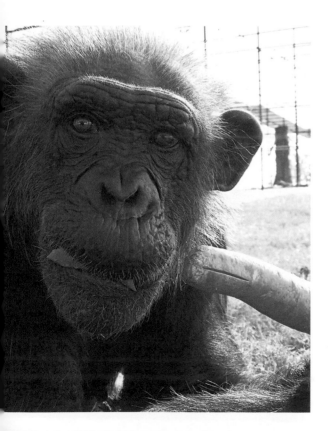

Kitty enjoying one of her favorite snacks
Photo by Diane Miller/The HSUS

RED LENTIL PÂTÉ

Enjoy one of my favorite recipes!

- 3 tablespoons (24 g) chopped pistachio nuts or toasted sunflower seeds
- 3 cups (705 ml) plus 2 tablespoons (30 ml) water, divided
- 1 large yellow onion, finely chopped
- 1 cup (160 g) finely chopped shallots
- 1 teaspoon (2 g) fennel seeds, crushed in a mortar or under a chef's knife
- ½ teaspoon dried thyme leaves
- 2 cloves garlic, minced
- 1 tablespoon (16 g) tomato paste
- ¼ cup (60 ml) dry white wine or sparkling apple cider
- 1 ½ cups (288 g) red lentils, picked over and rinsed
- 1 bay leaf
- ½ teaspoon salt or more
- Freshly ground black pepper
- Mint or basil leaves, for garnish (optional)

Brush a little olive oil on the bottom and sides of 1 large or 2 small loaf pans. Sprinkle the pistachio nuts on the bottom of the pan(s). Set aside.

In a large pot, heat the 2 tablespoons (30 ml) water. Cook the onion and shallots over medium-high heat, stirring frequently, until translucent, 5 to 6 minutes. Stir in the fennel, thyme, garlic, and tomato paste and cook, stirring constantly, for about 1 minute. Add the wine, and cook until most of the liquid evaporates, about 1 minute.

Add the remaining 3 cups (705 ml) water, the lentils, and the bay leaf and bring to a boil. Cover, decrease the heat to medium-low, and simmer for 20 minutes, stirring occasionally.

Add the salt and pepper and continue cooking until the lentils have melted into a coarse puree, 10 to 20 minutes longer. Remove the bay leaf and add more salt to taste.

Stir well, creating a smooth, thick mixture, with a texture similar to that of cooked oatmeal. If the purée is thin and soupy, boil it uncovered, stirring frequently, until it thickens.

Ladle the puree immediately into the oiled loaf pan(s). Smooth the top with a spatula. Let cool to room temperature. Cover and chill for at least 2 hours. Flip the pans over a platter and lift gently to reveal the pâté. Garnish with the mint leaves.

Yield: 1 large or 2 mini loaves

*Wheat-free, soy-free

Originally published in *The Vegan Table*

OLIVES

An ancient food, olives have been around since at least 3,000 BCE in the Mediterranean region. The olive itself in its natural state is not really edible; it needs to soaked and cured to remove the bitter taste. Traditional curing has been replaced with fast techniques that involve soaking the olives in a lye bath, but you can find olives that have undergone more old-fashioned methods. Look for those that have been "oil-cured," "brine-cured," "water-cured," or "dry-salted." Many of these can be found in olive bars in delis or "specialty" grocery stores.

There are more varieties of olives than I have space for here, but here are a few:

* Manzanilla: Thia small to medium-size green olive produced in Spain and California is brine-cured and has a firm, meaty texture. Also called a Spanish olive, it is typically pitted and stuffed with garlic or pimento.

* Kalamata: A good everyday black/deep purple olive that hails from Greece, it is harvested fully ripe and is brine-cured. I regularly add them to salads, tapenade, and pasta sauce.

* Niçoise: A small French black olive that often serves as a premeal snack, it is rich and nutty and often packed in oil and herbs.

* Liguria: A small black-brown olive native to Italy, it is typically brine-cured and has a somewhat salty flavor with a nutty almond aftertaste. It's a nice complement to add to homemade relish.

* Lugano: This medium-size Italian brownish-black olive is hearty and meaty and usually very salty. Sometimes packed with olive leaves, it makes a great hors d'oeuvre or as a complement to salads and pasta.

* Castelvetrano: The mother of all olives, in my humble opinion, it boasts an incredibly beautiful bright green color. Harvested when young, it is brine-cured, firm-textured, and mild-flavored.

As mentioned above, olives can be eaten in a variety of ways—on their own or as part of numerous dishes. Experiment by checking out an olive bar and trying different varieties.

Whole fat should be part of all of our diets. "Whole fat" is the fat that is contained in the food itself—not fat that has been processed out. Several years ago, the Mediterranean Diet was touted as one of the healthiest diets on the planet, and as a result, clever marketing campaigns convinced people to start consuming olive oil by the gallon. As discussed in Day 330 (Coconuts), fat is necessary in our diet, but oil is not. Fat helps our body absorb the fat-soluble nutrients such as vitamins A and D. Avocados, coconuts, olives, nuts, and seeds are great examples of whole fats.

ASKING FOR WHAT WE WANT

Because many vegans are concerned about not appearing difficult, their desire to be easygoing often turns into self-effacement. In attempting to not rock the boat with friends, family, or coworkers, they wind up accepting something that would be unacceptable in other aspects of their life.

This manifests itself in many ways, particularly when they are invited to dine with non-vegetarians, either at someone's home or at a restaurant. Afraid to ask for what they want, they often keep their opinions to themselves and then go hungry, eat unsatisfying food, or feel bad about not speaking up for themselves.

A common question people ask is, "How do I respond if someone serves me something non-vegan when I'm in her home?" The implication is that it's rude to decline anything that's offered. I don't often find myself in this situation, because I talk to the hosts before the event to ask if there's anything I can do to help with the food. I tell them I'm vegan, and we work something out ahead of time. People with food allergies do this all the time. Why should this be any different?

We tend to underestimate people's willingness to accommodate our needs, especially if they're friends and family. The glue that holds our relationships together is affection for one another, so why wouldn't people want to do something that reflects that affection? If they are not willing, if their blocks are more important to them

than their relationship with you, then that's a larger issue and perhaps the friendship needs to be examined. Mostly, I think you'll find that people are very amenable to our requests, but first we have to ask for what we want.

Why should someone else's comfort level be more important than our own principles—and our own desire for a satisfying dinner?

When we speak up for what we want with grace, joy, and integrity, people respond in kind.

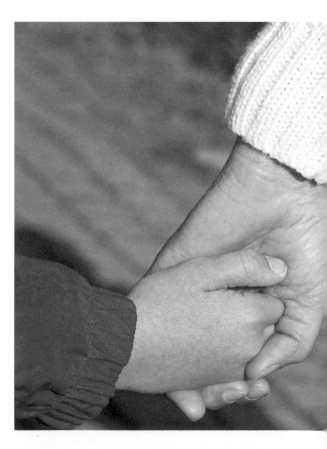

EATING MINDFULLY

Because we live in a culture that places more value on *doing* rather than *being*, it is no surprise that most people consider eating a secondary activity, squeezing it in as they're driving, working, and watching TV. Eating with awareness allows us to truly enjoy our food, engage in conversations with friends, and slow down. Eating is a sensual experience and should be appreciated as such. When we eat mindfully, we notice the texture and aroma of the food and savor the flavor of each bite. Eating mindfully draws our attention to our appreciation of the food—from our chewing to our swallowing.

Some simple tips can help us eat with awareness and pleasure:

* Plate your food in an appealing way, whether it's for yourself or friends and family.

* Eat with chopsticks.

* Eat with your nondominant hand.

* Chew your food thirty times per bite.

* Turn off the TV, cell phone, and computer while you eat.

* Eat sitting down.

* Say grace or have a moment of silence before digging in.

* Don't eat while driving.

* Identify the flavors in each bite.

* Don't follow each bite with a swig of a beverage. In fact, try eating without an accompanying beverage. Wait until the end of the meal to drink.

* Rest your fork, spoon, or chopsticks on your plate between each bite.

* Eat at a table (not on a living room chair with your plate on your lap).

EXCERPT FROM *AUGURIES OF INNOCENCE*
BY WILLIAM BLAKE

William Blake (1757–1827) was truly one of the greatest and most versatile artists ever to come out of England. Difficult to classify his work in one genre, he was a poet, a thinker, a painter, an engraver, and a printmaker—concerned largely with notions of good and evil, heaven and hell, and knowledge and innocence, as reflected in his most famous book, *Songs of Innocence and of Experience*.

An admirer of the writings and philosophy of Mary Wollstonecraft (see Day 81), Blake was interested in social justice and political events. Abhorrently opposed to slavery and in favor of racial and sexual equality, Blake extended his compassion and sense of justice to nonhumans, as evidenced by this powerful excerpt from *Auguries of Innocence*:

To see a World in a Grain of Sand
And a Heaven in a Wild Flower,

Hold Infinity in the palm of your hand
And Eternity in an hour.

A Robin Redbreast in a Cage
Puts all Heaven in a Rage;

A dove-house filled with doves and pigeons
Shudders hell through all its regions.

A dog starved at his master's gate
Predicts the ruin of the state.

The game-cock clipt and armed for fight;
Does the rising sun affright;

A horse misused upon the road
Calls to heaven for human blood.

Every wolf's and lion's howl
Raises from hell a human soul;
Each outcry of the hunted Hare
A fibre from the brain does tear;

A skylark wounded in the wing;
Doth make a cherub cease to sing.

He who shall hurt the little wren
Shall never be beloved by men;

He who the ox to wrath has moved
Shall never be by woman loved;

He who shall train the horse to war
Shall never pass the Polar Bar.

The wanton boy that kills the fly
Shall feel the spider's enmity;

He who torments the chafer's sprite
Weaves a bower in endless night.

The caterpillar on the leaf
Repeats to thee thy mother's grief;

The wild deer, wandering here and there,
Keeps the human soul from care;

The lamb misus'd breeds public strife,
And yet forgives the butcher's knife;

Kill not the moth nor butterfly,
For the last judgment draweth nigh.

The beggar's dog and widow's cat,
Feed them & thou wilt grow fat.

Every tear from every eye
Becomes a babe in eternity;

The bleat, the bark, bellow, and roar,
Are waves that beat on heaven's shore.

THE BEARS THAT RESCUE US: FAREWELL TO FRANZI

When Franzi first arrived at the sanctuary, we stood looking at the tiniest Moon Bear cringing in the corner of the smallest cage we had ever seen. Franzi had given up all hope—and small wonder.

Cruelly declawed and de-toothed, a large abscess under her chin, and a hole in her abdomen pouring out bile and pus, Franzi was a victim of the "bear farm" industry, milked daily for her bile.

Between China and Vietnam, 11,000 Moon Bears (and some Sun Bears) are caged on farms, where their bile is extracted and sold on the black market to dedicated bear bile consumers.

Little Franzi was a tragic example of "stress dwarfism." Possessing a "normal" bear-shaped head but a crudely stunted body, she had been in a cage for twenty-five years of her life.

She wouldn't look at us at all but stared at the bottom of her cage, her chest rising and falling as she breathed great gulps of fear. Suddenly, her nose quivered and her head turned toward me, as she caught the scent of something new but too tempting to ignore. Here was a fruity shake with strawberries, apples, mangoes, condensed milk, and jam, just in front of her nose—all for her.

Gingerly poking out her soft, pink tongue, Franzi took her first taste—and she closed her eyes and slurped, and slurped and slurped. As she neared the bottom, I poured the rest onto my fingers— not the most sensible thing to do with a newly rescued bear—and felt the softness of her velvety lips as she gently sucked the remainder of what was the best drink of her life.

From there it was all on her terms, with Franzi training us perfectly and knowing when to turn the screws. Her love of grapes saw her spitting out the skin and pips in contempt until she had taught us that they were never to be offered again without peeling and seeding them first.

As time went by, this rather choosy female, who had hated the presence of all other bears in "her" space, finally became attracted to brain-damaged Rupert—and a unique and loving friendship was born. They adored each other. Franzi, literally dwarfed by Rupert, who was three times her size, dominated him from beginning to end. She flirted and flounced in spring and then walked away when he appeared interested—leaving him to cozy up to a bag full of straw.

The only times she honored her love-struck toy boy with anything resembling affection was on the coldest of winter days as she snuggled next to him to keep her little body warm. The rest of the time she kept him on his toes and showed him exactly who was boss.

After seven years, it was time to let her go. Even with constant medication and veterinary care, her abdomen had become unnaturally distended from complications from the catheter that had been in her liver and uncomfortable because her heart and lungs were struggling to cope.

Franzi, who was in her nineties in human terms, made us laugh and cry in equal measure and her story touched thousands of people across the world. There are no words to say how much we'll miss her.

—Jill Robinson, founder of Animals Asia Foundation

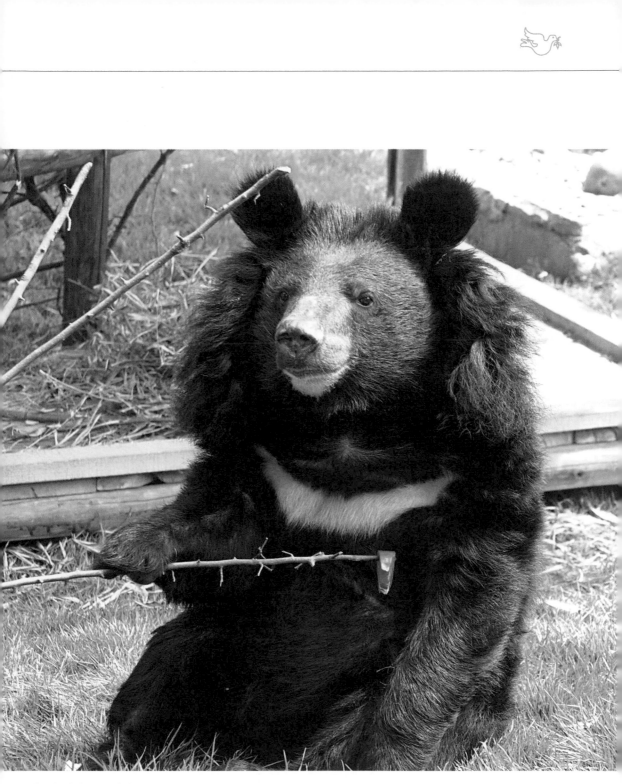

Franzi enjoying some fruit
Photo courtesy of Animals Asia

BLUEBERRY CRUMB CAKE

Thanks to podcast listener Sarah Clement in Perth, Australia, who veganized this old family recipe.

CAKE

- 2 cups (250 g) all-purpose, unbleached flour
- 1 cup (200 g) organic cane sugar
- 2 ½ teaspoons (11.5 g) baking powder
- Pinch of salt
- ½ cup (4 ounces, or 115 g) silken firm tofu (Mori-Nu is a popular brand)
- ⅔ cup (160 ml) nondairy milk (soy, rice, almond, hazelnut, hemp, or oat)
- 1 teaspoon (5 ml) vanilla extract
- ½ cup (112 g) melted nondairy butter, such as Earth Balance, or canola oil
- 1 to 2 cups (150 to 300 g) fresh or frozen blueberries

TOPPING

- ⅓ cup (40 g) all-purpose flour
- ½ cup (100 g) organic cane sugar
- 1 teaspoon (2.3 g) ground cinnamon
- ¼ cup (65 g) nondairy butter, such as Earth Balance, softened

Preheat the oven to 350°F (180°C, or gas mark 4). Lightly grease a 9-inch (23 cm) square baking pan and set aside.

To make the cake, in a large bowl, thoroughly combine the flour, sugar, baking powder, and salt. Set aside.

In a blender or food processor, blend the tofu, milk, and vanilla until creamy. You may need to turn off the machine and scrape down the sides to incorporate all of the ingredients together.

Create a well in the center of the flour mixture, and pour in the blended tofu and the melted butter. Stir until the dry and wet ingredients are just combined, and fold in the blueberries. I prefer to use frozen blueberries, because they tend not to "leak" their blue color into the cake itself.

Pour the cake batter into the prepared pan, and spread to even it out. (The batter will be thick.)

To make the topping, in a small bowl, combine the topping ingredients to create a wet crumb, and crumble it evenly over the batter.

Bake for 45 minutes, or until a toothpick inserted into the center comes out clean.

Yield: 8 servings

CHICKPEAS/GARBANZO BEANS

Also called garbanzo beans, chickpeas have been revered for centuries, eaten by ancient Romans but mostly considered "peasant food." This is borne out in a legend about the poet Horace, who, sick of life in the city, longs for a rustic dish of chickpeas and pasta.

The main ingredient in hummus, which literally means "chickpea" in Arabic, chickpeas can also be used to make flour; they can be added to soups, salads, and stews; they are the basis of the ubiq-uitous Indian dish called *chana masala*; and they are seen in dishes across many cuisines.

I eat beans several times a week, and chickpeas often top the list—not only because of the many things you can do with them but also because they're such a great snack. I usually just drain and rinse them from the can, throw them in a bowl, sprinkle them with salt and nutritional yeast, and pop them in my mouth.

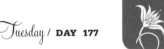

MORE COMPASSIONATE ALTERNATIVES TO VIOLENT CATTLE IDIOMS

Take the bull by the horns—With its allusion to bullfighting, this is an idiom we can do without and still express the bravery with which we tackle a problem head-on. Try "taking the bicycle by its handlebars," but if that's too playful, may I suggest some that already exist:

* Jump in with both feet

* Leap into the breach (yikes!)

* Take the plunge

* Run the gauntlet (eek!)

* March up to the cannon's mouth (ouch!)

* Meet head-on

* Take your life in your hands

That is not to say that calf- or bull-related idioms are always offensive.

Between 1,500 and 2,000 pounds (667 and 889 kg), bulls are pretty strong, and as autonomous beings with their own personalities, desires, and interests, they can be stubborn if forced to do something they don't want to. But so can people. Perhaps we should we say "human-headed" just as easily as we say "bull-headed."

VISITING ANIMAL SANCTUARIES

Sanctuaries are magical places—dare I say holy? The word *sanctuary*, after all, comes from the Latin word *sanctus*, which means "sacred." And when you visit animal sanctuaries, places where victims of abuse, neglect, or abandonment find refuge, solace, and safety, you will witness firsthand the many blessings bestowed upon resident and guest.

One of the things that is so remarkable when you spend enough time at a sanctuary is the changes you start to see in the animals. Having experienced abuse, neglect, or abandonment, they are justifiably wary of humans. With love and time, however, they begin to heal—physically and emotionally. In their strength, we can find hope.

Although the most important aspect of providing sanctuary for these animals is giving them space and time to heal, it's also important to tell their stories, even the saddest ones—not only to honor their lives but also to raise awareness and help prevent abuse for other individuals.

And that's a significant characteristic of sanctuaries: They emphasize the individual. In one individual's story, the stories of thousands—or billions—of animals are told. When people come to sanctuaries for the first time—particularly farmed animal sanctuaries—they see a dairy cow or beef steer or egg-laying hen or "meat" chicken for the first time as an individual with a personality—and it changes their perception of the entire species. Animals become individuals with names, whose eyes you can look into, whose face you can identify, whose body you can embrace.

I hear from a lot of people who feel distressed and even depressed when they first absorb what happens to animals at the hands of humans, and they ask me how to cope with that. My first suggestion is to focus on the hope, and sanctuaries enable us to do this. They offer the opportunity for people to bask in the beauty of the residents and to witness their healing.

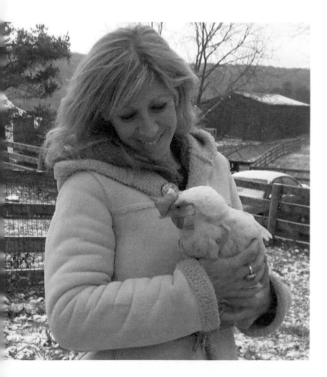

Colleen and Matilda, rescued from a live animal market and living out her life at Farm Sanctuary NY

KILLER OF SHEEP
WRITTEN AND DIRECTED BY CHARLES BURNETT

Reminiscent of the Italian neorealist films of Vittorio De Sica (see Day 305) and Roberto Rossellini, *Killer of Sheep* is a 1977 American film, written and directed by then–film student Charles Burnett. This stark drama, set in the Watts district of Los Angeles, follows Stan, who works in a sheep slaughterhouse and is utterly soul sick as a result.

There isn't necessarily a conventional linear narrative—the film is comprised of a series of related episodes—but what connects them all is the despondency with which Stan moves through his life. Though he vocally expresses his work-related depression in a conversation with a friend, he is otherwise an emotionally detached friend, husband, and father. With a far-off look and in a desperate tone in his voice, he says, "I gotta find me another job."

The slaughterhouse scenes were shot in an actual slaughterhouse outside of Los Angeles, and they mirror Stan's own experiences, becoming more intense as Stan's frustration increases. Initially, we just see an empty kill floor that Stan hoses down; the next time we're in the slaughterhouse, we see one of the workers sharpening the hooks the animals are hung on, and finally, we see the slaughtered sheep hanging and being skinned.

With many parallels between the plight of the sheep in the slaughterhouse and the character's experience of feeling trapped, the movie closes as Stan drives the frightened sheep up the chute, with Dinah Washington's heartbreaking song "This Bitter Earth" playing in the background.

OPEN EYES IN LITHUANIA

I grew up in Lithuania in a family of nonvegetarians and was taught that meat and dairy are good for you. My grandma used to keep pigs and chickens (just for family consumption), and when I was a kid I spent a lot of my summers at her country house. One day, I happened to see how she killed a hen—by cutting off her head—and once I heard the screams of a pig being killed. I couldn't understand those things when I was a child, but they left an impression on me.

I stopped eating beef and pork when I was thirteen or fourteen years old. I just couldn't stand the smell of the meat. I never felt the need to eat meat, but my parents would always convince me how important it is to eat chicken and fish, so I continued to do so—out of fear—until my

twenty-first birthday. That's when I became vegan.

Lithuania's traditional meals contain potatoes, meat, and a lot of grease (butter, sour cream, etc.). Although it may be a bit harder to be vegan in Lithuania, truly, I learned that it's not really *that* hard; we just don't have as much variety of food choices. So usually I just keep things simple (fruits, vegetables with grains, cereals, nuts).

I'm just so grateful my eyes are open.

—*Erika in Lithuania*

Grateful, open Erika

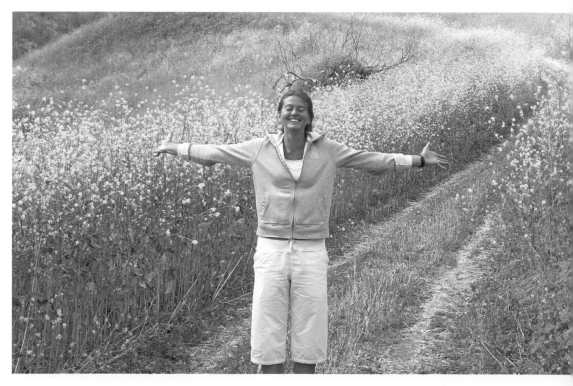

TROPICAL TEMPEH

This recipe is fantastic for serving in the summer, because of the tropical pineapple, but it's also a great cold-weather treat served piping hot over a bed of rice.

   16 ounces (455 g) tempeh, cubed
   1 tablespoon (15 ml) sesame oil
   3 tablespoons (45 ml) plus ¼ cup (60 ml)
      tamari soy sauce
   2 tablespoons (30 ml) mirin or rice vinegar
   1 tablespoon (20 g) agave nectar, maple
      syrup, or brown rice syrup
   ½ teaspoon red pepper flakes, divided
   2 yellow onions, sliced
   3 bell peppers of various colors, seeded and
      cut into ½-inch (1.3 cm) squares
   2 or 3 cloves garlic, minced
   1-inch (2.5 cm) piece fresh ginger, minced
   1 (20-ounce, or 560 g) can pineapple chunks,
      in juice (not syrup), or fresh pineapple
      chunks
   2 cups (470 ml) pineapple juice
      (use some from the can, if you reserved it)
   1 cup (235 ml) vegetable stock
      (store-bought or homemade)
   1 tablespoon (8 g) cornstarch
   ¼ to ½ cup (35 to 75 g) peanuts
   ½ head green cabbage, shredded

Place a steamer basket in a 3-quart (2.7 L) pot with water that just reaches the bottom of the steamer basket. Steam the tempeh for 10 minutes.

Meanwhile, whisk together the sesame oil, 3 tablespoons (45 ml) of the tamari, mirin, agave nectar, and ¼ teaspoon of the red pepper flakes in a medium-size bowl. Add the steamed tempeh, and toss to coat. Marinate for a minimum of 10 minutes.

While the tempeh is marinating, turn your oven to broil, and lightly coat your broil pan with some sesame oil. Remove the tempeh from the marinade (be sure to reserve the marinade), place on the pan in a single layer, and place under the broiler. Broil the tempeh for 5 minutes, toss, and broil for 5 minutes more, or until browned.

Spray a large sauté pan lightly with oil, and heat over medium-high heat. Add the onions, peppers, garlic, and ginger, and cook until the onions begin to turn translucent and the peppers brighten up. Next, add the remaining ¼ cup (60 ml) tamari, pineapple, pineapple juice, vegetable stock, and the remaining ¼ teaspoon red pepper flakes. Cook, while stirring, for 3 to 4 minutes.

Take about 3 tablespoons (45 ml) of the liquid from the pan, and combine it with the cornstarch in a separate bowl, stirring until the cornstarch is dissolved. Add it to the sauté pan, and stir. Now add the broiled tempeh and reserved marinade, stirring until it starts to glaze. Add the peanuts and cabbage, cooking for 1 to 2 minutes longer, or until the cabbage is somewhat wilted.

Remove from the heat and serve hot on a bed of brown rice.

Yield: 4 servings

*Wheat-free

GREEN LEAFY VEGETABLES

The evidence of the healthfulness of green leafy vegetables is overwhelming—from protecting against a number of different cancers and heart disease, strengthening our immune system, protecting our bones against degeneration, promoting lung health, and lowering cholesterol to enhancing our mental performance, lowering the risk for cataracts, protecting against rheumatoid arthritis, helping the colon function properly, reducing inflammation, and providing energy.

I aspire to consume 1 pound (0.45 kg) of greens every day. Even when I don't accomplish it, working toward it means I eat *a lot* of greens. There are more than 1,000 edible green leafies to choose from, including arugula, beet greens, bok choy, collard greens, cabbage, chard, chicory, dandelion, endive, escarole, fat hen, kale, mustard greens, purslane, romaine, sorrel, spinach, tatsoi, turnip greens, watercress—and so many others, including a vast array of edible flowers and herbs.

If any are unfamiliar, just give them a try. You may not like every single one, but you're bound to find an affinity for a few of them. Once you learn to prepare them properly, you might even find that you actually like those you once thought you hated.

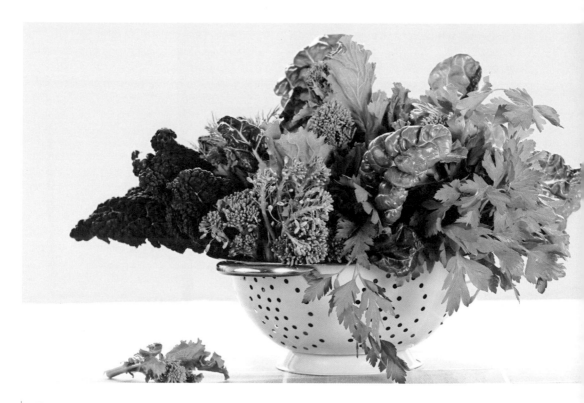

HOW DO YOU RESPOND TO, "WHY AREN'T YOU HELPING PEOPLE INSTEAD OF ANIMALS?"

Like other antagonistic questions, this one is not really meant to be a conversation starter. Rather, the people asking think they're catching animal activists in some a trap that is supposed to ultimately prove that animal activists care more about nonhuman animals than their "fellow humans." In our anthropocentric culture, this could very well be the worst thing you can accuse someone of.

Do some people truly believe that fellow humans aren't capable of caring about more than one thing at a time? Why assume that we're limited in our ability to care about everyone? Each of our hearts is large enough to hold everyone; some people choose to limit their compassion.

Any work that focuses on creating nonviolence and kindness in this world affects all other types of social justice. Compassionate people all have the same goal: the elimination of oppression, exploitation, and violence.

The link between cruelty to animals and violence toward people has been well established. It has long been demonstrated that domestic abuse and alcoholism abound in the homes of slaughterhouse workers. Also, studies of sociopathic behavior show that when people abuse animals, they are very likely to abuse humans, even commit murder.

The early founders of the animal rights movement in the United Kingdom and the United States recognized that their issue is connected with every human issue. Most of them were social justice activists also fighting for human rights, women's rights, children's rights, civil rights—and animal rights. They were hardly misanthropes.

The problem is *not* the people who are doing compassionate work in this world. There is a lot of work to be done, and there are a lot of people who sit back doing absolutely nothing. There are fewer who actually get up, speak out, and do something to make this a better world for *everyone*. Instead of criticizing animal advocates, why don't they instead ask the people who aren't doing *anything* why they do nothing?

BEING STILL

Ever since I arrived in this world, I've had a hard time being still. I've always had an abundance of energy but was labeled "hyper" instead of "lively," "high-strung" instead of "passionate," and "overactive" instead of "spirited." The vitality I had as a child followed me into adulthood and is what fuels my life and work. What was once considered a bane is now a gift that I embrace.

As someone who naturally places my value on being productive, I find it a constant challenge to be still and *unproductive*. Sure, I'm still when I finally collapse and watch a film or read a book, but even then, my mind is active.

Being truly still means turning off the music, putting down the book, turning off your thoughts, standing or sitting in one spot—and just breathing. Just listening. This can be done anywhere, anytime.

When you are still, you don't think about what you have to do or what you've done already. You are in the here and now. You listen better, you're more observant, and your thoughts are clearer.

For some, this stillness takes the form of sitting meditation; for others, it simply means stepping away from all the external computerized stimuli and retreating to a quiet place. When you understand that stillness comes from within, you realize you can even be still in a roomful of people.

> I'm best at being still when I'm in nature or in the presence of animals. They are my inspiration. Looking at my cats or watching the birds and squirrels in my yard grounds me immediately.

Colleen learning to be still from Dawn at Farm Sanctuary
Photo by Connie Pugh

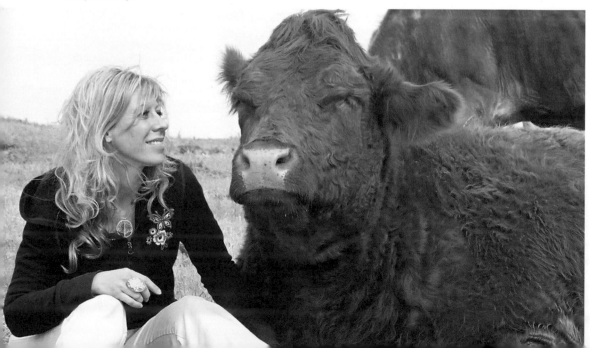

FRANKENSTEIN
BY MARY SHELLEY

Mary Shelley was born in England as Mary Wollstonecraft Godwin on August 30, 1797. She knew her mother, Mary Wollstonecraft (see Day 81), for only eleven days before she died of an infection she contracted while giving birth to her. Shelley, who took the name of her husband (writer Percy Bysshe Shelley), was a novelist, a short story writer, an essayist, and a dramatist, most famous for her novel *Frankenstein, or The Modern Prometheus*.

The story behind the conception of *Frankenstein* is now legendary. In the summer of 1816, Percy, Mary, Lord Byron (see Day 165), and John William Polidori were all vacationing in a villa in Switzerland, where they spent three days indoors because of torrential rainstorms. They began devising their own ghost stories, and as a result, Mary wrote *Frankenstein*. (Polidori wrote the short story *The Vampyre*, which influenced an entire genre of gothic horror fiction, including Bram Stoker's *Dracula*.)

Frankenstein is a favorite book of mine for a number of reasons, including the emphasis on the "monster's" compassion and vegetarianism. Of course, it is the monster who is sympathetic and Victor Frankenstein who is the real monster, reflected in his affinity for meat and animal experimentation. Embodying the ultimate God complex as he obsesses over creating life, just as Prometheus of Greek mythology did, Dr. Frankenstein seems to take pleasure in whatever means are necessary to accomplish his aims: "Who shall conceive the horrors of my secret toil as . . . I dabbled among the unhallowed damps of the grave or tortured the living animal to animate the lifeless clay."

Portraying Victor Frankenstein as a modern-day Prometheus is also interesting, because it was Prometheus who stole fire from heaven and gave it to humans, inspiring them to hunt, kill, and cook animals.

Frankenstein's creation, on the other hand, is benevolent and kind and abhors the killing he does in order to feed his master.

> "My food is not that of man," says the creature. "I do not destroy the lamb and kid to glut my appetite. Acorns and berries afford me sufficient nourishment. My companion will be of the same nature as myself, and will be content with the same fare. We shall make our bed of dried leaves; the sun will shine on us as on man, and will ripen our food. The picture I present to you is peaceful and human, and you must feel that you could deny it only in the wantonness of power and cruelty."

Although many of us read this novel in high school, I highly recommend rereading it through the lens of animal consciousness and vegetarianism. I think you'll be impressed and inspired.

FROM UNABASHED MEAT-EATER TO ENTHUSIASTIC VEGAN

When I met my fiancé, Brian, one of the first things he shared was that he is vegan. I admit to being a bit scared. I love to cook and assumed I would not be able to cook anything for him. I was mostly scared about what this would mean for my life. Would he judge my menu picks at a restaurant? Share slaughterhouse horror stories in an effort to get me to stop eating animals?

Our first date was at a vegetarian restaurant. We had the best falafels, and it felt like we'd already shared many meals together rather than just a short lunch. A date that was only supposed to last a few hours stretched well into dinnertime and nighttime tea.

I started reading vegetarian and vegan cookbooks and recipe sites in an effort to further my way into his heart by way of baked goods. I wasn't planning to change the foods I ate; I was just going to expand my repertoire.

One doesn't read about vegan food without also reading about why veganism is necessary in the first place. I always proudly labeled myself an animal lover. I wanted to be a vet when I was little so I could help hurt and sick animals. I loved Luckie, my dog of fourteen years, beyond reason. The rare moments of clarity I had about the connection between food and animal cruelty were quickly wiped away with a shrug.

I would sometimes apologize to Brian for eating animals; he never once judged me or preached. But he didn't mince words, either. When he said there was no difference between eating foie gras, which I abhorred, and other animal products, which I was still eating, I flinched but knew he was right.

One day, I ate roasted chicken for dinner while reading an article on factory farming in an issue of the Humane Society of the United States members' magazine. There was a picture of a pig with his nose sticking out of a metal crate. I stopped eating. I was horrified that I could read this article and still eat a dead animal. From that moment on, I immediately stopped eating all land animals. After some time and exploration, I became vegan.

It's now been more than two years. My bookshelf is full of vegan cookbooks, and Brian and I—who adopted our dog Benji together—are getting married. I volunteer with the Animal Welfare Society and am preparing to attend nursing school to become a nurse-midwife. In addition to my passion for empowering women to be active participants in their health, I look forward to being the "vegan midwife" and serving as a support to and advocate for women who are sold misinformation about nutrition.

I feel as though I was always vegan and just needed to awaken to who I truly am.

—*Joselle in Philadelphia, Pennsylvania (U.S.)*

CHICKPEA TACOS

A staple in the home of my friends Cadry Nelson and David Busch, this dish packs a flavorful punch whose ingredients can be found in most of our cupboards.

   1 tablespoon (15 ml) olive oil or water, for sautéing
   1 small yellow or red onion, finely chopped
   2 cloves garlic, minced
   1 (15-ounce, or 420 g) can chickpeas, drained and rinsed
   1 teaspoon (2.5 g) ground cumin
   1 teaspoon (2.6 g) chili powder
   1 teaspoon (2.5 g) paprika
   1 teaspoon (1 g) dried oregano
   Juice from ½ lemon
   1 cup (30 g) raw spinach or Swiss chard, coarsely chopped
   8 hard corn taco shells or whole wheat tortillas
   2 tomatoes, diced
   1 avocado, pitted and diced
   Hot sauce (optional)
   Chopped fresh cilantro, for garnish

Add the olive oil to a large sauté pan over medium heat. Add the onion and garlic, and sauté until the onion turns translucent, about 5 minutes.

Add the chickpeas, cumin, chili powder, paprika, oregano, and lemon juice to the pan, and stir to combine. Mash the chickpeas with a fork or spoon, so that they don't roll out of the taco shell.

Add the spinach, and stir to combine. As the chickpea mixture cooks, add more water to the pan in small increments to keep the ingredients from sticking and to make it a bit saucy. Cook for about 7 minutes longer, or until the sauce is your preferred thickness and the dish is heated through.

Fill the taco shells with the chickpea mixture, tomatoes, avocado, and the hot sauce. Sprinkle with cilantro, and serve.

Yield: 8 tacos

*Soy-free, wheat-free if using corn tortilla

SEA VEGETABLES

A more accurate (and more appetizing) term than "seaweed," sea vegetables are consumed in high quantities in Japan (more than anywhere else) and play a large role in that coastal country's cuisine. Despite their impressive nutritional profile, sea vegetables are not found on many menus in the United States.

Sea vegetables can essentially be categorized into three groups, according to their color (though this can vary):

Green and Blue-Green

Spirulina was so highly valued by the Aztecs that it was used as a form of currency. Retaining many minerals from the water, it is rich in potassium, calcium, zinc, magnesium, manganese, selenium, iron, and phosphorus. It can be found as a food supplement in natural food stores and is often added to fruit smoothies for color and nutrients.

Brown

Kombu is the best-known species of kelp, having been cultivated in Japan for about three hundred years. Kombu is often used to make a nutrient-rich and delicious soup stock. Many people also add it to a pot of cooking beans to help them cook faster and to increase the digestibility of the beans.

Wakame, also a type of kelp, is eaten both dried and fresh and has the highest amount of calcium after seaweed—ten times that of cow's milk. It also has four times the iron in beef. Often added to soups, it also makes a delicious foundation for salads.

Red

Dulse flourishes in the cold coastal waters of both the Atlantic and the Pacific, but it is cultivated along the coast of Brittany in France. Considered the most delectable of the sea vegetables, dulse has been used by the people of Scotland, Ireland, and Iceland for centuries.

Nori is a general term for an edible seaweed belonging to the genus Porphyra; despite its deep green-black color, it is considered a red algae. It will be familiar to anyone who has ever had sushi, because it is integral to this Japanese staple. Use it to make your own sushi rolls at home or to make vegetable wraps. Cut into strips, it can be added to salad.

Irish moss or carrageen is actually a seaweed and not a moss. Found along the coasts of the North Atlantic in both Europe and North America, it is sourced mainly in Ireland, where it is steamed and served with potatoes or cabbage. Outside of Ireland, its most common use is in the making of vegetarian gelatin (carrageen).

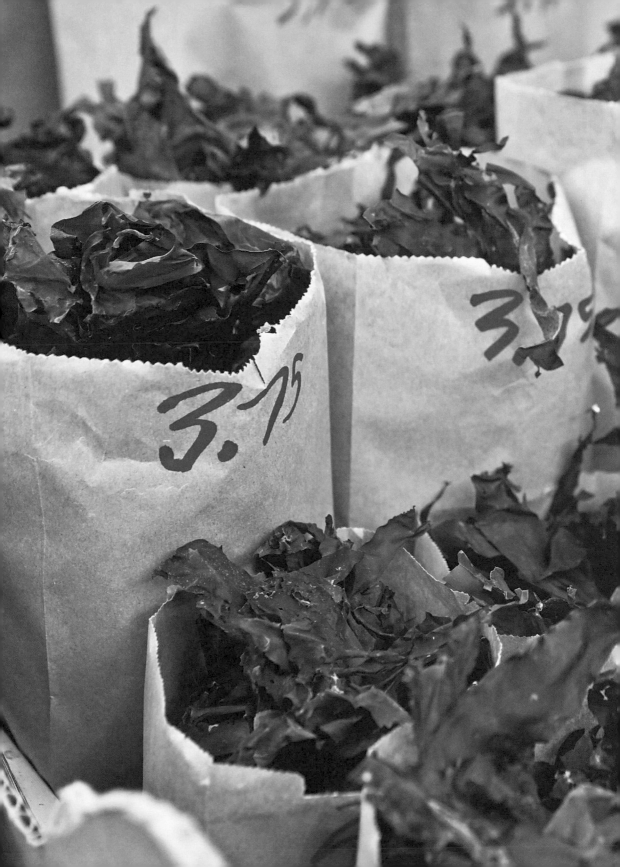

HOW DO YOU RESPOND TO, "WHAT ABOUT THE INSECTS THAT ARE KILLED GROWING VEGETABLES"?

The absurdity of this type of question is often masked by what appears to be genuine, logical concern for insects. And yet, what it really is is an effective strategy for putting vegans on the defensive while appropriating the moral high ground: "It seems hypocritical to me that vegans (or vegetarians) don't care as much about insects as they do about other animals. What about *them*?"

Of course, this question is always posed by a meat-eater. I find it troubling that someone who consciously eats mammals and birds is trying to find fault with people who consciously don't eat mammals and birds.

We happen to live in an imperfect world where animals are killed in ways we really don't have control over. Yes, insects are killed in the growing of vegetables. But insects, mammals, *and* birds are killed in the growing of vegetables for the "raising" and killing of mammals and birds. You have to raise crops to feed the animals we eventually kill so humans can eat them. So, in reality, you're actually killing more insects when you're eating both plants and animals.

We can respond to this person with a few questions in return: "Are you saying that because we can't do everything that we should do nothing? Are you saying that you've found some kind of flaw in the philosophy of someone who is trying to live a life of nonviolence—as much as is possible in our imperfect world?"

When these types of questions come up, we should respond not to the absurd questions but rather to the real issue. Otherwise, we get sucked into arguments about hypothetical scenarios and get distracted from the fact that by choosing *not* to eat animals, we're making a real, measurable difference in the reduction of animal suffering.

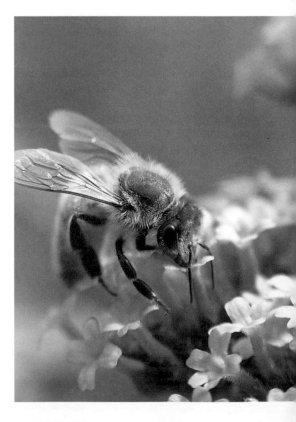

CREATING A SACRED SPACE

The word *sacred* is derived from the Old Latin word *saceres*, which means "to bind, enclose, protect." What I love about the origins of the word is the image I have when I think of creating a safe, special, sacred space: it is indeed a place where I feel protected and cozy and far from the clutter of everyday life.

We all crave a place of retreat—where we can be quiet and still, where we can just listen, where we can be alone. It's the reason children build forts, tree houses, and clubhouses. Within those walls, the world is smaller and manageable and not so overwhelming. As we grow into adults, however, we abandon our forts and infrequently build them anew, often feeling swallowed up by the vastness of the world.

It doesn't take much to create a place of solace. It can be done in a corner of your home, outside on your balcony or in your yard, or in a room you've designated as your own. The idea is to build a space to which you can withdraw—to drink tea, to meditate, to ruminate, to listen to music, to write, to do whatever you need to do to rejuvenate and relax.

* Make it your own—by filling it with personal objects that hold a special meaning for you.

* Make it comfortable—by providing a comfortable place to sit, be it a cushion, a chair, or several pillows.

* Make it intimate—by enclosing it with flowers or fabric or by making it cozy with soft lighting.

* Make it enticing—by including sounds and scents that attract you.

My retreat space inside includes photos of animals, the sound of water, and plants. It's nothing elaborate—but it's mine. For me, the most important aspect of my space is keeping my computer far, far away from it. As long as it's near me, I will work. My sacred space is where I am not doing anything but just being.

May you create for yourself a place of your own where you can be still and unproductive.

"BLOOD"
BY ISAAC BASHEVIS SINGER

Like "The Slaughterer" (Day 39), Isaac Bashevis Singer's short story "Blood" is an indictment against ritual slaughter and is full of harrowing images. Set in rural Poland, "Blood" centers around the adulterous affair between Risha, married to the elderly Reb Falik, and Reuben, the ritual slaughterer she hires.

Their first mating dance is a sign of what's to come, as Risha becomes aroused by the deftness with which Reuben slaughters the chickens she brings to him.

Conducting their illicit affair in the slaughtering shed, Risha and Reuben begin to derive pleasure from the death that is all around them; soon Risha joins in the slaughtering and then takes over completely, grossly violating Jewish law and absolutely perverting natural law. Risha's sexual passions are driven only by the blood she sheds.

The town's butchers, who've been forced out of business by Risha's success, enlist a man to spy on her, and he witnesses Risha taking off her clothes and stretching out on a pile of straw in the middle of the animals who are bleeding to death.

An angry mob forms and returns to the estate armed with bludgeons, knives, and ropes, and Reuben runs away in fear. Mad and remorseless, Risha curses the crowd and turns them away.

In her dreams, the animals get some revenge: "Bulls gored her with their horns; pigs shoved their snouts into her face and bit her; roosters cut her flesh to ribbons with their spurs."

The story ends several years later when the people of Laskev are "terrified by a carnivorous animal lurking about at night and attacking people." When they finally catch and kill this mysterious beast, they discover that it is Risha.

LIFE CHANGE IN A BOOKSTORE

I am a transplant to New England, a bucolic place of rolling farmland and expansive meadows. I moved here a decade or so ago from (Old) England, from a small agricultural area that is, in many respects, an environmental mirror. From a young age, I was surrounded by the farming community—dairy and meat—and fully absorbed its message of the animals' place in my world: They were the product; I was the consumer.

Fast-forward a couple of decades. I had stopped eating sheep ("Lambs are too cute!" I said) and pigs ("Studies indicate they're as intelligent as dogs," I declared). But still I ate cows, chickens, turkeys, ducks, and all manner of aquatic life. I also loved cheese and dairy products.

One Sunday, my husband and I were whiling away a pleasant afternoon in a bookshop. I'd picked a stack of books to browse through, including a work with the rather distinctive title *Skinny Bitch*. I liked its commonsense message—eat food, not junk. Skimming through, I reached a section on the treatment of animals—on how they are turned from warm, sentient creatures into cold, shrink-wrapped flesh. I read quotations from slaughterhouse workers about their disdain, brutality, and lack of compassion as they tortured and killed these terrified creatures. The world stopped spinning, time slowed, and all of the air was sucked out of the room. I couldn't breathe, I couldn't move, and I was overwhelmed with nausea, fear, despair, and complicity.

That day, I became vegetarian. Immediately, without a second thought. My husband had only one question: "What will we eat?" And at the time, it seemed like a good question. Now, to us both, it seems ridiculous!

In the days that followed, through the *Vegetarian Food for Thought* podcast, I learned more about the realities of animal exploitation.

Within three short weeks, I was *vegan*. I expanded my repertoire, trying new foods in new ways. I felt a new peace, a sense of becoming centered and aligned, a part of a growing movement. In the weeks and months that followed, I became calmer and more hopeful than ever before and gained a new purpose.

My life has changed remarkably. The things I worried I could never live without have no hold on me. My diet has improved, I have lost some weight and am fitter and stronger. But the greatest gift is the peace of mind that comes with knowing I am no longer contributing to the horror and suffering of animals. I have always loved animals, but only now am I able to live up to my own ideals, to apply them consistently, to live fully, to live compassionately.

—*Amanda in Westfield, Massachusetts (U.S.)*

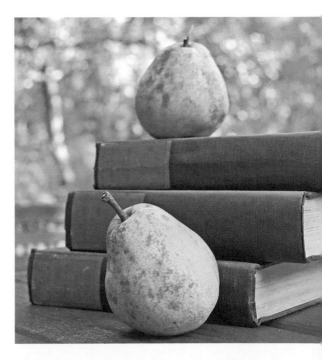

GREEN BEAN AND CHICKPEA SALAD

The ubiquitous chickpea, along with red onion, finds its way into all sorts of Mediterranean salads.

- 3/4 **pound (341 g) long green beans, washed and trimmed**
- 1 ½ **cups (360 g) cooked or 1 (15-ounce, or 420 g) can chickpeas, rinsed and drained**
- 1 **small red onion, chopped**
- 2 **tablespoons (30 ml) vegetable broth (homemade or store-bought)**
- 1 **tablespoon (15 ml) balsamic vinegar**
- 1 **tablespoon (2.4 g) fresh thyme leaves, or 1 teaspoon (1 g) dried**
- **Salt and freshly ground black pepper**

Prepare a large bowl of ice water and set aside. In a medium-size stockpot or saucepan large enough to accommodate a 9-inch (23 cm) steaming basket, put 2 to 3 inches (5 to 7.6 cm) of water. Place the steaming basket in the pot and add the green beans.

Bring to a boil over high heat. Cover tightly, reduce the heat to medium, and steam until crisp-tender, 5 to 7 minutes. Carefully remove the steaming basket and refresh the green beans in the ice water for 5 minutes. Drain well.

Cut the beans into 2-inch (5 cm) lengths and place in a large shallow bowl, along with the chickpeas and onion.

In a small bowl, whisk together the broth, vinegar, thyme, salt, and pepper. Add to the green bean mixture, tossing thoroughly to combine. Let stand at room temperature for 15 minutes to allow the flavors to blend. Toss again.

Serve at room temperature. Or cover and refrigerate for at least 1 hour and serve chilled.

Yield: 4 servings

*Oil-free, soy-free, wheat-free

WATERCRESS

One of the many healthful green leafy vegetables, watercress contains four times the calcium of cow's milk. (I only use cow's milk as a measuring stick because we've been bombarded with messages about cow's milk and calcium since we were tots.) What watercress *doesn't* have that cow's milk has, however, is saturated fat, animal protein, dietary cholesterol, lactose, and blood (which is inevitably part of the animal's milk).

Interestingly, watercress is a member of the brassica family, which also includes broccoli, cabbage, kale, kohlrabi, and Swiss chard, and like its cousins contains a high amount of anticancer properties.

Although it's most frequently eaten raw in green salads, it can also be enjoyed cooked. When cooked, it becomes sweet but also reduces in size by three-fourths, so you might want to start with a large volume.

There are a number of things you can do with watercress:

* Add watercress to green salad. It gives a delightful bitterness.

* Garnish soups, such as miso and barley, with watercress.

* Combine watercress, chopped avocado, grapefruit or orange slices, olive oil, lemon juice, and vinegar for a delicious starter or side salad.

* Make watercress tea sandwiches with nondairy cream cheese, snipped chives, and minced parsley leaves.

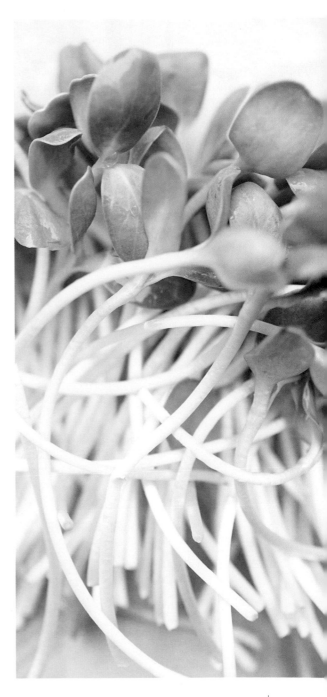

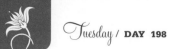
COMPASSIONATE ALTERNATIVE:
DON'T PUT THE CART BEFORE THE HORSE

This popular expression means "let's not reverse the accepted order of things." The first reference to this phrase in English comes in George Puttenham's "The arte of English poesie" in 1589. Now, the phrase itself isn't necessarily as violent as, say, "kill two birds with one stone" (see Day 2), but it is referring to horses being used for our purposes, so perhaps we can simply change it to: "Don't put your shoes on before your socks" or "Don't slice the bread before it's baked."

LOOKING AT IMAGES OF ANIMALS

Not only are there health benefits to living with and spending time with nonhuman animals, but there is also evidence that simply gazing at an image of an animal can decrease heart rate, increase endorphins, and decrease blood pressure and anxiety.

Based on my own small one-person anecdotal study, I can say this is true. I surround myself with images of animals in my life and animals I've never met, and just a glance in their direction calms me and involuntarily puts a smile on my face.

* Print some photos of your own animals or of friends' animals; frame them, hang them, and look at them often.

* Sponsor an animal from a shelter or sanctuary, and hang his or her photo where you can see it plainly—on your monitor, wall, or desk.

* Visit your favorite animal organizations' websites for a quick dose of beauty.

* Bookmark such sites as cuteoverload.com, dailypuppy.com, dailykitten.com, and yes, dailycoyote.com. Visit often.

* Spend some time at petfinder.com admiring all the dogs, cats, and bunnies—especially once you know you're ready to adopt—and find your new family member.

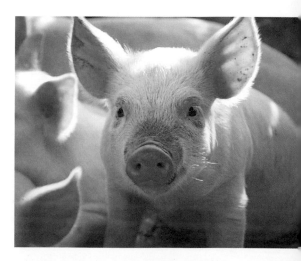

THE VEGETARIAN PHILOSOPHY OF PYTHAGORAS
AS TOLD BY OVID IN *THE METAMORPHOSES*

Pythagoras of Samos is believed to have been born somewhere between 580 and 572 BCE and died somewhere between 500 and 490 BCE. Among other things, he was the founder of a religious movement that came to be called Pythagoreanism, most known for its theory of the transmigration of souls.

Just as we have no primary texts by Socrates, we have none by Pythagoras either. Instead, we have to rely on the writings of people who came after him to learn anything about him.

One of these sources lived hundreds of years after Pythagoras died: Publius Ovidius Naso, known simply as Ovid. Ovid was a Roman poet who lived from 43 BCE to 17 CE; his most famous work is called *The Metamorphoses*, an epic poem that draws on Greek mythology. In it, he devotes a number of chapters to Pythagoras's teachings, and one is dedicated to his philosophy of vegetarianism.

Early vegetarians were called Pythagoreans, and Pythagoras is considered the "father of vegetarianism" in that he taught it as a formal ethical tenet to follow. Vegetarianism has been part of a religious lifestyle in the East for thousands of years, but Pythagoras formalized it in the West for the first time—or at least as far as we are able to document.

His moral objections to eating animals seems to stem from his religious conviction that the human soul transmigrates (or reincarnates) after physical death, so he warned that if you're consuming an animal, you may very well be consuming a human soul. Subsequent followers of his teachings took this less seriously than the fact that the killing and consuming of animals desensitizes humans to animal suffering, a theory that stems from Pythagoras's teachings, which is apparent in Ovid's poem.

There are many translations of Ovid's *The Metamorphoses,* though my favorite is the one by Rolfe Humphries, which is reprinted in a little-known but very well-researched, well-edited book called *Ethical Vegetarianism: From Pythagoras to Peter Singer.*

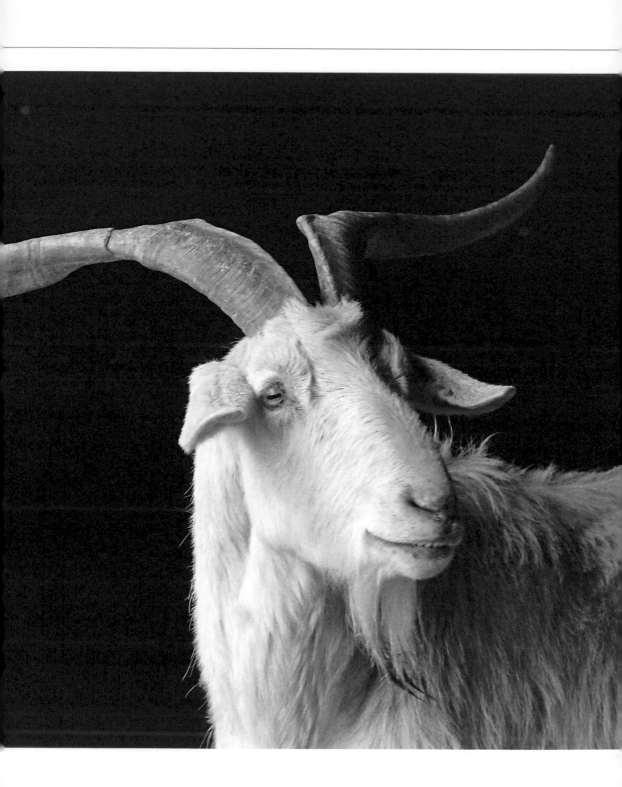

NEPTUNE, A MAGICAL BEING

Anyone who doesn't believe animals have souls never met Neptune, a beautiful white goat brought to Farm Sanctuary in 1995. Neptune's story prior to his rescue is a sad one, but I have no doubt that his life at the sanctuary healed his wounds. His powerful presence was apparent to everyone who met him—or just saw him. He was filled with radiance and beauty and gentleness and love and wisdom, and I was often moved to tears just being near him. I kid you not. His presence was that powerful.

I had the privilege of spending many, many quiet hours with Neptune, watching the sunset and basking in his glow. He would hold his face up and feel the breeze on his face and seem to meditate as he basked in the setting sun.

He arrived at Farm Sanctuary after having endured a most hideous abuse. He was kept by a man who lived in a rural area and had several animals. A neighbor was concerned about their living conditions, including that of Neptune and another goat, Neptune's female partner. This neighbor wanted to help the animals without raising ire in the animals' "owner," but it was often to no avail. The situation never improved.

In fact, it worsened when the neighbor intervened and called the authorities. Unfortunately, it was this turn of events that would be bittersweet for Neptune. The "owner" of the animals was angry that the neighbor had "meddled" and retaliated in a cruel, hateful way. He decided to relocate and left some of his animals behind. Before he departed, he cut the throat of Neptune's companion and left her hanging on a fence. Worse yet, he tethered Neptune to this fence with only 1 foot (30.5 cm) of rope. Neptune endured this for several days before the neighbor found him and brought him to Farm Sanctuary.

Despite having been mistreated by a particularly cruel human, Neptune never held it against the other humans he met. And he met thousands. He benevolently and confidently ruled over the other goats, maintaining a seriousness that set him apart from many of the others. A happy and radiant being, he also carried a sadness with him from his past that never entirely left him.

During my more recent visits, it was apparent Neptune wasn't doing very well. His arthritis was worsening rapidly, and the pain medication wasn't giving him the relief he needed. When I received a call that his quality of life was compromised to the degree that he would not make it more than a few more days, I immediately made my way to the sanctuary to say good-bye.

As I grieve for the loss of his physical presence, my heart is filled with his spirit, his grace, and his beauty, and my memory is filled with countless, priceless shared moments.

—CPG

Magical, majestic Neptune at Farm Sanctuary
Photo by Derek Goodwin for Farm Sanctuary

WATERMELON AND ORANGE SALAD

A healthful dish to whip up in a flash, this salad holds up nicely in the fridge for at least a day.

¼ cup (60 ml) fresh orange juice
¼ cup (60 ml) grapeseed or canola oil
Juice of 1 lime
1 tablespoon (15 ml) red wine vinegar
1 tablespoon (11 g) Dijon mustard
1 shallot, minced
¼ teaspoon salt
⅛ teaspoon freshly ground pepper
2 oranges, peeled and cut into slices
    or coarsely chopped
6 cups (900 g) cubed watermelon
¾ cup (30 g) finely minced fresh basil
½ cup (55 g) toasted slivered almonds

In a small bowl, combine the orange juice, oil, lime juice, vinegar, mustard, shallot, salt, and pepper. Whisk to thoroughly combine all the ingredients.

To a large bowl, add the oranges and watermelon. Add the vinaigrette, and toss to combine. Divide among 6 bowls, and sprinkle the basil and almonds over each serving.

Yield: 6 servings

*Wheat-free, soy-free

MUSTARD GREENS

Part of the cabbage family, the mustard plant provides the seeds to make the condiment mustard as well as edible leaves to be enjoyed in a variety of ways.

Mustard greens are the most pungent of the greens and lend a peppery flavor to food. They originated in the Himalayan region of India more than 5,000 years ago. Like most greens, they're very versatile and are used in cuisines throughout France, China, Japan, India, and the southern United States.

Here are a few ways to use them:

* Finely chop mustard greens, and add them to a salad.

* Add chopped mustard greens to a soup.

* Sauté them in olive oil with walnuts, and squeeze a little lemon juice on near the end of cooking. (The acid from the lemon juice tends to cut the bitterness; the vitamin C from the lemon juice increases the absorption of iron.)

* Add chopped mustard greens to a pasta salad, or cook them the way you would collard greens (see Day 274).

Good substitutes for the delicate green leaves include escarole, kale, spinach, and Swiss chard.

A RHETORIC REVOLUTION

Although I don't support censorship, there are some words you will never hear me utter: words that denigrate "vegan food" and that elevate the status of meat, dairy, and eggs. When properly used, they cause no real harm, but when paired in certain phrases, their meaning becomes downright destructive.

The culprits are none other than "faux," "fake," "mock," "substitute," and "imitation." Other altogether unappetizing-sounding variations include "analogue," "alternative," and "replacement"—words that make vegan food seem strange and unappealing. Who wants to eat an "analogue"?

Milk

Not only should we call plant-based milks what they are (e.g., soy, almond, rice, oat, hazelnut— *never* "milk substitute" and *never* "mylk"), but we should also do the same when referring to animal-based milk. It's "cow's milk," not simply "milk" or "regular milk."

Butter

We already use the word *butter* to refer to *nut* and *fruit* butters (peanut, almond, cashew, apple) and other fats that are solid at room temperature, such as cocoa butter and shea butter. Choose, then, to say "nondairy butter"— *never* "imitation" and *never* "butter substitute."

Meat

I even propose we take back the word *meat*, which comes from the Old English word *mete* and originally referred to something that was *eaten* and not *drunk*. We already say "coconut meat" and "nut meat," so why shouldn't we embrace "grain meat," "soy meat," and "wheat meat" and reject "faux meat" and "fake meat"? Burgers or deli

slices made from these plant foods are not *fake*; they're made from *real* ingredients.

When we use words that make plant-based foods seem *unreal* and *unappetizing*, we foster the public perception that these foods are just that. If we reclaim the language around plant-based foods, we can go a long way in mainstreaming the vegan ethic.

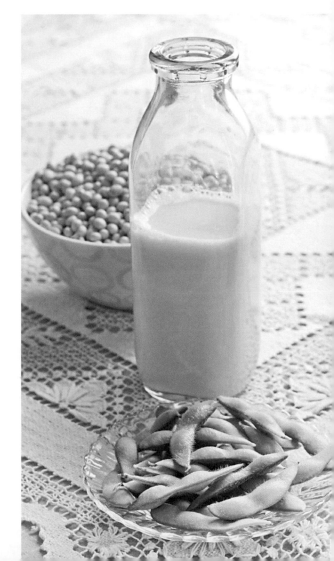

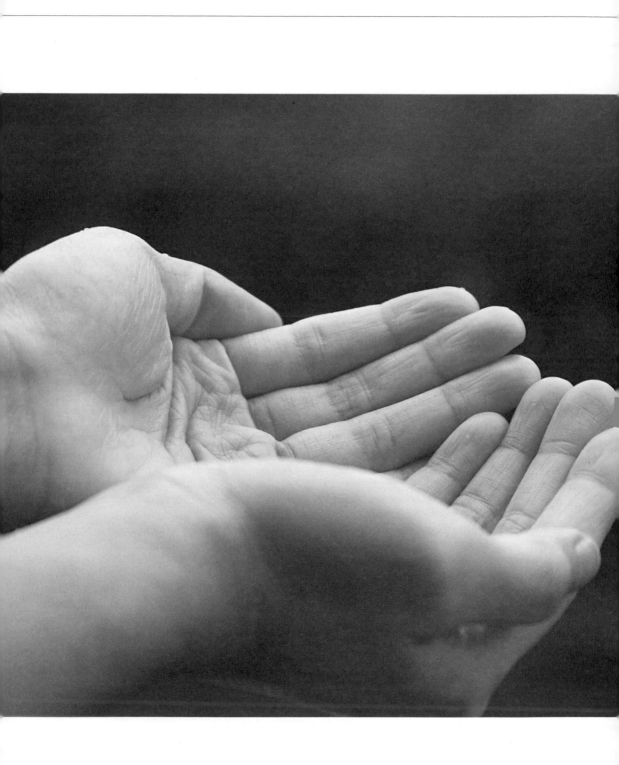

GIVING BACK

The Judeo-Christian practice of tithing has always being interesting to me. The root of the word comes from an Old English word, meaning "tenth," the idea being that you make a voluntary monetary contribution to support an organization that equals 10 percent of your income. The amount is less important than the principle, whose origins date back to biblical times.

The reason I appreciate this practice is because I believe that to keep abundance flowing, you have to keep money moving. Money, just being one form of energy, needs to be circulated in order to proliferate, and giving some of my money to charitable causes is one way to do this.

Ten percent may not work for everyone, so create a percentage that works for you. Once you decide how much to give, the next decision is how often and through what medium to give.

* Do you want to make a monthly donation? Most organizations let you set up an automatic bank transfer or credit card charge.

* If you want to donate annually, find out about a particular program you'd like to support throughout the year.

* Plan for special fundraising events or disasters that may occur throughout the year, and set money aside for such a purpose.

* If you donate online or by credit card, some administrative costs may be incurred for the organization. Perhaps you want to write a check instead.

* Ask your company if they offer a direct donation option, whereby a certain amount of your paycheck each month can be directed to your chosen nonprofit.

* The fun part is deciding who to give to. I usually make one large annual donation to one organization and then send a smaller amount to a different organization each month, including my local animal shelter. I love choosing which organization to donate to each month and have several animal and vegan organizations I choose among.

* If donating to health organizations, be sure to first find out if they fund animal research. Visit caringconsumer.com for a list of cruelty-free charities.

* If donating to environmental organizations, make sure they are aligned with your values. Many larger ones (World Wildlife Fund, Sierra Club, Nature Conservancy) advocate and fund various forms of hunting.

* Create a charity gift or charity wedding registry at JustGive.org.

EXCERPTS FROM *EMILE, OR ON EDUCATION*
BY JEAN-JACQUES ROUSSEAU

Perhaps the work for which philosopher Jean-Jacques Rousseau (see also Day 109) is most remembered, *Emile, or On Education* was published in 1762 and immediately burned. Tackling the nature of education in a person's life, *Emile* also addressed the very small subject of the nature of man, exploring the relationship between an individual and the larger society.

Instead of writing his ideas in the form of a treatise, he expounds his philosophy in a novel, which enables him to illustrate—through his fictional main character, Emile—exactly what he envisions to be the ideal education of children, including how they should be fed. Aside from making some gross generalizations ("The English are noted for their cruelty"), Rousseau provides keen insight about the natural food preferences of children and the negative effects of consuming animal products.

The indifference of children towards meat is one proof that the taste for meat is unnatural; their preference is for vegetable foods, such as milk, pastry, fruit, etc. Beware of changing this natural taste and making children flesh-eaters, if not for their health's sake, for the sake of their character.

For however one tries to explain the practice, it is certain that great meat-eaters are usually more cruel and ferocious than other men. This has been recognised at all times and in all places. The English are noted for their cruelty while the Gaures are the gentlest of men. All savages are cruel, and it is not their customs that tend in this direction; their cruelty is the result of their food. They go to war as to the chase, and treat men as they would treat bears. Indeed in England butchers are not allowed to give evidence in a court of law, no more can surgeons. Great criminals prepare themselves for murder by drinking blood. Homer makes his flesh-eating Cyclops a terrible man, while his Lotus-eaters are so delightful that those who went to trade with them forgot even their own country to dwell among them.

VEGAN IN THE UK

I had never really been a particularly healthy person growing up. I guess I ate mostly what the rest of New Zealand society ate: meat and a lot of dairy.

As I grew older, I paid more attention to my eating habits and health in general, although I did, however, still believe that there was nothing wrong with lean red meat and dairy in a well-balanced diet.

The plight of animals never really crossed my mind. Sure, they were killed for our consumption. Of course they were; that's what they were raised for! And anyway, if I didn't pick up that chicken breast at the supermarket, someone else would, or it would be wasted.

After graduating from school, I traveled to all sorts of places and tried a range of cuisines. Seeking desperately to avoid the "fussy" label I had earned as a child, I ate all manner of delicacies served for my consumption, including sea snake, puffer fish, raw horse meat, raw chicken, liver, and cartilage. None of this bothered me at the time. It is only now, when I look back on myself at those moments, that I am saddened.

I've been vegan for two years now, and it has changed my life completely. I can't say there was a definitive moment that led me to adopt a more compassionate lifestyle or that I woke up one morning and it all fell into place like the pieces of a puzzle. Things happened gradually. I was aware of issues surrounding the consumption of animal products in a peripheral sense; they were always there, but I had never chosen to focus on them.

Veganism is not a journey that ends once you've completely rid your life of animal products. It is an ongoing journey and one that you will be able to travel with throughout your life, like a good companion. Veganism is the voice that asks you to reconsider, to live your life in accordance with your beliefs, and to aspire to be better.

—*Sarah in London, England*

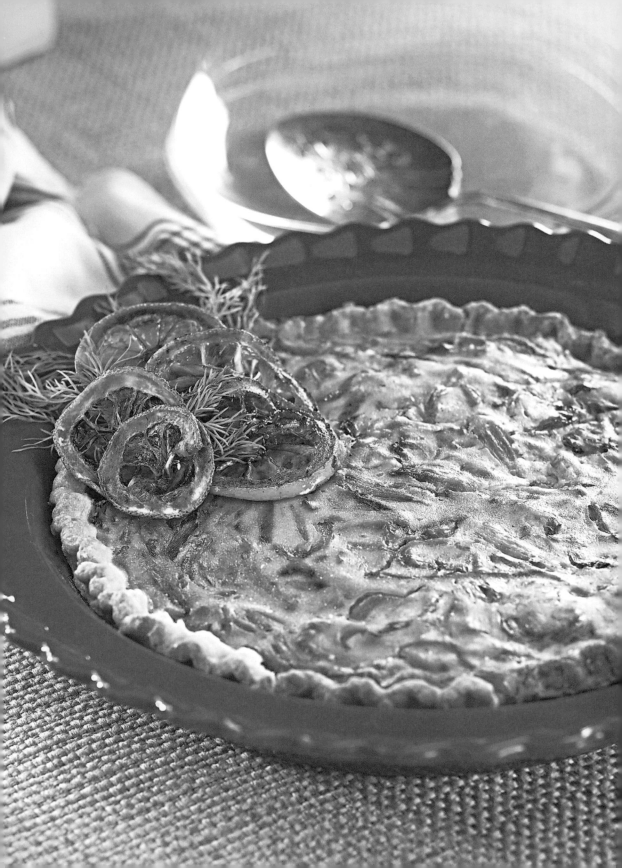

FRENCH ONION PIE

Although I had been making (and teaching) this elegant yet simple dish for years, it first appeared in print in my second book, *The Vegan Table*.

> 2 uncooked pie shells, thawed
> 5 large yellow or white onions, thinly sliced
> 4 cloves garlic, minced
> 1 tablespoon (14 g) nondairy butter, oil, or water, for sautéing
> 1 teaspoon (4 g) granulated sugar
> ½ teaspoon salt, plus a little extra
> 1½ cups (355 ml) nondairy milk (soy, rice, almond, hazelnut, hemp, or oat)
> 15 ounces (420 g) extra-firm tofu (*not* silken)
> ½ teaspoon black pepper
> ½ teaspoon nutmeg
> 5 tablespoons (40 g) unbleached flour
> 2 tablespoons (25 g) nutritional yeast flakes (optional)

Preheat the oven to 350°F (180°C or gas mark 4). Bake the pie shells for 10 minutes, and remove from the oven. Set aside.

In a large sauté pan, cook the onions and garlic in the nondairy butter, stirring occasionally, until the onions become translucent. Add the sugar and a little salt to taste. Cook for 15 to 25 minutes (or longer if you'd like the onions some-what caramelized, which happens more easily with oil than with water).

In a blender or large food processor, combine the milk, tofu, remaining ½ teaspoon salt, pepper, nutmeg, flour, and nutritional yeast until the mixture is smooth. In a large bowl, add the contents of the blender to the sautéed onions.

Stir all the ingredients together and distribute evenly between the 2 partially cooked pie shells. Bake for 45 minutes, or until the crust is golden brown and the filling is set. Serve immediately.

Yield: Two 9-inch (23 cm) pies, 10 to 12 servings each

Originally published in *The Vegan Table*

BLACK-EYED PEAS

Characterized by their white color and black dot on the side, black-eyed peas are widely cultivated in India and Africa and can be added to salads, soups, and chilis. An excellent source of calcium, folate, and vitamin A, black-eyed peas are traditionally eaten on New Year's Day in the southern United States and are the basis for a traditional dish called "Hoppin' John" made of black-eyed peas cooked with rice and Cajun seasonings. The traditional New Year's meal also features collard or mustard greens, which is supposed to bring good luck and financial enrichment. (The peas represent coins, and the greens symbolize paper money.)

Rice and black-eyed peas is a popular dish in Jamaica and other Caribbean islands, and in Vietnam, black-eyed peas are used in a sweet dessert called *chè đậutrắng* (black-eyed peas and sticky rice with coconut milk).

* Small in size, black eyed-peas are available fresh, canned, dried, or frozen and generally don't have to be soaked before cooking them.

* Turning somewhat creamy when cooked, they are a good candidate for hearty bean salads and casseroles.

* I love the varying textures of a bean salad made with black-eyed peas, corn, green beans, and chopped tomatoes. Toss with lemon juice, a splash of vinegar, a touch of olive oil, and chopped fresh herbs.

Originally, black-eyed peas were called *mogette*, which is the French word for "nun." The black eye in the center of the bean (where it attaches to the pod) reminded some of a nun's head attire and named it thus. That name is now out of use, though they are also called cowpeas and California blackeyes.

EASING PEOPLE IN

I love talking to people about being vegan, but I accept that some people are afraid of the V-word. They might have known someone who was vegan who turned them off to it altogether; they might not know how to pronounce the word; they might harbor their own stereotypes. With this awareness, when I bring up the topic—and I make a point to bring it up whenever I can—I do so with the intention of making the other person comfortable. I *ease* into it, if you will.

When I meet new people, I bring up that I'm vegan, but sometimes I start by saying I'm

vegetarian. I gauge the situation first before just saying "vegan"; I may first venture into more familiar territory.

I firmly believe that people want to talk about this issue (veganism, animal rights, food ethics), but they just don't know how. When you perceive people as being open-minded and friendly, that's what you tend to find. When you find ways to ease the topic into the conversation so they feel *they* brought it up and that it wasn't just thrust upon them, you may be pleasantly surprised by the results.

ESSENTIAL FATTY ACIDS—FINDING BALANCE AND INCREASING ABSORPTION

Omega-3 (also known as alpha-linolenic acid, or ALA) is one of the two primary essential fatty acids. The other is omega-6 fat (also known as linoleic acid, or LA). (When something is called "essential," it means our body cannot manufacture it, so it's required in our diet.)

Both omega-6s and omega-3s are polyunsaturated fats, and optimal health depends on the proper balance between these two fatty acids. However, people are getting too many of the omega-6 fatty acids because they're cooking with omega-6-rich corn, safflower, and sunflower oils (commercial "vegetable oil" is usually a combination of these) and because these fats are used to extend the shelf life of processed, packaged foods, which people tend to consume a lot of. Omega-6 fats are also found in meat, dairy, and eggs in the form of arachidonic acid.

Two components of omega-3 fatty acids are EPA and DHA, which are found mostly in sea vegetables, such as the algae that fish eat. Ultimately, what we want to do is increase our conversion of short-chain omega-3 ALA acids into these longer chain fatty acids: EPA and DHA. We can do this by lowering our consumption of omega-6s and increasing our consumption of those omega-3s through such foods as flaxseeds and walnuts.

Some people (diabetics, for instance) don't convert omega-3 fatty acids into DHA sufficiently, and they may be more prone to depression, allergies, and inflammatory skin disease, such as eczema. Other factors that inhibit the conversion are excessive saturated fat, cholesterol, and trans fats in the diet. The rate of conversion is limited in infants and declines as we get older.

So, the big question is: Do we need to supplement with a direct source of DHA? As far as the research indicates:

* If you have diabetes or are over sixty-five, it would be prudent to take DHA directly.

* If you're pregnant or lactating, you might consider supplementing to help pass it on to your infant.

* Low levels of DHA are associated with several neurological and behavioral disorders, such as depression, attention deficit hyperactivity disorder (ADHD), schizophrenia, and Alzheimer's disease, so if you suffer from any of these or know someone who does, you might consider supplementing with some DHA directly. Stores tend to be increased after a few months.

* If you don't fall into any of these categories—and that's most people—the conversion seems to occur with no problem, and you can obtain essential fatty acids through food. About once a year, however, I take a direct DHA supplement for a month or two—just for insurance.

"TO A YOUNG ASS"
BY SAMUEL TAYLOR COLERIDGE

Living from 1772 to 1834, Samuel Taylor Coleridge was an English poet, literary critic, and philosopher, who, with William Wordsworth, founded the Romantic Movement in England. Considered one of the "Lake Poets" (referring to those who lived in the Lake District of northwestern England), Coleridge is most known for his long poem "The Rime of the Ancient Mariner," his poem "Kubla Khan," his critical work on Shakespeare, and his influence on American transcendentalism.

His poem, "To A Young Ass," which I've also seen called simply "The Donkey," was written in 1794 and beautifully expresses immense sympathy and compassion for a small, abused donkey.

> Poor little foal of an oppressed race!
> I love the languid patience of thy face:
> And oft with gentle hand I give thee bread,
> And clap thy ragged coat, and pat thy head.
> But what thy dulled spirits hath dismay'd,
> That never thou dost sport along the glade?
> And (most unlike the nature of things young)
> That earthward still thy moveless head is hung!
> Do thy prophetic fears anticipate,
> Meek child of misery! thy future fate?
> The starving meal, and all the thousand aches
> Which patient merit of the unworthy takes?
> Or is thy sad heart thrill'd with filial pain
> To see thy wretched mother's shorten'd chain?
> And truly, very piteous is her lot
> Chain'd to a log within a narrow spot
> Where the close-eaten grass is scarcely seen,
> While sweet around her waves the tempting
> green!

> Poor Ass! thy master should have learnt to show
> Pity—best taught by fellowship of Woe!
> For much I fear me, that he lives, like thee,
> Half-famish'd in a land of Luxury!
> How askingly its footsteps hither bend?
> It seems to say, "And have I then one friend?"
> Innocent foal! thou poor despis'd forlorn!
> I hail thee *Brother*—spite of the fool's scorn!
> And fain would take thee with me, in the Dell
> Of Peace and mild Equality to dwell,
> Where Toil shall call the charmer Health his bride,
> And Laughter tickle Plenty's ribless side!

> How thou wouldst toss thy heels in gamesome
> play,
> And frisk about, as lamb or kitten gay!
> Yea! and more musically sweet to me
> Thy dissonant harsh bray of joy would be,
> Than warbled melodies that soothe to rest
> The aching of pale Fashion's vacant breast!

Waylon, one of Colleen's best friends at Farm Sanctuary

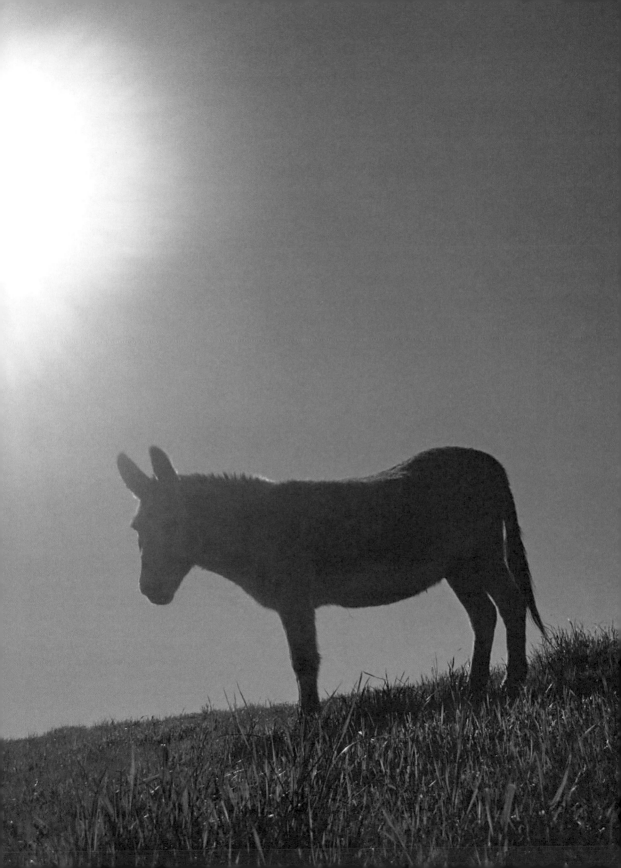

ALEXANDER, THE BEAUTIFUL BLACK LEOPARD

Since 1984, the Performing Animal Welfare Society (PAWS) has been dedicated to the protection of performing animals and to providing sanctuary for abused, abandoned, and retired captive wildlife.

Pat Derby tells her story in her autobiography, *Lady and Her Tiger*, the first exposé of the harsh training methods and minimal care standards in the entertainment industry. She had worked with exotic animals as a trainer on the set of many films and popular television shows in the 1970s. Pat was shocked to discover a profession rampant with neglect and abuse. Stories of abusive training on movie and television sets prompted her and her husband Ed Stewart to found PAWS.

Alexander, a beautiful black leopard, is just one of thousands of victims of the exotic pet trade. He was purchased as a cub for $2,500 by a family in Texas, and kept chained out in the family backyard. Houston Animal Control seized him but returned Alexander to his owners after they agreed to take him outside city limits.

Shortly after, he scratched a toddler and was confiscated once again by Animal Control. Because this was his second seizure, Houston City ordinance mandated that he be euthanized. The Houston SPCA appealed the decision and the animal was released to their care. Houston SPCA then contacted PAWS, where he will live permanently and safely. He arrived March 11, 1999, after spending seven months at the Houston SPCA.

He spends his days in a spacious natural habitat full of natural grasses and trees, a pond, and lots of area to explore.

—CPG

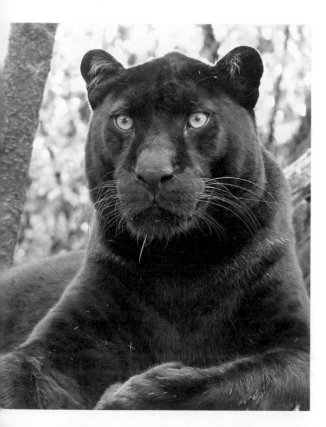

Alexander at PAWS

Photo courtesy of Performing Animal Welfare Society

BEET BURGERS

This recipe is a result of having wanted to replicate a favorite beet burger from a local restaurant for a long time. I'm totally tickled to have done so.

2 cups (240 g) grated beets (about 2 large beets)

1½ cups (300 g) cooked bulgur wheat (or quinoa or millet)

1 cup (130 g) toasted sunflower seeds

½ cup (120 g) toasted sesame seeds

½ cup (80 g) minced onion (about 1 small onion)

½ cup (60 g) bread crumbs

¼ cup (60 ml) olive or canola oil

3 tablespoons (24 g) all-purpose flour

3 tablespoons (12 g) finely chopped fresh parsley

4 cloves garlic, finely chopped

2 to 3 tablespoons (30 to 45 ml) tamari soy sauce

¼ teaspoon cayenne pepper, or to taste

Salt

Preheat the oven to 350°F (180°C, or gas mark 4). Line a baking sheet with unbleached parchment paper.

In a large bowl, combine the grated beets, bulgur, sunflower seeds, sesame seeds, onion, bread crumbs, oil, flour, parsley, garlic, tamari, and cayenne. Add salt to taste.

At this point, test if you can create a patty that will stay together. These are definitely softer-type burgers, but you should still be able to form a patty with no problem. If it still falls apart, add a little more bulgur or flour until you have a firm patty that won't fall apart while cooking/baking.

Continue forming uniform-size patties. I make mine a little bulky and get about 12 patties out of them. You can also make them a little smaller and less dense.

Bake for 25 minutes, or until firmer and the vegetables are cooked through. Carefully flip halfway during the cooking time.

Serve each burger on a whole wheat bun, topped with sliced tomatoes, grilled red onions, avocado slices, and eggless mayonnaise. (Wildwood's Garlic Aioli and Follow Your Heart's Vegenaise are my favorites.)

Yield: 10 to 12 patties

Originally published in *Color Me Vegan*

VINEGARS

Having a variety of vinegars in your cupboard means instant flavor in whatever dish you add them to. Because there are so many different kinds, I can't cover them all here, but I encourage you to spend some time in the vinegar section of your grocery store—especially a store that may stock more special varieties.

Discovered by chance more than 10,000 years ago, vinegar gets its name from the French *vin aigre*, which means "sour wine." Vinegar is the result of the fermentation of ethanol, which varies according to the liquid the ethanol is fermented in.

Here is a brief overview of a few delicious, versatile vinegars, all of which should be easy to find in a store near you.

Apple cider is great to have on hand for making a quick dressing for various salads, whether greens-based or pasta-based. Relatively inexpensive, it's available in raw (unpasteurized and unfiltered) and processed forms. I would choose the former for flavor and nutrition.

Balsamic is the mother of all vinegars—in my humble opinion. There is true balsamic (fermented/aged for a long time) and short-cut balsamic (designated by the words "from Modena" on the label). Real balsamic vinegar is thick, sweet, and syrupy, and you can practically eat it right off the spoon!

Wine vinegars, both white and red, are "everyday" vinegars—nothing special but good to have on hand. Good for salad dressings and marinades, red wine vinegar complements heartier dishes, such as mushrooms and winter vegetables; white wine vinegar is best for lighter fare.

Rice is the mildest of all the vinegars, which I use abundantly in Asian recipes, including when I make sushi. Seasoned rice vinegar has added sugar, which lends a little sweetness, and sprinkling a little on my favorite greens is often enough for me. A basic vinegar that lacks the complexity of balsamic, it's good to have on hand.

Store all vinegars in a cool, dark place. They will last for about a year after opening; after that time, the flavors will diminish.

COMPASSIONATE ALTERNATIVES TO VIOLENT CHILDREN'S SONGS

In our culture, it is considered radical to tell the truth. I remember someone asked me once, very innocently, "If you had children, would you impose your viewpoints and values on them and not feed them meat?"

First of all, parents impose their viewpoints and values on their kids all the time. It's called parenting. I don't know of many people who actually raise their children with values that don't coincide with their own. And as for the choice *not* to feed children meat, I can't think of a more consistent message to give to children. I grew up learning that my dog was worthy of love but the bodies of animals who covered my dinner plate were worthless—or, rather, killed for *me*! I was (implicitly) taught that the bird with the broken wing who was lucky enough to fall in my yard was worth saving, but the chickens and turkeys who "give their lives for me" were valuable only insofar as their flesh was tender and juicy.

I also grew up singing the most violent songs. By the time I was three, I knew the words to "A Hunting We Will Go," "The Bumblebee Song" ("I'm squishing up a baby bumblebee"!), "Three Blind Mice" ("They all ran after the farmer's wife, who cut off their tails with a carving knife"!). Granted, I was taught some nice songs about eency weency spiders climbing up waterspouts and about a mouse who ran up and down a clock, but I didn't know that so many of my favorite songs were reinforcing the lowly status of animals.

Now, it's such a joy to watch my vegan friends give consistent and compassionate messages to their children, aware though they are that we live in a culture that doesn't support these messages of truth but that encourages instead messages of domination and control.

We've had so much fun making up new words to animal-unfriendly songs:

* "Baa baa black sheep, have you any wool? Yes sir, yes sir, three bags full; one for the master, one for the dame, and one for the little boy, who lives down the lane" became instead: "Baa baa black sheep, have you any wool? Yes sir, yes sir, but it's not meant for you. I have none for the master, none for the dame, and none for the little boy, who lives down the lane." You have to sing it to appreciate the beauty of it!

* The little piggy who had roast beef has roasted veggies instead.

* And the teacher doesn't actually kick Mary's lamb out of the school, as she does at the conventional ending of that nursery rhyme.

Some people label as "politically correct" any attempt to reframe the familiar. Every message we teach to children becomes part of them, and any attempt to teach children compassion is not, in my mind, politically correct; it is simply *correct*.

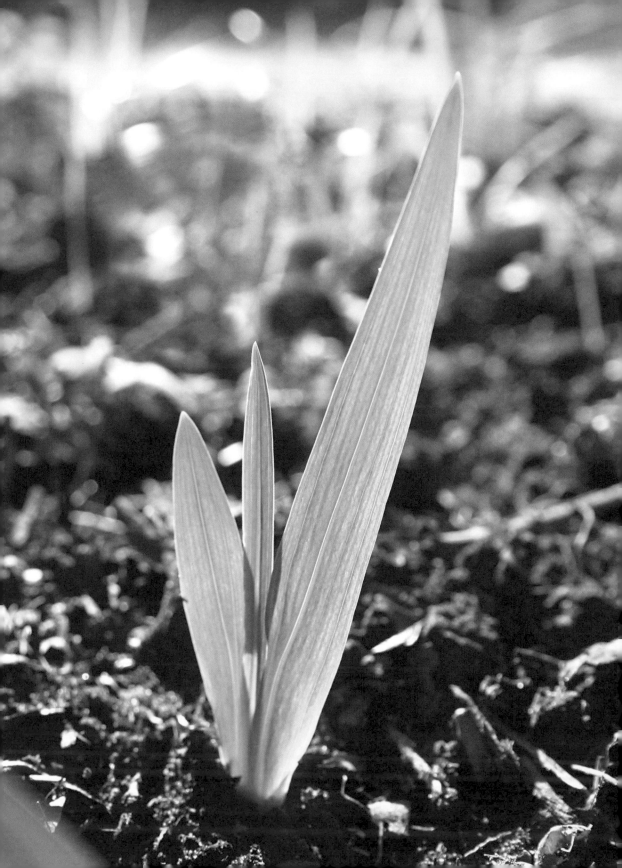

FERTILIZING YOUR GARDEN—VEGAN STYLE

When it comes to human nutrition, the bottom line is: the nutrients we need are plant- (and bacteria-) based—not animal-based. The same is true when it comes to healthy soil. The nutrients that plants need to grow come from the ground—not animals. Aside from secondary and trace nutrients, the three major plant nutrients are nitrogen, phosphorus, and potassium, often expressed as N-P-K. (N for nitrogen, P for phosphorus, and K for potassium, referring to its Latin name on the periodic table.) On every box of commercial fertilizer, you'll see there are three numbers, such as 24-6-6. This refers to that the amounts that particular fertilizer contains—by weight—24 percent nitrogen, 6 percent phosphorus, and 6 percent potassium.

These different minerals promote different types of growth, so you'll want to know what your goal is before you use one of these single fertilizers. Here's how it breaks down:

* **Nitrogen** promotes leaf and stem growth. An excess of nitrogen will cause a lot of foliage growth at the expense of flowers and fruit, so unless there really is a nitrogen deficiency, be careful not to overload fruit- and flower-bearing plants with it. Nitrogen fertilizers include cottonseed meal, alfalfa meal, flaxseed meal, and soybean meal.

* **Phosphorus** is very important for root growth. Flowering bulbs and root crops can always use some phosphorous, so you might want to consider adding phosphorus when you're planting bulbs in the fall. Typically, bone meal is used as phosphorus, but that's not necessary. Rock phosphate is a much better, humane choice; it's not from slaughtered animals.

* **Potassium** promotes disease resistance and is needed for overall plant health. Potassium deficiency produces very tall plants with weak stems as well as leaf tips and edges turning yellow, then later brown. Great sources of potassium include kelp meal, seaweed, and wood ashes.

Although fertilizer blends are available, they often contain slaughterhouse waste products such as blood meal, bone meal, hoof meal, horn meal, feather meal, fish emulsion, and fish heads. Obviously, I avoid the blends and just buy the single mineral-based amendments.

Remember, though: There is a difference between adding nutrients to plants and keeping the soil nourished. Sometimes plants need a boost—like we all do—but just as we cannot live on supplements alone, so too plants need a strong, healthy foundation. And that can come only from strong, healthy soil, which comes from organic matter. (See Day 241.)

ELIZABETH COSTELLO
BY J. M. COETZEE

Elizabeth Costello is a 2003 novel by South African–born, Nobel Prize–winning vegetarian J. M. Coetzee. Elizabeth Costello, who first appears in his 1999 novel *The Lives of Animals,* is the character through which Coetzee addresses animal rights. Some might even say that she is the mouthpiece for the author himself.

In *Elizabeth Costello*, the titular main character is a renowned writer who is invited to speak at a variety of universities, conferences, and events as a guest lecturer. Using the opportunity to espouse her views on animal rights and factory farming, Costello echoes her creator's own speech when she calls meat production a "crime of stupefying proportions."

A quintessential academic, Costello has spent her life questioning, theorizing, and fashioning opinions from the world around her. But now— older and somewhat weary—her ideas threaten her relations and reputation. Instead of giving a lecture on writing, she decides to talk about the mistreatment of animals and her aversion to it. Two of her lectures, one called "The Philosophers and the Animals" and the other "The Poets and the Animals," make up the longest section of the book and create the most discomfort in her audience of intellectuals.

Conversations at post-lecture dinners gravitate toward the topics of animal rights, making her son—a professor at one of the colleges she speaks at—embarrassed and uneasy, especially when he anticipates someone asking, "What made you become vegetarian, Ms. Costello?"

His mother has [the response] by heart; he can reproduce it only imperfectly. "You ask me why I refuse to eat flesh. I, for my part, am astonished that you can put in your mouth the corpse of a dead animal, astonished that you do not find it nasty to chew hacked flesh and swallow the juices of death wounds."

Offending those around her when she makes comparisons between factory farming and the Holocaust, Costello echoes Coetzee's own words from the same speech he gave in 2007:

Of course we cried out in horror when we found out what they had been up to. We cried: What a terrible crime, to treat human beings like cattle! If we had only known beforehand! But our cry should more accurately have been: What a terrible crime, to treat human beings like units in an industrial process! And that cry should have had a postscript: What a terrible crime, come to think of it—a crime against nature—to treat any living being like a unit in an industrial process!"

VEGAN PEACE

When I was a kid I ate whatever my parents put in front of me and rarely questioned it. As I got older and began to question things, I remember one night when we had hamburgers for dinner, my sister teased me by mooing and reminded me I was eating a dead cow. I continued to eat it, though.

I met Matt (now my husband) a few years after living on my own. He was picky about meat and not a fan of pork or beef and really only ate hamburgers when we ate out. The majority of what we cooked and ate at home was precooked chicken.

My desire to go vegetarian was getting stronger, but being introverted, I held back. I was too worried about what people would say. I did not want to inconvenience them and knew eating out would be an issue.

This did not last too long, however, and one day I just decided to go for it. About six months after

I had gone vegetarian and about two weeks before our wedding, my husband told me he was going to go vegetarian as well.

Although going vegetarian was a choice I was proud of and made me feel I was doing some good, I always had a persistent nag in the back of my mind regarding veganism.

This nag eventually broke down my resistance and I started doing research and reading everything I could on veganism and animal rights. I realized that the dairy and egg industries were no better and probably worse than the meat industry. I stumbled upon the *Vegetarian Food for Thought* podcast, which pushed me off the fence I'd been sitting on for so long. It is bar none the best decision I've ever made!

—*Crys in St. Louis, Missouri (U.S.)*

MANGO PAPAYA PUNCH

A refreshing hot-weather beverage, this punch provides oodles more nutrition than any store-bought juice.

- 1 cup (175 g) frozen mango chunks
- 1 cup (140 g) frozen papaya chunks
- 1 cup (235 ml) fresh orange juice
- ¼ cup (60 ml) lime juice (1 medium-size lime)
- 3 to 4 cups (705 to 940 ml) cold water, or to desired thickness
- 1 teaspoon (2 g) grated orange zest
- Crushed ice, for serving
- Fresh mint leaves, for garnish

Place the mango and papaya in a blender. Cover, and puree until smooth. Add the orange juice, lime juice, water, and orange zest. Blend well, and taste. Serve over crushed ice and with fresh mint leaves in pretty glasses.

Yield: 8 servings

*Soy-free, wheat-free, oil-free

Originally published in *Color Me Vegan*

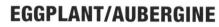
EGGPLANT/AUBERGINE

Although the origins of the eggplant seem to be rooted in India, the first surviving mention of this vegetable (well, botanically, it's a fruit) is in a fifth-century Chinese book about agriculture, called the *Ts'i Min Yao Shu.*

Having bounced all around the world, what is called eggplant in North America and aubergine in Europe is different from what is called eggplant in Asia. In Western countries, it is large and purple and often called the Italian or globe eggplant. In Asia, there is a wide variety: some are pale green, some are white, some are lavender; some are long, some are spherical, and some are egg-shaped.

Always popular in cuisine in Asia and the Near East, eggplants were dismissed as inedible by Europeans for a long time. Only during the fifteenth century did it gradually gain popularity. The Spanish and Portuguese colonists took it to America, where it is a beloved vegetable.

Most of us have been taught to salt (Italian/ globe) eggplants to remove their bitterness, but this is not really necessary if you buy fresh eggplants in season. If you do salt your eggplant, simply slice it into disks, cover them with salt, and let sit for at least an hour. When ready to use, simply rinse off the salt and proceed with your recipe or cooking method.

I have found that so many recipes call for vats of oil when cooking eggplant, because it famously soaks up so much oil when cooking. There's a great legend behind the Turkish dish called *imam bayildi,* which means "the imam (priest) fainted." This dish consists of aubergines stuffed with onions and cooked with olive oil. There are several tales about how the dish got its name. One is that the imam fainted because of how tasty it was; another is that his wife fainted because of how expensive the ingredients were; and the other is that the priest fainted because of how much oil was in it!

Finding truth in that last tale, I do what I can to reduce the oil in my eggplant recipes, and I have found that steaming the eggplant makes a huge difference. It makes it tender and juicy without all the added oil.

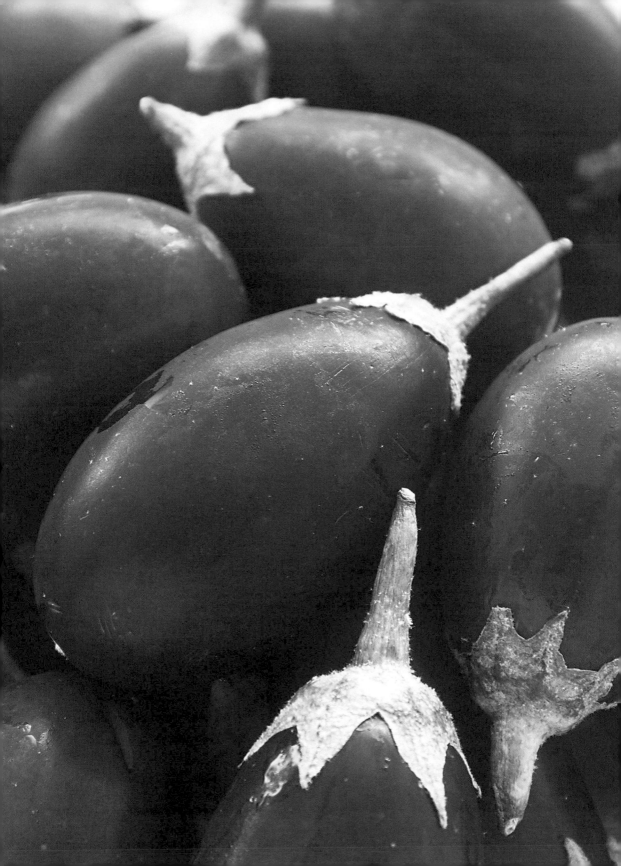

COMPASSIONATE ALTERNATIVE: **KILL THE FATTED CALF**

The fatted calf is the symbol of an exuberant celebration upon someone's long-awaited return. It is derived from the parable of the prodigal son in the New Testament; in biblical times, people would often reserve one of their animals and feed him a special diet to fatten him up. Slaughtering this animal was to be done on rare and special occasions, such as when the prodigal son returns.

With enthusiasm upon the arrival of a special guest, you could say:

* Break out the best china!

* Pour the best wine!

* Strike up the tunes!

* Prepare an elaborate feast!

* Bring forth the cornucopia!

You get the idea. The point is to celebrate without harming anyone—in our language or behavior.

LIMITING PROCESSED FOODS

The most healthful diet we can eat is one based on whole foods—foods that are as close to their natural state as possible. That doesn't mean you should feel guilty for eating something "processed"; it means when you make the foundation of your diet whole foods, you have a little wiggle room for some less-than-perfect foods.

The truth is, however, the more whole foods you eat, the more whole foods you crave. When you eat a diet based on whole foods, you stop craving the richness of many packaged, processed foods, which tend to be laden with salt and fat.

But it's also important to keep in mind that within the category of "processed foods," there is a huge spectrum. Canned beans, frozen vegetables, and dried fruit, for example, have gone through minimal processing, but they're perfectly acceptable alternatives to "fresh," which isn't always available.

Even when it comes to more highly processed foods, such as vegetarian meats, there is a spectrum. Some are made with whole ingredients; some are made with highly processed ingredients. Take a look at the ingredients list to determine this.

Although we have yet to discover what negative effects—if any—such highly processed foods will have on our health (never has a society consumed such a high amount of processed foods—vegan or not), each time we eat something processed, we're displacing a healthful whole food, and the latter should be our goal each time we eat.

EYES WITHOUT A FACE/LES YEUX SANS VISAGE
DIRECTED BY GEORGES FRANJU

In this 1960 film by French director Georges Franju, a surgeon obsessed with restoring his daughter's face, which was mutilated in a car accident, kidnaps young women and makes them victims of his hideous experiments, much like the tortured animals he keeps in his basement. With the help of his affectless assistant Louise, Doctor Génessier lures women to his countryside estate, where he removes their face and grafts it onto Christiane's. He then disposes of their body and continues this cycle until the transplant works. One can only imagine the torment he has inflicted upon his imprisoned dogs and birds in preparation for his human experiments.

And imagination is exactly what Franju inspires. Although there is one graphic scene in particular that upset 1960 audiences and critics and is still disturbing today, the film depicts the gruesomeness with subtlety and—quite frankly—beauty.

To the credit of Franju and his talented team of screenwriters, this monster is very human, motivated by guilt and love, which makes his actions all the more disturbing. However, even the doctor's daughter is plagued with remorse over the lengths to which her father goes and the depths to which he sinks in order to recover her once-beautiful face. Spending most of the time in a mask that renders her face emotionless, Christiane is sympathetic to the fellow victims of her father's "science."

In one particularly beautiful scene, a silent Christiane visits the dogs her father confines in cages in his underground laboratory. She approaches each one and tenderly embraces them, momentarily subduing their cries with her affection. Resigned to disfigurement and unwilling to allow her father to hurt any more women, a steadfast Christiane frees not only a woman who was to be her father's next victim but also the dogs and doves her father experimented on.

In the harrowing final scene, knowing exactly who their tormentor is, the dogs exact their own justice, and Christiane, herself now free (albeit emotionally as well as physically scarred), walks slowly into the woods with one of the freed doves alighted on her hand.

This rare film can finally be seen in its original splendor, having been lovingly restored and released by the Criterion Collection. The DVD also includes Franju's 1949 documentary short *Blood of the Beasts (Le sang des bêtes)*, depicting Paris slaughterhouses, primarily those that killed horses. Intercutting footage of animal slaughter with shots of children at play, it is an incredibly disturbing peek into real-life, everyday horror.

KIKI JACKSON: FROM STARVATION TO SANCTUARY

In the spring of 1999, Dr. Sheri Speede discovered Kiki Jackson and a female companion in a small concrete cell at a hotel in the coastal town of Kribi, Cameroon. Both chimpanzees were adults and estimated to be about fifteen years old at that time. Kiki and his companion were being fed regularly, and despite their dismal living conditions, they were in better health than two other adults who needed to be rescued. Dr. Speede made a promise to rescue Kiki and his companion as soon as possible.

The next opportunity to visit Kiki came in November 1999, when Dr. Speede sent a volunteer to check on the two chimpanzees. What she discovered was devastating. The person who had been paid to feed the chimpanzees left Kribi in September and no replacement had been hired. Kiki's companion starved to death.

Kiki, himself horribly emaciated and barely alive, had refused to let anyone remove her body from the filthy concrete cage for days. From that day in November 1999, we took charge of Kiki's care until he could be brought to the Rescue Center.

By June 21, 2000, when Kiki was finally brought to the sanctuary, he had gained 40 pounds (18.1 kg).

His sweet, gentle disposition makes him a wonderful leader of his adoptive family. Kiki lives with adult male Chouki, who is blind, and six juveniles. Kiki and Chouki are loyal and devoted best friends and together they take good care of the younger chimpanzees. Their forested enclosure is equipped with special accommodations to help Chouki navigate.

—Dr. Sheri Speede, founder of Sanaga-Yong Chimpanzee Rescue Center, Cameroon, Africa

Kiki Jackson at Sanaga-Yong
Photo courtesy of Sanaga-Yong Chimpanzee Rescue Center

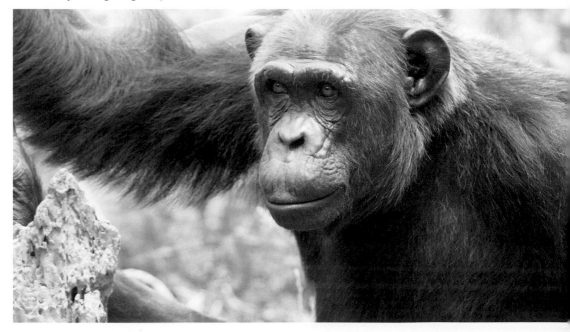

SAFFRON RICE WITH CURRIED APRICOT DRESSING

This recipe, adapted from San Francisco's Millennium Restaurant's cookbook, has been in my repertoire for years. Personalize it by adding your favorite root vegetables, such as carrots, sweet potatoes, turnips, and rutabagas.

- 1 tablespoon (15 ml) water or vegetable stock, for sautéing
- 1 medium-size yellow onion, finely diced
- 2 cloves garlic, minced
- 1 teaspoon (2.5 g) ground cumin
- 1 teaspoon (2 g) fennel seeds
- ¼ teaspoon freshly ground pepper
- ½ teaspoon salt, or to taste
- 2 cups (380 g) uncooked brown basmati rice
- ½ teaspoon saffron steeped in ¼ cup (60 ml) warm water
- 3½ cups (823 ml) water or vegetable stock
- 2 cups (220 g) cubed garnet or jewel yams, steamed and cooled
- 1 tart apple, diced and tossed with lemon juice
- 3 scallions, thinly sliced
- ½ cup (68 g) toasted pine nuts

CURRIED APRICOT DRESSING
- ¼ cup (75 g) apricot preserves
- ⅓ cup (80 ml) rice vinegar
- 1 tablespoon (6 g) curry powder
- ¼ teaspoon ground cardamom
- ¼ teaspoon cayenne pepper
- ⅓ cup (80 ml) water
- ¼ cup (60 ml) oil
- Salt
- 2 tablespoons (12 g) finely shredded mint leaves, for garnish

In a medium-size saucepan, heat the water or stock over medium heat and sauté the onion and garlic until just softened, about 5 minutes. Add the cumin, fennel seeds, pepper, and salt. Sauté for 1 minute. Add the rice and stir constantly for 2 minutes, or until the rice smells fragrant. Add the saffron in the water as well as the 3½ cups (823 ml) water, bring to boil, and cover. Reduce the heat to low and simmer for 40 to 45 minutes, or until the liquid is absorbed. Remove from the heat and transfer to a large bowl.

To the bowl, add the yams, apple, scallions, and pine nuts. Set aside.

To make the dressing, combine all the ingredients in a blender or food processor and blend until emulsified. Taste and adjust the seasonings. Combine most of the dressing with the rice/veggie mixture, and mix thoroughly. Taste, and add the rest of the dressing, if desired, or reserve for another use. Arrange on a serving platter. Garnish with the mint.

Yield: 6 to 8 servings

*Wheat-free, soy-free

Originally published in *Color Me Vegan*

SUSHI

Despite misconceptions to the contrary, sushi does not mean "fish." The word *sushi* comes from an archaic grammatical form that is obsolete in other contexts; technically, the word *sushi* means "sour," which reflects its early fermented roots.

A proper definition of sushi can be found in your standard dictionary: "cold rice dressed with vinegar, formed into any of various shapes." Though raw seafood is definitely a traditional topping, so are vegetables. The point is that sushi has more to do with the rice, its shape, and that something is placed on top of it (or rolled with it) than with fish, per se.

The different rice forms—not fish—distinguish one type of sushi from another.

* Nigiri sushi is an oblong, bite-size rice brick topped with wasabi and a vegetable.

* Maki rolls include rice and chopped ingredients wrapped as a log in a sheet of dried seaweed, then cut into bite-size circular pieces.

* Temaki sushi is comprised of rice and multiple other ingredients held in a large crispy cone of dried seaweed.

* Inari is sushi made with toppings stuffed into a small pouch of fried tofu.

* Chirashi-zushi, or scattered sushi, is made with toppings served scattered over a bowl of sushi rice.

Once you realize that sushi has everything to do with the shape of the rice and not fish, your imagination and creative juices can run wild preparing various vegetables for your sushi.

Various condiments make up the sushi-eating experience, including:

* Soy sauce is often used to dilute the wasabi.

* Wasabi is the grated root of the wasabi plant. Although its heat resembles that of the European horseradish rhizome, it is a different plant altogether. A little goes a long way, so if you're sensitive to spicy flavors, go easy on the wasabi.

* Sweet pickled ginger (*gari*) is eaten both to cleanse the palette and to aid in the digestive process.

When making sushi at home, you'll need a few utensils unique to this special cuisine.

* Special Japanese knives (*hocho*) are used by the pros, but you can get away with a good, sharp chef's knife.

* Bamboo rolling mats are essential for making maki rolls and can be found in any large kitchen supply store.

* Hopefully you already have a pair of chopsticks, but if you want to really impress your friends, you can buy a pair of cooking chopsticks, called *ryoribashi*.

* Although a flat spatula will enable you to get the job done, a wooden rice paddle (*shamoji*) really does make it easier—and more authentic.

Distinct from sushi, sashimi consists of raw seafood and a dipping sauce and other condiments. The word itself means "pierced body," and it's *not* sushi because it doesn't contain any rice—only a piece of the "pierced body" of a fish.

HOW DO YOU RESPOND TO, "IF EVERYONE STOPPED EATING THEM, FARM ANIMALS WOULD TAKE OVER"?

Although it's an intriguing thought, a farmed animal is not freed whenever someone becomes vegan. The effect is not that direct.

However, as demand goes down, so will supply.

More and more people are *going vegan*, but it is not happening at a rate that will cause cattle to create traffic jams or chickens to replace squirrels in people's yards. It is simply not rational to think that the entire world will go vegan all at once.

Each year, billions of animals are bred all around the globe just to be killed. Because they're not allowed to reproduce naturally, they're bred artificially for the sole purpose of making a profit off of their body.

The more we stop eating them, the fewer animals we'll produce.

Having said that, I don't believe that people walk around genuinely concerned that the world will be overrun with farmed animals as we stop eating them. It's a red herring that distracts people from the real issue.

"Are you serious?" is certainly an appropriate response to this statement (see Day 114), but so is simply stating the fact that when we stop breeding them, there will be fewer animals to begin with.

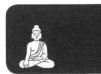

UNDERSTANDING PALM OIL

As the anti-trans-fat movement emerged (see Day 318), alternative shelf-stable fats took their place—namely oils from the palm tree. Different from coconut palm oil, palm oil is semisolid at room temperature, making it an alternative to unhealthful, unnatural partially hydrogenated oil.

Widely used as a cooking oil in West African countries for centuries, palm oil has become a hot commodity over the years. Late in the nineteenth century, it was exported by the British for use as a lubricant when the industrial revolution surged. It was also used as an ingredient in soap, including in the well-known brand Palmolive—which contained both palm and olive oils, hence the name.

There is much concern over the harvesting of palm oil in that it has been linked to deforestation and habitat destruction where endangered animals already face a tenuous future. The best solution is to choose whole foods as much as possible; the second solution is to make inquiries to the companies who use palm oil to find out where they source it from. Some—certainly not all—companies have committed to buying palm oil only from locales and companies that harvest it humanely, without violating human rights or animal habitat.

Although palm oil is healthier than partially hydrogenated oil, it is still present in foods considered processed, so keep that in mind when making food choices: The more whole, the better.

THE FANTASTIC PLANET
DIRECTED BY RENÉ LALOUX

La Planète Sauvage is a 1973 French science fiction animated film whose literal translation is *The Savage Planet*. Based on a 1957 novel called *Oms en série (Oms by the Dozen)* by Stefan Wul, the film, directed by René Laloux, takes place in the far future on a distant planet called Ygam, where a race of giants (Draags) breeds and domesticates what are essentially human beings (called Oms) and keeps them as pets, as playthings, and as beasts of burden.

Several times larger than the puny Oms, the Draags—blue in appearance with bulbous red eyes—treat their playthings with cold impunity, despite their technological sophistication and supposed spiritual advancement. (Sound familiar?)

The domesticated Oms, a play on the French word *homes*, meaning "men," are forced to wear collars; the "wild Oms" are allowed to range free in nature, though they are exterminated every so often to control their population. Some of these wild Oms create a plan to thwart this de-Oming; they partner with the domestic Oms, adventure ensues, and the Draags and Oms eventually learn to live in peace.

Winning the Grand Prix Award at the Cannes Film Festival in 1973, this short allegorical seventy-two-minute film can be viewed through any lens that reflects the exploitation of one group over another, whether these groups are human or not. Recalling Swift's *Gulliver's Travels,* the theme and tone of *Fantastic Planet* unabashedly reflect the hypocrisy of humans' treatment of nonhuman animals—whether it's our consumption, breeding, domestication, or extermination of them.

LOVE TRIANGLE

That Hannah the sheep is in love with Rambo the sheep is no secret at Catskill Animal Sanctuary. Indeed, it's most obvious as Hannah bolts from her stall each morning in search of her Romeo. If she finds him immediately, all is well. But if Rambo is out of sight, she is initially disturbed, then worried, finally panic-stricken and uttering a heart-wrenching, baleful "baa-aah" as the time it takes to find her soul mate increases. Once she locates him, all is again right in her world. It is a relationship that she needs desperately, and one that Rambo tolerates.

Trouble is, Barbie loves Rambo, too.

Barbie is a "broiler," the term used by the poultry industry to describe chickens intended for meat. She's one of hundreds who've arrived over the years, lucky escapees from live poultry markets, slaughterhouses, transport trucks, and the ritual sacrifices of Santeria. Bred to grow huge quickly, "broilers" who are lucky enough to escape slaughter and find sanctuary often die of violent heart attacks in a year or two; their weight is literally too much for their bodies to bear.

This one, our little Barbie, was found in Brooklyn, hiding under a blue Honda.

Like many of our animals, Barbie free ranges during the day. She's still young, so before activity simply becomes too painful, the exercise is good for a body that will quickly grow morbidly obese. So, Barbie snuggles into her home in the main barn each night, but each morning she and her hen friends come out to explore the barnyard and cozy up to whomever she chooses.

Unfortunately, Barbie has chosen Rambo. For several weeks, Barbie napped right next to Rambo, sometimes so close that surely even through his wool Rambo felt the heat emanating from her big bird body. For a while, Hannah tolerated the new friendship. After all, Barbie was merely *a chicken*.

But when Barbie decided that Rambo was a wonderful sofa, it was just too much for Hannah. No longer fully mobile, Barbie nonetheless managed to climb atop Rambo's back, the saintly sheep motionless. After taking a moment to decide whether to face the back of his head or his rear, Barbie settled into wooly bliss and fell asleep. Time after time, Rambo took her overtures in good stride.

The first time I saw this, I ran to grab my camera. And then I heard it: the rapid click-click-click of sheep hooves moving toward us. It was Hannah. *She had spotted them.*

The ball of brown wool pushed past me as if I weren't there and strode within 6 inches (15 cm) of the offending pair, neither of whom budged. She glared at them, then she looked at me. She looked back at them, then she looked at me. There was no need for words here, as *"Are you going to help me here, or what?"* was etched into every gesture.

"I'm sorry, Hannah," I whispered, approaching her with consoling words. But Hannah pooped and marched outside, wanting nothing more of Rambo, the interloper, or me.

—*Kathy Stevens, founder of Catskill Animal Sanctuary, Saugerties, New York (U.S.)*

Barbie and her boyfriend, Rambo, at Catskill Animal Sanctuary

Photo courtesy of Catskill Animal Sanctuary

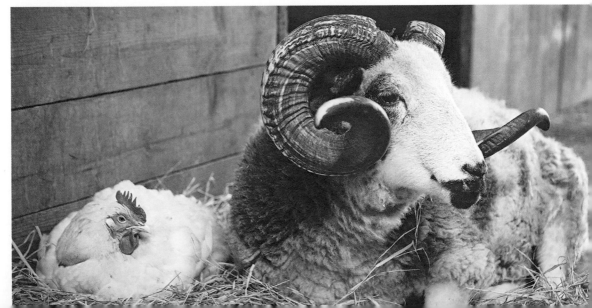

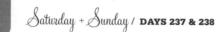

CITRUS COLLARD GREENS WITH RAISINS

I'm grateful to friend and colleague Bryant Terry for allowing me to reprint this recipe from his fantastic cookbook, *Vegan Soul Kitchen*.

- **1 tablespoon (18 g) and ½ teaspoon (3 g) coarse sea salt**
- **2 large bunches collard greens, ribs removed, cut into a chiffonade, rinsed, and drained**
- **1 tablespoon (15 ml) olive oil**
- **2 cloves garlic, minced**
- **⅔ cup (96 g) raisins**
- **⅓ cup (80 ml) fresh squeezed orange juice**

In a large pot over high heat, bring 3 quarts (2.7 L) of water to a boil and add 1 tablespoon (18 g) of the salt. Add the collards and cook, uncovered, for 8 to 10 minutes, until softened. Meanwhile, prepare a large bowl of ice water to cool the collards.

Remove the collards from the heat, drain, and plunge them into the bowl of cold water to stop the cooking and set the color of the greens. Drain by gently pressing the greens against a colander.

In a medium-size sauté pan, combine the olive oil and garlic over medium heat. Sauté for 1 minute. Add the collards, raisins, and remaining ½ teaspoon (3 g) salt. Sauté for 3 minutes, stirring frequently.

Add the orange juice and cook for an additional 15 seconds. Do not overcook (collards should be a bright green). Season with additional salt if needed and serve immediately. (This also makes a tasty filling for quesadillas.)

Yield: 6 servings

*Soy-free, wheat-free

MAITAKE MUSHROOMS

According to lore, maitake are named *such* ("dancing mushrooms" in Japanese) because foragers danced with glee whenever they discovered them.

They are also called hen of the woods, and they're prized for their earthy flavor and firm texture. They can be used in any dish that calls for mushrooms, though they're best in dishes that take a longer time to cook. If you're using them for a quick-cooking dish, simply braise them for 30 minutes in a low-simmering broth.

* Add maitake mushrooms to a soup. Bring 2 cups (470 ml) vegetable or mushroom broth to a low simmer. Add 3 or 4 cleaned, stemmed, and sliced maitake, sliced scallions, a dash of tamari soy sauce, and hot sauce.

* Chop 1 pound (0.45 g) cleaned and stemmed maitake in a food processor. Sauté over medium heat for about 5 minutes. Add 2 cloves chopped garlic, 2 tablespoons (30 ml) olive oil, and salt and pepper to taste. Sprinkle with parsley, and add to pasta or toss with sautéed greens.

* Grill maitake mushrooms, and use as a topping for pizza or bruschetta.

HOW DO YOU RESPOND TO, "YOUR BEING VEGAN DOESN'T MAKE A DIFFERENCE"?

Being vegan does make a difference—it makes a huge difference to the animals you're not eating! Hundreds of animals—probably thousands, if we include all the sea creatures—that one person would otherwise eat in his or her lifetime are spared by one person being vegan.

The potential number of people inspired by you living your truth and your values is vast. More people inspired means fewer animals eaten, and so on. For someone to criticize you for being part of the solution says more about that person than it does about being vegan. The first question I have for them is: "What are *you* doing?" Why is it that the people who seem to have the most to say aren't doing anything at all?

If someone were to say that to me, in the spirit of effective advocacy and gentle truth, I'd look at her sympathetically and confidently and say that I'm doing the best I can, that I am part of the solution, and that to the animals, it makes all the difference in the world.

There are a few ways to understand people who make a statement like this:

* They may not want to believe that making behavioral changes has an impact; if they did, then they would be compelled to change their own behavior.

* They may think that *your* positive actions reflect badly on *their own* negative actions. Rather than examine or change their behavior, they tell you yours is inconsequential.

* They may be insecure and figure if they bring you down to their level, they'll feel better about themselves.

* They may suffer from cynicism, and—next to cruelty and arrogance—there's nothing less pleasant.

* Or they're just plain insensitive.

Whatever motivates such a pessimistic outlook, be confident that your committed compassion is indeed having an impact.

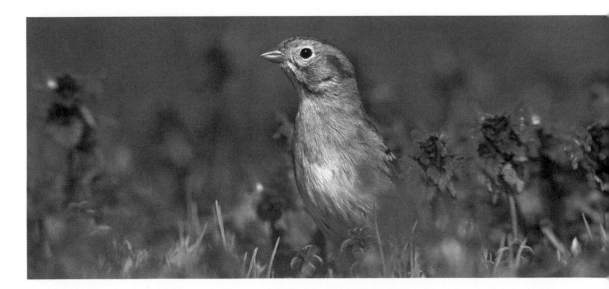

COMPOSTING

Composting reduces waste, returns vegetable scraps to the cycle of nature, and enables gardeners to use the best nutrients to enrich our flower beds, fruit trees, and vegetable gardens.

Organic plant matter is the best thing for your garden—the cheapest and the most nutrient-dense, providing your soil with a strong foundation for your plants to grow and thrive.

One way to compost is to gather garden and yard waste (leaves, acorns, etc.) and create a pile of them in one corner of your yard. Combine it with some soil and stir it every so often to aerate it so the waste breaks down and generates nutrients.

Another way to compost is to save all those fruit and veggie scraps that we vegans have a lot of (or should have a lot of!), assuming everyone is eating their fruits and veggies. It takes a while to create a system in your home so you don't attract fruit flies or any other uninvited critters, but once you figure it out; it's a breeze.

You can keep a large bowl on your counter and cover it with a large lid, or buy a compost scrap bin for the kitchen from a kitchen, garden, or online "eco store." Dump it every day; otherwise, it will smell up the house.

You can purchase compost bins at garden stores (or online "eco stores"), but I recommend first checking with your city's waste management department. Many cities provide compost bins at a low cost.

Having said that, after many years and many different kinds of bins, we've settled on the round varieties, which resemble large drums lying on their side and sitting on a runner that we spin every few days to get the oxygen flowing. They're the easiest to work with and the most efficient in terms of turning the scraps into actual compost.

FILMS THAT DEPICT THE "ANIMAL-LOVING" CRIMINAL

The depiction of the "sensitive criminal" is seen in many films in order to effectively humanize a character who might otherwise be violent or immoral. While the quiet hit man in Luc Besson's 1994 film *Léon* (*The Professional* outside of France) showed his soft side by tenderly caring for a houseplant, and then a little girl, more often the companion is an animal.

Both Elia Kazan's 1954 *On the Waterfront* and Jim Jarmusch's 1999 *Ghost Dog: Way of the Samurai* feature loner protagonists who find solace only in the homing pigeons they raise, certainly a metaphor for their own trapped existence. The tenderness with which they care for their birds says a lot about the size of their heart—and their enemies know this, too. In each film, the main character's opponents kill his birds in order to hurt him where he feels it the most.

Terry Malloy, Marlon Brando's character in *On the Waterfront*, affectionately tends to his pigeons and instructs his young protégé to be careful about spilling any water when he cleans their coops: "I don't want them to catch cold," he says. Terry, impressed by their behavior and habits, tells Edie Doyle, a beautiful girl he's wooing, that pigeons are very faithful, that they "get married" and stay together until one of them dies. We also learn from Edie's father that *she* is a protector of animals, too, when he gruffly but lovingly complains that his daughter brings in every stray animal she sees—and always the ones who have six toes and are "cockeyed."

Forest Whitaker's Ghost Dog (he's given no other name in the film) is equally attentive to his birds. A mysterious, quiet (almost totally silent) hit man, he follows the ancient code of the samurai, as outlined in *The Book of the Samurai*, which he carries with him wherever he goes. His connection to animals extends beyond his concern for his pigeons. Twice a dog appears in the film, each time staring directly at Ghost Dog; when a sparrow lands on his sniper rifle, he takes a moment to admire him before returning to his work; and when he encounters two hunters who have brutally killed a black bear, he exacts justice.

Many other films use this same trope:

* John Frankenheimer's *Birdman of Alcatraz* dramatizes the true story of convict Robert Stroud (played by Burt Lancaster), who finds redemption through his relationship with birds.

* In the 1942 noir, *This Gun for Hire*, Alan Ladd is hit man Philip Raven, who is kind to animals—and children.

* Jef Costello (played by Alain Delon), the main character in Jean-Pierre Melville's 1967 film *Le Samourai*, is detached in every way, except for the affection he shows for his little canary, caged though he is.

Having hardened their hearts in order to live a life of corruption and murder, these men need animals to represent the innocence they can still return to, the redemption that is still possible for them, and the love they can still feel.

WHAT WINGS ARE FOR

Ruby was a Buff Orpington hen whom we'd had since she was a chick. She lived among our main flock with her hen friends and a rooster. When Ruby was three years old, she molted her feathers early and seemed a little slower than usual, so we placed her in one of our "special needs" areas for a few days.

The next day I drove past an industrial chicken shed, and when I looked closer, I saw two small chickens, abandoned among the manure.

I brought the two chickens out of the shed and into a carrier in the car. It was a nice, sunny day, so when I arrived home, I put the carrier in the backyard and opened the door. Being used to "broiler" chickens being slow and handicapped, I was surprised when one chick came out right away and headed for the woods, straight into the poison ivy. It wasn't easy for me to catch her.

We named her Poison Ivy and the other one Oak. Unfortunately, when Oak stood still, her right leg stuck out at a 45-degree angle, with her foot in the air. She had sores from scrambling around to survive inside the shed. She spent two days with us before being euthanized. Every movement seemed to cause her pain. Releasing her from this world seemed the kindest thing we could do for her.

Leaving Ivy alone made for more sadness, so we moved her in with Ruby and watched them closely. Seeing that they shared food and water and seemed fine with each other, we hoped they'd become friends and keep each other company.

A day or two later when we went to check on them, we discovered Ruby sheltering Ivy under her wing.

Ruby and Ivy soon moved in with the small, ever-changing flock of rescued industrial chickens, and continued on as mother and chick. Sometimes the two of them would spend the day in the flower garden, digging in the grass and dirt. As Ivy grew bigger, she would still try to tuck herself under Ruby's wing, even though she was soon larger than Ruby. Eventually, only her head could fit under Ruby's wing. Even so, they both appeared very happy resting together like this.

Ivy died of heart failure within a year, but she and Ruby remained friends her whole life, even after Ruby stopped mothering her.

—*Kay Evans and Jim Robertson for United Poultry Concerns, Machipongo, Virginia (U.S.)*

Ruby sheltering Ivy under her wing
Photo courtesy of United Poultry Concerns

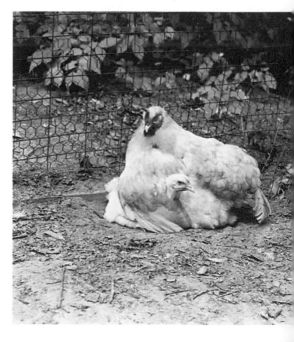

STUFFED ARTICHOKES

Too many people are intimidated by this gorgeous, folate-rich vegetable (actually a flower bud). The truth is, once you learn the ins and outs (literally!) of working with an artichoke, it becomes second nature.

4 large artichokes
3 tablespoons (45 ml) oil, divided
1 yellow onion, chopped
4 cloves garlic, minced
1 cup (58 g) bread crumbs
½ cup (60 g) walnuts, toasted and finely chopped
4 tomatoes, seeded and diced
1 teaspoon (6 g) salt
Freshly ground pepper
3 tablespoons (12 g) minced fresh herbs (parsley, basil, oregano, thyme)
1 teaspoon (5 ml) lemon juice
Melted nondairy butter or eggless aioli (such as Wildwood's Garlic Aioli), for serving

With a sharp knife, cut the stems off the artichokes so they sit flush. With scissors, cut the pointy tips off the outer artichoke leaves. In a large pot with a steamer basket, steam the whole artichokes for 25 to 45 minutes, or until the leaves pull easily away and are tender at the base. The cooking time varies according to the size of your artichokes, type of steamer you use, amount of water, etc.

Meanwhile, in a large sauté pan, heat 1 tablespoon (15 ml) of the oil, and sauté the onion and garlic over medium heat for about 5 minutes, until the onion is soft and translucent.

Add more oil as necessary along with the bread crumbs and walnuts. Combine thoroughly with the onion and garlic mixture.

Add the tomatoes and salt, stirring them into the mixture, and season with pepper to taste. Stir in the fresh herbs and the lemon juice, adjust the seasonings, and remove from the heat.

When the artichokes are done and cool enough to handle, pry open the tops with your fingers and expose the cavity into which you will spoon the mixture, divided evenly among the artichokes. Don't worry about the fact that the stuffing will touch the choke. Once you get to the bottom and finish the stuffing, you'll be able to differentiate between the stuffing and the choke, eating the former and removing the latter to get to the heart.

Because you will be waiting for the artichokes to cool before adding the stuffing, these will be at room temperature by the time you serve them. If you make everything ahead of time (or are eating leftovers), just pop the stuffed artichokes into a microwave, preheated oven, or steamer basket for a few minutes to serve warm or hot.

For information on how to eat an artichoke, see Day 148.

Yield: 4 servings

*Soy-free, wheat-free if using wheat-free bread crumbs

Originally published in *Color Me Vegan*

CORNMEAL

Corn is a cereal grain that is cultivated through-out the world. Because genetically modified varieties now make up a significant proportion of the total harvest, choose organic.

* Cornmeal is dried corn kernels ground to a fine, medium, or coarse texture. (Sometimes corn-meal is called "polenta" in the grocery store.)

* Corn flour is finely ground cornmeal.

* Cornstarch (also called corn flour) is quite literally the starch of the corn grain, used as a thickener for sauces and gravies.

* Polenta, a staple of northern Italy, is a mush made from cornmeal.

* Hominy is dried white or yellow corn kernels from which the hull and germ have been removed.

* Grits is a common dish in the southern United States. Similar to polenta, grits are usually made from coarsely ground hominy as op-posed to cornmeal.

Typically in the United States, cornmeal is steel-ground, which means the husk and germ of the corn kernels have been completely removed. Less nutritious, it can be stored in an airtight container in a cool, dry place almost indefinitely.

Stone-ground cornmeal retains some of the hull and germ, providing more flavor and more nutri-tion. More perishable than steel-ground, it will keep longer if stored in the refrigerator.

Steel- and stone-ground cornmeal can be used interchangeably.

* Some popular cornmeal dishes include grits, cornbread, spoonbread, johnnycakes, and hushpuppies.

* Use cornmeal when making pizza to coat the pizza stone so the dough slides easily on and off.

* Cornmeal makes a wonderful crust for tofu and mushrooms.

* Add some cornmeal to your favorite pancake batter.

* Make polenta, a staple in Italy, using white or yellow cornmeal. In ancient Rome, chestnut meal or farro (a barleylike grain) was used in-stead, but today ground cornmeal is common.

You can find cornmeal in the bulk section of most grocery stores or in boxes where the flours and sugars are shelved.

HOW DO YOU RESPOND TO, "AREN'T ANIMALS KILLED WHEN FARMERS CLEAR LAND FOR CROPS?"

The bottom line: A lot of animals are killed each year by humans to satisfy our appetites:

* About 10 billion land animals, and about 45 billion animals total including aquatic animals, are killed per year in the United States.

* Around 5 million wild animals are killed by the U.S. government (with taxpayer dollars) per year on behalf of private ranchers.

* Add to that the number of birds and fish who die because of the pollution of the ecosystems from the tons of manure and urine produced by "livestock," and these numbers are even higher.

These animals are killed directly and indirectly just to satisfy our habitual appetite for animal flesh and secretions. By ceasing to eat them, we reduce the number of animals killed.

The person who accuses vegetarians of being responsible for the death of unintentionally killed animals during plant production is grasping at straws. (Truth be told, we contribute to even higher numbers of these animals killed when we eat meat, because you have to grow plants to feed the animals.)

We don't live in a perfect world, and we cannot claim to be perfect people, but being vegan isn't about striving for perfection.

Our intention is to do the best we can to not intentionally harm any other living being. Being vegan is one way to do that. Hence, my motto: "Don't do nothing because you can't do everything. Do something. Anything."

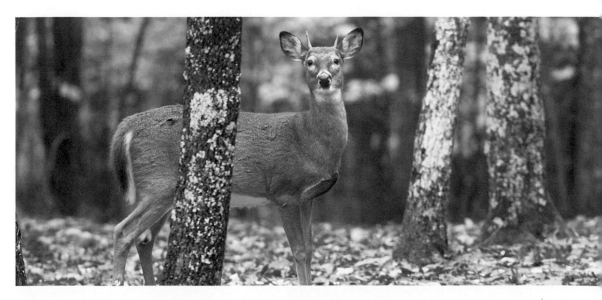

KNOWING YOUR LIMITATIONS

I believe that bearing witness to animal atrocities is essential to staying connected to the truth, but the trick is finding the balance so you become empowered rather than despondent.

Bearing witness to the inherent cruelty inflicted upon the innocent victims of our appetites can be very painful, and I encourage people to know themselves well enough to know how much they can handle. The idea is to be an effective advocate who can speak to the truth—not endure self-inflicted abuse for its own sake. The effect of bearing witness can be traumatic, but that's not always a bad thing.

Many years ago, I used to do a lot of "Street TV," where I would bring a portable TV/DVD player to a public street, play videos of animal exploitation, and hand out "Why Vegan?" pamphlets and *Vegetarian Food for Thought* podcast sampler CDs.

One day, I asked a good friend of mine, who was vegan, if she wanted to join me in setting up the TV and distributing information. An hour before I was to leave to pick her up, she called to say that she was going to cancel but wanted to tell me why.

She said she thought that the images themselves produced trauma in people—in passersby, in children, in anyone who saw those images—and that she didn't feel comfortable being part of creating trauma. After she had thought about it, she had had a revelation: Several years before, those very same images of animal abuse were indeed very traumatic for her and it was that trauma that awakened her and led her to become vegan in order to reduce animal suffering.

I thought that was a really wise perspective. Of course this stuff is traumatic, and it's what many of us need to knock ourselves into consciousness and become part of the solution.

If you feel that watching something will hinder you rather than energize you, then be true to yourself. Learn where your line is, and be honest, but don't be so afraid of feeling sad that you avoid what is also a very human emotion.

28 DAYS LATER
DIRECTED BY DANNY BOYLE

Danny Boyle's movie is enjoyable from beginning to end—especially if you're a fan of zombie movies (but even if you're not, don't let that deter you from watching it), though it's by and large the beginning of the movie that is most relevant to our subject of animals—and a consciousness about animals—in film and in the arts.

28 Days Later starts with a montage of human violence. The camera pulls back to see that this violence is on a screen—on one of many screens—all of them mounted in front of an unwilling ape. S/he is strapped to a table and forced to watch all of the human violence.

Masked members of an animal liberation organization break in, and a researcher stumbles upon them as they are breaking free the animals—mostly nonhuman primates. The researcher tells them that the apes are infected. When the activists ask what they're infected with, the researcher tells them: "Rage."

Beyond this, animal rights don't necessarily play heavily into the rest of the story. Essentially, the infected animals escape and spread the virus throughout London, which becomes a veritable wasteland, except for a few uninfected survivors that remain. The animal liberationists are never mentioned again and are not blamed for the outbreak. Society at large reflects the violent footage the apes were forced to watch, and the Rage virus enables even those who aren't infected to act without any regard for life.

This is most bluntly illustrated by the soldiers we meet halfway through the film, who keep an infected man chained up and treat him "like an animal." They also decide that in order to rebuild society, they'll start by making sexual slaves of the heroine and a young girl.

This is a movie worth watching for many reasons, not the least of which is pure entertainment. But its social commentary is ever present.

GILDA, THE TURKEY

I never knew that a turkey would purr like a cat as our Gilda does. She lies lazily in the sun on her side with one leg stretched out. As we stroke the soft white feathers on her head, her eyes close, and she purrs with serenity and contentment.

Gilda was born into a mechanized hatchery, the daughter of "breeder" parents who never knew her or each other. The first thing she did when she touched the ground at our home was to look around for a long time. She stared intently at every new thing, constantly tilting her head from one side to the other so as not to miss a single detail about us, the yard, the sky, anything. It was like watching a baby seeing the world for the very first time.

Six months later, Gilda knows our place as if she's been here all her life. In a way, she has, because her life started when she came here.

The other day I spied on her as she intensely worked on a very private project. With her stub toes (her toes were cut off on the day she was born), she meticulously dug out a hole in some soft earth for a nest and shaped it just so. She then canvassed the yard, carefully selecting just the right grass and twigs (with her cut-off beak) to line her precious nest with. I went back a short time later to find her sitting in the new nest, and jealously guarding a lovely egg.

—*Karen Davis, founder of United Poultry Concerns, Machipongo, Virginia (U.S.)*

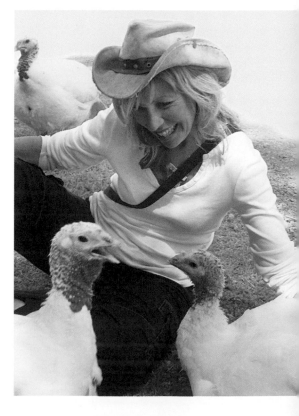

Colleen with rescued turkeys

Photo courtesy of Michael Scribner

WHITE BEANS WITH SWISS CHARD AND RICE

When I was still eating and cooking chickens, I specialized in one dish in particular called chicken à la king. This hearty stew reminds me of that dish, though it's infinitely better! It can be made as thick or thin as you like, depending on how much water you add.

> 1 bunch Swiss chard, finely chopped
> 1 tablespoon (15 ml) olive oil or water, for sautéing
> 1 yellow onion, chopped
> 2 to 4 cloves garlic, minced
> 5 cups (1,175 ml) vegetable stock
> 1 (15-ounce, or 420 g) can cannellini beans
> 1 cup (190 g) uncooked brown rice
> 1 bay leaf
> ½ teaspoon salt, or to taste
> Freshly ground pepper

Unless the ribs of the chard are uncharacteristically tough or thick, there is no need to remove the leaves from the stems. They can all be chopped together, especially because the leaves and stems are cooking long enough to become very tender.

Heat the oil in a soup pot over medium heat. Add the onion and chard, and cook, stirring often, until the onion softens and the chard wilts, about 5 minutes. Add the garlic, and stir together for 30 seconds to 1 minute, or until fragrant.

Add the stock, beans, rice, bay leaf, and salt, and stir to combine. Bring to a gentle boil, cover, lower the heat, and simmer until the rice is fully cooked. Stir occasionally, and add more water, if necessary.

By the end, the mixture should be soupy but thick. Remove the bay leaf, and season to taste with additional salt, as needed, and fresh black pepper.

Yield: 4 servings

COMPASSIONATE COOKS TIP
When reheating this the next day, you might want to add a little water first.

*Soy-free, wheat-free, oil-free if sautéing in water

FOOD LORE: "THE STRAW, THE COAL, AND THE BEAN"

A delightful little tale about why beans have a black seam—by the Brothers Grimm.

An old woman lived in a village. She had gathered a serving of beans and wanted to cook them, so she prepared a fire in her fireplace. To make it burn faster she lit it with a handful of straw. While she was pouring the beans into the pot, one of them fell unnoticed to the floor, coming to rest next to a piece of straw. Soon afterward a glowing coal jumped out of the fireplace and landed next to them.

The straw said, "Dear friends, where do you come from?"

The coal answered, "I jumped from the fireplace, to my good fortune. If I had not forced my way out, I surely would have died. I would have burned to ash."

The bean said, "I too saved my skin. If the old woman had gotten me into the pot I would have been cooked to mush without mercy, just like my comrades."

"Would my fate have been any better?" said the straw. "The old woman sent all my brothers up in fire and smoke. She grabbed sixty at once and killed them. Fortunately, I slipped through her fingers."

"What should we do now?" asked the coal.

"Because we have so fortunately escaped death," answered the bean, "I think that we should join together as comrades. To prevent some new misfortune from befalling us here, let us together make our way to another land."
This proposal pleased the other two, and they set forth all together.

They soon came to a small brook, and because there was neither a bridge nor a walkway there, they did not know how they would get across it.

Then the straw had a good idea, and said, "I will lay myself across it, and you can walk across me like a bridge."

So the straw stretched himself from one bank to the other. The coal, who was a hotheaded fellow, stepped brashly onto the newly constructed bridge, but when he got to the middle and heard the water rushing beneath him, he took fright, stopped, and dared not go any further. Then the straw caught fire, broke into two pieces, and fell into the brook. The coal slid after him, hissed as he fell into the water, and gave up the ghost.

The bean, who had cautiously stayed behind on the bank, had to laugh at the event. He could not stop, and he laughed so fiercely that he burst. Now he too would have died, but fortunately a wandering tailor was there, resting near the brook. Having a compassionate heart, he got out a needle and thread and sewed the bean back together.

The bean thanked him most kindly. However, because he had used black thread, since that time all beans have had a black seam.

TURNING THE TABLES

There seems to be an unspoken societal expectation that vegans be as silent about their food choices as possible. Written into this expectation is the following clause: "Vegans (and vegetarians) must be considerate, respectful, and sensitive to meat-eaters at all times. They must not speak of their reasons for being vegan unless asked first. But when they are asked, they must make their answers as brief and sanitized as possible so as not to upset the meat-eater while he/she finishes lunch."

There is a stereotype that vegans talk about being vegan all the time. The irony is, once people find out I'm vegan, I quickly become their confessor, counselor, and sounding board.

Unsolicited, they tell me how often they eat "meat," how much they've cut back, or how they've considered becoming vegetarian. They tell me they eat only "humanely killed" animals (an oxymoron at best), or they challenge me to solve other great hypothetical dilemmas.

Every encounter with animal-eaters is an opportunity to offer a perspective they may not have encountered before. However, every vegan/animal advocate I know treads ever so gently.

But treading gently doesn't mean we shouldn't challenge the status quo through outreach and education, and this can be accomplished by turning the tables:

* Nonvegetarians unabashedly ask vegetarians and vegans why they don't eat animals and their products. When is the last time you heard a vegan ask a meat-eater to defend why she eats animals?

* How many blessed times can vegans answer the question, "Where do you get your protein?" but you never hear them say to a meat-eater: "Oh my word! You're a meat-eater? Where do you get your folate, fiber, vitamin C, vitamin E, and selenium?" Or "You really eat that stuff? Have you heard that it's linked with cancer, heart disease, and diabetes?"

Vegetarians *should* start asking our friends and family members these questions, because left unchallenged, our species will continue to allow billions of animals to be born every year only to be killed—for appetite, habit, and tradition.

We should take our roles very seriously and continue to be as respectful, considerate, and sensitive as we can be. But we will also inevitably upset comfort zones—just by turning the tables and proudly being the vegan in the room.

EATING RAW

Although I believe that an abundance of raw vegetables and fruits should be part of everyone's diet, I am not convinced that 100 percent of our diet needs to consist of raw food. "Raw foodism" is based on the principle that cooking food destroys the healthful enzymes of plant foods, and though cooking does destroy some enzymes, most of these enzymes are destroyed by the acid in our stomach anyway. What's also true is that there are just certain healthful properties of plant foods we cannot absorb without the cell walls being broken down a bit—that is, through cooking.

Here's what Jack Norris, RD, at veganhealth.org has to say. I agree with his perspective:

> Cooking has both negative and positive effects. Cooking, for long periods especially, can damage some vitamins. Boiling and steaming causes vitamins and minerals to seep out of the food. Chemicals thought to cause cancer are formed when food is burned or oils are heated above the point at which they smoke. Deep-frying foods causes trans fats to form, which increases cholesterol levels.

On the plus side, cooking can break down food components that would otherwise bind minerals and prevent their absorption. It can soften fiber, which allows more food to be eaten. Cooking liberates some nutrients, such as beta-carotene and other antioxidants, for easier absorption. It denatures proteins, essentially flattening them out, which can aid in digestion. Cooking destabilizes toxic components of some foods, such as goiter-promoting properties of broccoli. It makes many foods, such as beans and many grains, edible.

In summary, fresh fruits and vegetables should be eaten regularly. I suggest several servings of raw foods a day. Above that, listen to your own body: If you feel like eating a higher proportion of your foods raw, or all your foods raw, go for it! (But make sure you get a regular supply of vitamin B_{12}.)

I also highly recommend the book *Becoming Raw* by Brenda Davis and Vesanto Melina.

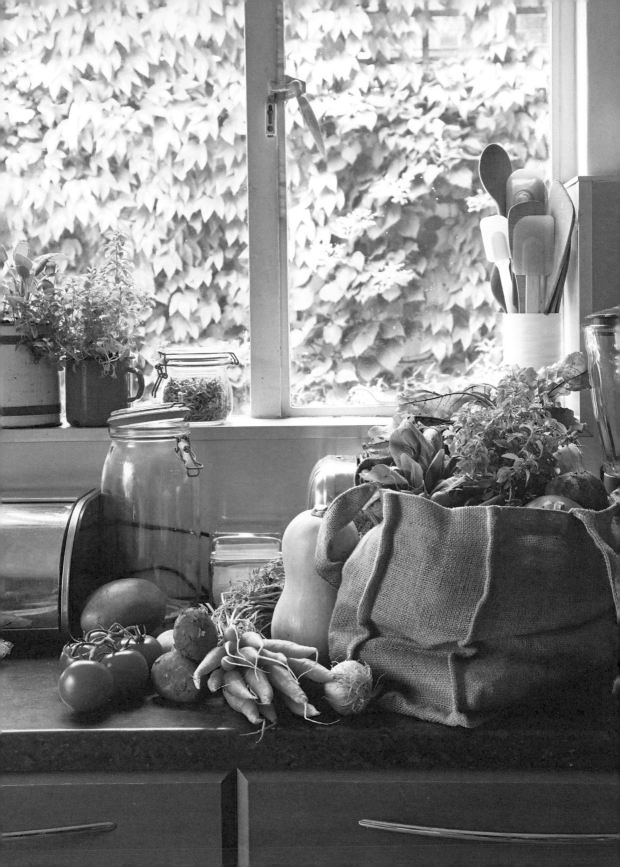

ANIMALS
BY DON LEPAN

Animals is a contemporary first novel by Don LePan, which takes place in a future era after the "great extinction" when all the animals that humans once consumed have been wiped out. Consequently, society has created a category of sub-humans, those who are "defective" in some way, known as the mongrels. Initially kept as pets (and referred to as "chattels"), they eventually begin to be farmed by humans, who fatten them up and use them as sources of labor until they're killed at ten or eleven years old for meat.

Using keen insight—as well as hindsight and foresight—LePan creates simple but disturbing parallels between our own treatment of animals and this future society's treatment of the "mongrels." Centered around one mongrel boy named Sam, a sympathetic and sweet boy abandoned by his mother and adopted as a pet into the Stinson family, the narrative is often interrupted with interjections by Sam's biological brother, who explains the events that led to the current state of things.

One of my favorite passages illustrates how well LePan understands the role language plays in the process of desensitization. Broderick, the brother, explains that "the product was not called *mongrel* or *mongrel meat.* Just as in the old days people had distanced themselves from the animals they were eating by calling a cow *beef* and a pig *pork*, so too did they find other names for mongrel meat. In North America it became known as *yurn*, in Britain and Australia as *fland*—though in Britain it was often also referred to as *new mince*, after the most popular ground form."

If it sounds disturbing, it is, which is precisely LePan's goal.

At the end of the novel, LePan includes an Author's Afterword, in which he unabashedly admits that he hopes his novel will "provide fodder for philosophical debate on the wider arguments concerning whether or not humans should kill and eat non-human animals." The impetus for creating his character Sam, he explains, "is to inquire into the particular reality for a sentient creature…[and what it would be like] to face something akin to today's factory farming."

That may not have a lofty artistic ring to it, but for me, it places Animals in the tradition of other works over the centuries—namely *Uncle Tom's Cabin* and *The Jungle*—in which the author's first aim was to expose a social ill rather than write a great work of fiction. He no doubt did the former, and I'll leave it up to you as to whether he accomplished the latter.

EGG-EATING VEGETARIAN BECOMES VEGAN

Vegetarian for ten years, I had always been proud of my choice not to eat animals, but the notion of being vegan was always in the back of my mind.

When I made the connection between the veal and dairy industries, my mind changed. The veal industry is the result of all the males discarded by the dairy industry. I had long felt that veal was one of the most reprehensible things you could eat, and yet I was supporting that very industry every time I put [cow's] milk in my coffee.

Growing up in a rural area, we had our own cow, Moo. My parents would have the vet artificially inseminate her—a process we knew she was none too fond of, because she would always try to hide when she heard his van coming down the driveway. She was able to make the connec-

tion between the sound of his engine and the nasty procedures that were done to her.

Clearly, Moo was a lot better at making connections than I was: She had to have babies in order to give milk. It amazes me that I lived forty years without considering the implications of millions of cows constantly giving birth to calves that would be 50 percent male, and just what would happen to all those male calves.

Becoming vegan has profoundly affected me. It's a much deeper change than becoming vegetarian ever was and feels a lot more significant. Looking around, I see the world through new eyes. It feels like a homecoming, like I'm finally living a life that's true to who I really am.

—*Alexandra in Vancouver, Canada*

APPLE, CRANBERRY, CHERRY, AND POMEGRANATE SALAD

This simple and light dish is a winner for its flavor and its textures: chewy, creamy, crunchy, and crispy.

- 4 red-skinned apples, chopped (not peeled)
- ¼ cup (27 g) blanched slivered almonds, toasted
- ¼ cup (30 g) chopped dried cherries, or ½ cup (78 g) pitted and halved fresh cherries
- ¼ cup (30 g) dried cranberries
- ¼ cup (44 g) chopped dates
- 1 cup (245 g) nondairy vanilla yogurt
- 1 tablespoon (15 ml) lemon juice (optional)
- ¼ cup (27 g) pomegranate seeds

In a medium-size bowl, stir the apples, almonds, cherries, cranberries, dates, yogurt, and lemon juice until all the ingredients are combined.

Divide the salad among 4 plates, and sprinkle each with the pomegranate seeds. This salad will hold up well in the fridge overnight.

Yield: 4 servings

*Oil-free, soy-free with soy-free yogurt, wheat-free

DANDELION GREENS

In much of the Northern Hemisphere, dandelion is a perennial and persistent lawn weed. Homeowners who curse these yellow flowers should take heart: You can weed and get a dose of greens at the same time! Seriously, you can harvest the greens that are growing around your house, but I advise against this if your lawn is chemically treated. If you know that the area around your house is pesticide-free, grab a paring knife and hunt for the greens. Look for smooth, small leaves 3 to 5 inches (7.6 to 12.7 cm) in length.

The English name *dandelion* is a corruption of the French *dent de lion*, meaning "lion's tooth," referring to the coarsely toothed leaves. Closest in flavor to mustard greens, dandelion leaves can be eaten cooked or raw in various forms; usually the young leaves and unopened buds are eaten raw in salads, while older leaves are cooked. Raw leaves can have a slightly bitter taste, but modern varieties have been bred to be much leafier and far less bitter.

* Dandelion greens are wonderful eaten raw as part of a salad, where their spiciness is apparent.

* Lightly boiled and sprinkled with salt and a bit of cider vinegar, they make an easy and delicious side dish.

* In France, where dandelion greens are still very popular, they are often lightly sautéed with garlic and salt.

* They can be used as a substitute for spinach, Swiss chard, and kale in almost any dish.

* Sauté them with a little garlic, olive oil, red pepper flakes, and salt, and you just can't fail.

The closest relative to dandelion greens is wild chicory, though you can replace both of them with endive, watercress, or arugula.

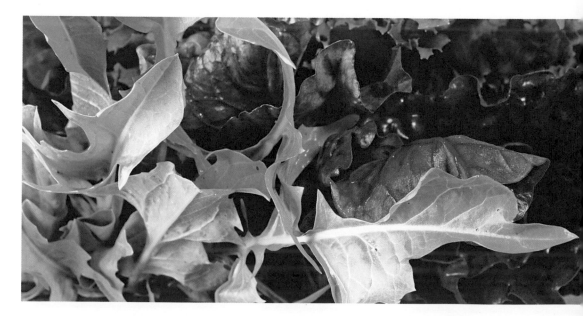

HOW DO YOU RESPOND TO, "MY GRANDFATHER GREW UP EATING MEAT EVERY DAY, AND HE LIVED TO BE NINETY-FIVE YEARS OLD"?

The subtext of this question is usually: "Clearly, there is no connection between diet and life expectancy."

Of course there are always exceptions to the rule, but there are undisputed conclusions, such as the American Dietetic Association's position on vegetarianism:

> Vegetarian diets offer a number of nutritional benefits, including lower levels of saturated fat, cholesterol, and animal protein as well as higher levels of carbohydrates, fiber, magnesium, potassium, folate, and antioxidants such as vitamins C and E and phytochemicals. Vegetarians have been reported to have lower body mass indices than nonvegetarians, as well as lower rates of death from ischemic heart disease; vegetarians also show lower blood cholesterol levels; lower blood pressure; and lower rates of hypertension, type 2 diabetes, and prostate and colon cancer.

Decades of research demonstrate that a diet rich in plant foods and free of animal products is healthier than one based on meat, dairy, and processed foods. And longevity isn't the only thing to consider when it comes to living a healthy life: There's a lot to be said for *quality* of life. We're living to a ripe old age now—not simply because we're evolving to cope with our destructive lifestyle but because artificial interventions are keeping us alive longer. Are we better off living with stents in our chest, taking pills every day, having our chest cut open to reroute our arteries, eating until we're so overweight that we have our stomach stapled?

When people say they know people who lived until ninety-five who ate meat, smoked, and didn't exercise, I guess I would ask them if they had been on any medications or had any surgeries, and inquire about the quality of those ninety-five years.

Just because we live long doesn't mean we live well.

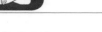
BEARING WITNESS

Although I do think it's important for vegans to bear witness to animal suffering by looking at photos or watching videos that have been shot by undercover investigators, I do not make this suggestion merely to encourage masochism. Because animal suffering is hidden from view in our society—allowing the perpetrators to continue their abuse behind bolted doors— a small dose every once in a while is enough to remind us why we were moved to boycott violence against animals in the first place.

The abusers are so afraid of the public seeing the truth about how animals are treated that it's virtually impossible to document the everyday occurrences in animal factories, in laboratories, and in the animal entertainment industry. The people who go undercover to document abuses are unsung heroes, in my book, quite literally risking life, limb, and liberty to bring the dirty secrets of the animal exploitation industries into public view; to look at the fruits of their labors is to honor their work.

But that is not the only reason I think it's important to bear witness. I know of a few people who were effective and consistent voices for the animals for a number of years until life's circumstances removed them far enough away from the realities of animal exploitation and they forgot who they were. Without a community of like-minded people to remind them and without a periodic visual dose of the truth, they fell out of touch and reverted back to eating animals or animal secretions.

Footage and photographs of animal abuse are especially important when you do not have a community of like-minded people around you—or even one fellow vegan in your life. They provide a necessary link when you feel isolated and disconnected.

The worst thing we can do to the abusers and the best thing we can do for the animals is to bear witness to the abuses and document them for others to see. The power of the image cannot be diminished, and the truth of it cannot be denied.

THE UNBEARABLE LIGHTNESS OF BEING
BY MILAN KUNDERA

This philosophical novel, written in 1984 by Milan Kundera, is set in Communist Prague in 1968 during the Soviet invasion of Czechoslovakia. The main characters are Tomáš, a brain surgeon; his wife, Tereza, a photographer; and Sabina, a free-spirited artist and lover of Tomáš.

Another character named Karenin plays a central role in the novel and in the relationship between Tereza and Tomáš, though he is not human. He is their beloved dog. Although Karenin's presence plays a pivotal role in Tereza and Tomáš' relationship—and our understanding of them—Kundera also utilizes him to make a larger statement about the healing role of animals in our lives and as a kind of contrast to humans. Whereas many of the characters in this novel lack self-control and act on instinct (characteristics typically attributed to nonhuman animals), the animals behave as the humans should: caring, loyal, and steadfast.

These themes are epitomized in the seventh chapter, called "Karenin's Smile." Tereza and Tomáš move to the country, where Tereza taps into her love of animals, Karenin enjoys the undivided attention he receives from the couple, and he even befriends a pig named Mefisto. It is at this time that Tereza discovers a tumor on Karenin, and he's diagnosed with cancer, leaving Tereza heartbroken.

While he is dying, Tereza perceives a "smile" on Karenin's face, which unites the couple who had been drifting apart. They guide Karenin out of his suffering, leaving the author to comment on the mercy we are able to show animals when they are in pain: "Dogs do not have many advantages over people, but one of them is extremely important: euthanasia is not forbidden by law in their case; animals have the right to a merciful death."

Many other similarly poignant passages throughout the book are memorable even outside of the context of the narrative:

> Mankind's true moral test, its fundamental test … consists of its attitude towards those who are at its mercy: animals. And in this respect mankind has suffered a fundamental debacle, a debacle so fundamental that all others stem from it.
> …
> The very beginning of Genesis tells us that God created man in order to give him dominion over fish and fowl and all creatures. Of course, Genesis was written by a man, not a horse. There is no certainty that God actually did grant man dominion over other creatures. What seems more likely, in fact, is that man invented God to sanctify the dominion that he had usurped for himself over the cow and the horse.

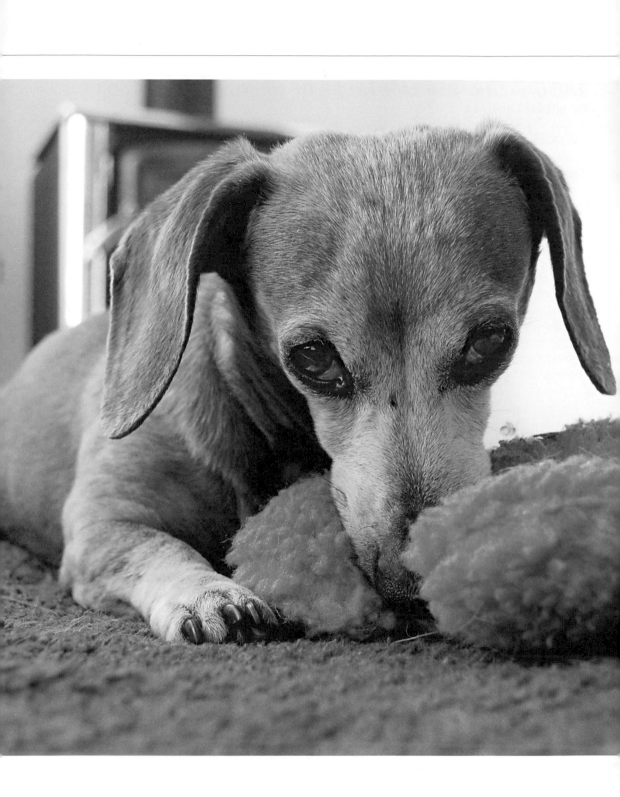

BAILEY, THE SURVIVOR

A Deputy County Attorney called us about a handicapped miniature dachshund named Bailey who was caught up in a court case. Bailey was one of more than 100 dogs found at an animal hoarder's property.

Two years earlier, a veterinarian had treated Bailey for disk problems, but the surgery didn't work. Bailey sometimes "fishtailed" when he walked. Other times his rear legs would cycle rapidly, leaving him hopping in place. If he turned too fast, his hindquarters would collapse.

Bailey's owner had decided she didn't want to deal with him any longer. She handed Bailey off to the animal hoarder.

Fast-forward two years. The County Attorney's office asked the same vet to evaluate the dogs at the animal hoarder's property. There, hiding in the corner of a pen with fifteen other dogs, was a miniature dachshund with a damaged spine. The other dogs were running over him and falling on top of him.

The vet recognized Bailey as one of his former patients. It was the first time the vet knew his client had abandoned Bailey to an animal hoarder. The vet told us Bailey looked like he had given up. He said, "You could see it in his eyes. There was no hope. He just wanted to die."

So we expected a sad little thing to arrive at the sanctuary, but instead we got an 11-pound (5 kg) bundle of spirit and playful energy.

We took him to a specialist for an exam and also consulted with our veterinary surgeon. The conclusion: Any more surgery would not be an option for Bailey. The important thing was that he did not seem to us to be in any pain, and our specialist detected no sign of it either during his exam.

Today this plucky little survivor lounges all day on a bed in our living room, and at night he sleeps in front of the woodstove. And oh, how Bailey loves his toys! He'll grab a soft toy with his mouth, toss it into the air, then hop over to retrieve it and toss it again.

During his first few days here it seemed like Bailey couldn't believe his luck. He kept looking around the house in wide-eyed wonder, as if it were too good to be true and wasn't going to last. Now he has a look that says, "This is home and I'm here to stay!"

—*Rolling Dog Ranch Animal Sanctuary, Lancaster, New Hampshire (U.S.)*

Bailey at Rolling Dog Ranch Animal Sanctuary

Photo courtesy of Rolling Dog Ranch Animal Sanctuary

ASIAN-INSPIRED LETTUCE WRAPS

A favorite recipe, this is one of my go-to week-night meals. A very firm tofu with some of the water squeezed out is the best tofu to use for this.

4 tablespoons (60 ml) water, divided
2 tablespoons (20 g) minced garlic
1 tablespoon (6 g) grated or finely minced fresh ginger
1 red bell pepper, seeded and finely chopped
1 large carrot, finely chopped
16 ounces (455 g) extra-firm tofu
1 tablespoon (16 g) chili paste
2 tablespoons (30 g) light brown sugar
2 tablespoons (32 g) light miso paste
2 teaspoons (5 g) sesame seeds
10 Boston, Bibb, or butter lettuce leaves, rinsed and patted dry
10 basil leaves
2 small cucumbers, peeled and julienned

Heat 2 tablespoons (30 ml) of the water in a sauté pan over medium heat. Add the garlic and ginger, and cook for 2 minutes, until they soften. Add the red pepper and carrot, and cook for another minute.

Meanwhile, crumble the tofu in a separate bowl until pretty small, resembling bread crumbs. Add to the sauté pan, and cook for 10 minutes, thoroughly combining with the vegetables. Add the chili paste, and stir to combine.

Place the brown sugar and remaining 2 table-spoons (30 ml) water in a saucepan, and dissolve over medium-low heat. Remove from the heat, and stir in the miso paste and sesame seeds. Add to the tofu mixture, and thoroughly combine.

To make the wraps, trim the edges of the lettuce leaves to make them uniformly circular. Add a basil leaf and some julienned cucumber to each "cup." Add the tofu mixture, and enjoy!

Yield: 10 wraps

*Oil-free, wheat-free

Originally published in *The Vegan Table*

EAT MORE BEANS!

Too many people avoid including beans in their diet.

* Some people avoid them because they think you have to cook them from scratch.

* Some people avoid them because—being unwilling to cook them from scratch—they have mistakenly understood canned beans to be inferior in nutrition.

* Some people avoid beans because they cause them physical discomfort.

You absolutely don't have to cook them from scratch if you don't want to, but see Day 99 for easy tips. Canned beans may be more expensive than dried beans, but that is the only drawback. You're not losing *anything* in terms of nutrition. Some people complain about the salt content of canned beans; the solution is to buy salt-free canned beans, or rinse and drain the beans before you eat them.

To increase digestibility of beans:

* Again, eat more beans! The more you eat, the more your digestive system becomes accustomed to them.

* Take an anti-oligosaccharide enzyme (oligosaccharides are the sugar in beans). Since a normal human digestive tract doesn't contain any anti-oligosaccharide enzymes, taking one just as you're eating beans increases digestion of these sugars. This enzyme is currently sold in the United States under the brand name Beano, but because it contains gelatin, I recommend Bean-zyme, a vegetarian version found in large natural food stores and in my store online.

* Add a little vinegar to the beans just after they're cooked, or add kombu seaweed to the beans while they're cooking.

* Eat canned beans, which tend to be easier for people to digest, mainly because the sugars have been cooked out, and the beans have been rinsed really well, making these oligosaccharides less prevalent.

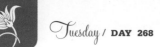

ETYMOLOGY OF "COMMUNICATION"

When I'm communicating with a nonvegan about the joys and benefits of being vegan, my intention is to have a dialogue—not create a dichotomy between me—the vegan—and the nonvegan.

My intention is to stay focused on the issues at hand; to ask questions with authenticity; and to answer with honesty, integrity, and humility. I try to be clear about where I end and another person begins. I'm not afraid to speak for animals.

If I'm talking to someone, my intention is to really *talk* to her to communicate, and so I think it's worth keeping in mind the etymology of this word.

Communicate is built from the word *common*, which literally means "shared by all." And I like that. This issue isn't about me against you, vegan against non-vegan. My moral superiority over your moral superiority. It's about all of us being unified against animal cruelty and suffering. It's about all of us being empowered to live as healthfully as possible. These are values "shared by all."

Instead of standing against one another, we need to stand together on common ground—communally.

SPENDING TIME IN NATURE

Time spent outdoors can be restorative and rejuvenating, whether you're just walking in the woods or strolling on a beach. Spending time in nature connects us with the most fundamental cycles of life, where they are most apparent in the birth, death, and rebirth of life all around.

In nature, our senses are engaged, and we are humbled, as we become aware of how small we are and how fleeting our lives are relative to the vastness and perpetuity of the Earth and her constant seasons.

The rhythms of nature can provide a model for our own lives, as we slow down and retreat during the dark winter days or find rejuvenation in the emergence of spring. The cycles of the moon can lead us toward our own need to shed a part of ourselves (during its waning), expand who we are (during its waxing), and fully manifest our desires (during her fullness).

Nature has much to offer if we spend but a little time there. Even in our fast-paced, industrialized, modern world, we can find ways to retreat into nature:

* Do outside whatever you usually do inside, whether it's eating, cooking, yoga, meditation, reading, or working.

* Create a backyard wildlife sanctuary.

* Take a walk in the woods or on the beach.

* Kayak or canoe on a river.

* Walk in your neighborhood and notice the trees, gardens, and flora.

* Watch the sunset.

* Watch the sunrise.

* Visit national parks and support their preservation.

* Volunteer to clean up parks and beaches.

* Take a moonlight stroll.

* Picnic in your backyard.

* Take up bird-watching.

Colleen and a friend on one of her favorite hiking trails
Photo by David Busch

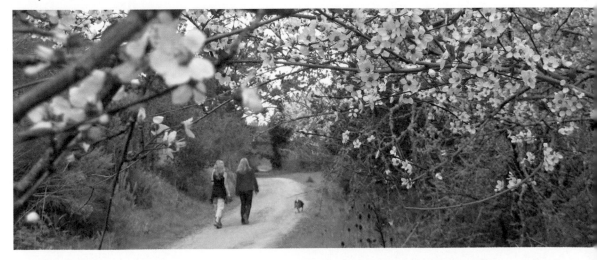

"I LIKE ANIMALS"
BY LAURA MORETTI

This is an excerpt of an essay, reprinted with the permission of its author, Laura Moretti, founder and editor of *The Animals Voice*.

"Why do you suppose you like animals so much?" was the million-dollar question put to me Christmas Eve (and one I hadn't provoked). I knew my family was expecting me to say something like, "I like animals because they're cute and cuddly and furry and fun to play with."

But instead I said, "I like animals because they are honest."

My observation triggered a facetious comment from one of my brothers. "About what?"—as if honesty were merely about telling the truth, and everyone knows animals can't talk! His notation was met with hearty laughter; for once, they thought they'd repaid me for all the discomfort I'd caused them at other family gatherings.

"I like that animals don't pretend to be someone they're not," I continued in my reply, hushing the crowd. "To quote a phrase, 'Dogs don't lie about love.' Animals don't fake their feelings. I like that they're emotionally fearless."

"I like animals," I added, "because they only take out of life what they need. They don't abuse their environment, annihilate species, pollute their water, contaminate the air they breathe. They don't build weapons of mass destruction and use them against others—particularly members of their own species. I like animals because they have no use for those things, or for war or terrorism. They don't build nations around genocide."
"That's because they don't know any better," a brother-in-law argued. "They don't do those things because they don't know how."

"A pride of lions doesn't get together," I countered him, "and decide how to exterminate zebras—their very source of nourishment. I don't think it's because they don't know how. I think it's because it's counter-productive."

"I also like animals," I continued, "because they don't punish themselves for their perceived inadequacies. They don't dwell on things of the past, nor use them as excuses for behavior in the present. And they don't plan to live some day in the future, they live today, this moment, fully, completely, and purely. I like animals because they live their lives with so much more freedom than humans live theirs."

"That's because they don't think," one of my cousins offered.

"Is that the difference?" I wondered. "'I think therefore I'm cruel, destructive, insecure, abusive?' You meant to say they don't think the way *we* think." The room had become strangely quiet. I was amazed at how closely my family was listening, despite the occasional grunt to the contrary.

"I like animals because they don't bow down to imaginary gods they've created, nor annihilate each other in the name of those gods; I like animals because they only know how to give unconditional love and implicit trust. I mean, animals either extend those things to you or they don't; there are no shades of gray. They have the best of what makes us human and none of our vices."

"And thank God," someone injected.

"Lastly," I added, "animals are the most victimized living creatures on earth; more than children, more than women, more than people of color. Our prejudice enables us to exploit and use them, as scientific tools and expendable commodities, and to eat them. We do to them any atrocity our creative minds can summon. We justify our cruelties; we have to or we can't commit them. I like animals because they don't do to themselves or to others the things we do to them. And they don't make excuses for unethical actions because they don't commit unethical acts."

"And finally," I finished, "I like animals because they're not hypocrites. They don't say one thing and do another. They are, as I've said, honest. Animals—not humans—are the best this planet has to offer."

And, interestingly enough, despite my soapbox rant, not a one of them made a snide comment or a hint of laughter. The conversation actually rolled into shared stories of animals they've known, stories of animal loyalty and intelligence, their humor and innocence. And it was me who'd become the listener.

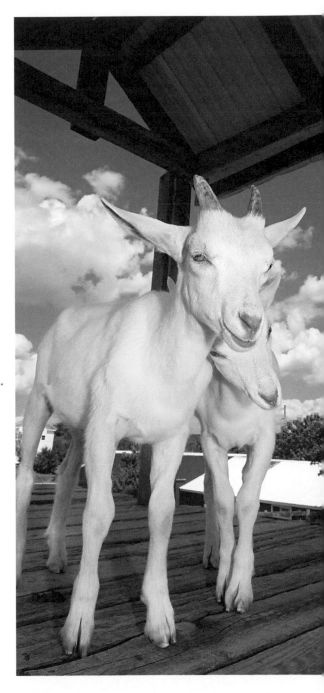

Rescued goats ZuZu (left) and Otto (right) at Farm Sanctuary

Photo by Connie Pugh for Farm Sanctuary

JOURNEY TO AWAKENING: STEP BY STEP

When I was a child I loved animals, or so I thought. For, while I really felt a kinship with and a great deal of affection for all animals, I hadn't made the connection between their lives and who it was I was eating every day.

Growing up we always had pets; I was an only child, and our animals were really a part of our small family of two humans. I wanted to be a

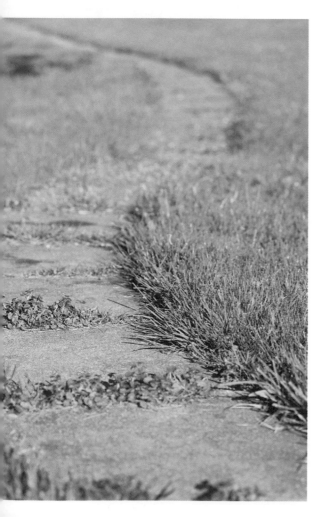

zoologist or an oceanographer. I moved worms that had washed up on the sidewalk after rain back onto the soil.

I was raised by my mother, who was a hippie in the 1960s, so I was more than familiar with health food stores and vegetarianism. We were lacto-ovo vegetarians for a while when I was young, but we ended up on a meat-based diet.

When I was eleven, I went to a friend's house for dinner. They were preparing lobster, which I had never had before. I watched in horror as my friend's father put a live lobster into a huge pot of boiling water. A few long minutes later, the lobster threw the lid of the pot onto the floor in a valiant attempt to save his life. One claw was poking out, reaching. He was still alive in there, somehow. The father slammed the lid back on and walked away.

I didn't have any lobster that day.

When I was twenty-two, I saw *Diet for a New America*, the incredible documentary by John Robbins about how what we eat affects ourselves, animals, and the planet. I watched, amazed, as everything I had been taught about animal products in my life and diet was expertly dismantled by this kind, compassionate person. I sat rapt, with tears in my eyes. I became vegan— and never looked back.

—*Linda in San Francisco, California (U.S.)*

GINGER-SESAME TEMPEH STEAKS

The longer you marinate the tempeh, the more flavorful it is.

8 ounces (225 g) tempeh
1 tablespoon (15 ml) olive oil
2 tablespoons (30 ml) sesame oil, divided
2-inch (5 cm) piece of fresh ginger, minced or thinly sliced
2 cloves garlic, minced
4 sprigs fresh parsley
2 tablespoons (30 ml) tamari soy sauce
1 tablespoon (20 g) agave nectar
2 tablespoons (30 ml) water
Freshly ground black pepper

Cut the tempeh into fourths, and then create thinner steaks by slicing through the thickness of each piece of tempeh with a sharp knife. You should have about 8 relatively square slices of tempeh.

In a small bowl, combine the olive oil, 1 tablespoon (15 ml) of the sesame oil, fresh ginger, garlic, parsley, tamari, agave, water, and pepper. Stir to blend, and pour into a shallow baking pan. The pan should be large enough to hold the tempeh but small enough so the marinade covers the bottom.

Place the tempeh slices on top of the marinade, cover, and marinate for at least 1 hour, flipping every 15 minutes.

When ready to cook, heat the remaining 1 tablespoon (15 ml) sesame oil in a large sauté pan over medium heat. When hot, add the tempeh slices, and drizzle with 1 tablespoon (15 ml) of the marinade. Cook until browned on the bottom side, about 5 to 7 minutes.

Turn, drizzle with 1 tablespoon (15 ml) more of the marinade, and cook until browned on the other side, about 5 to 7 minutes. Drizzle with the remaining marinade, and cook just a couple minutes longer.

Serve hot or at room temperature.

Yield: 2 to 4 servings

*Wheat-free

COLLARD GREENS

Dating back to prehistoric times, collard greens are a member of the cabbage family and thus closely related to kale. In fact, the ancient Greeks grew kale and collards and made no distinction between them.

When choosing collard greens, look for firm, unwilted leaves that are deep green in color (almost olive) with no signs of yellowing or browning. Store *unwashed* collard greens in a damp paper towel in a plastic bag. Store in the refrigerator crisper bin, where they will keep for three to five days, though the sooner they are eaten, the less bitter they will be.

When you're ready to use them, wash the leaves very well, because they tend to collect sand and soil, and pat dry.

Some of my favorite ways to prepare collard greens:

* Chop the greens and slowly simmer in salted vegetable stock with a dash of liquid smoke or one or two chipotle peppers. The salt and smokiness not only add flavor but also temper their tough texture and bitter flavor. Cook until they are soft and serve with fresh baked cornbread. (Dip the cornbread into the remaining liquid from the cooked greens, called the pot likker. Pot likker is the highly concentrated, vitamin-rich broth that results from the long boil of the greens.)

* Boil or steam chopped collard greens and then drizzle with olive oil and lemon juice.

* Steam chopped collard greens, then add to a pot of black-eyed peas and brown rice for a Southern-inspired meal. Traditionally, collards are served with black-eyed peas on New Year's Day, to promise a year of good luck and financial reward. (The greens represent paper money, and the peas represent coins.)

* Use raw or lightly steamed collard greens as a wrap, instead of using a tortilla or nori sheet.

* Spread peanut or almond butter on a collard leaf and roll it up.

* Sauté collard greens with a little olive oil, garlic, and crushed chile peppers.

COMPASSIONATE LANGUAGE: **COCK-AND-BULL STORY**

You've most likely uttered a complaint about someone telling you a "cock-and-bull" story, but why would a rooster and a bull symbolize a fictional tale meant to delight or amuse?

There are competing theories about the origin of this phrase, including one that claims it is a corrupted version of "a concocted and bully story." "Bully" itself is a corruption of the Danish word *bullen*, "exaggerated."

Another theory from StraightDope.com suggests that the phrase "came about when coaches would carry travelers to one of two inns that were close to each other on the old London Road at Stony Stratford near Buckinghamshire, England. Rivalries arose between the groups of travelers who favored one inn over the other, and boastful tales were exchanged. The names of the two inns? The Cock and the Bull, of course."

Yet another proposes that the expression refers to old fables that feature magical, talking animals, a notion that the early seventeenth-century French phrase "cock to donkey" (*coq-a-l'ane*) refers to, which nicely fits the definition penned in Randle Cotgrave's *A Dictionarie of the French and English Tongues* in 1611:

> An incoherent story, passing from one subject to another.

The first known use of the idiom was in John Day's 1608 play, *Law-trickes or Who Would Have Thought It*: "What a tale of a cock and a bull he told my father," says one character. Apparently, however, the phrase was already in use by then.

In short, no animals were harmed in the making of this phrase!

AVOIDING FOODBORNE ILLNESSES

When humans began domesticating cattle, pigs, sheep, goats, and chickens and turkeys, it meant living in close proximity with animals, breathing, eating, and drinking their germs. Despite the rituals performed to ward off disease, it spread through zoonosis, the transmission of infectious disease from nonhumans to humans.

Being animals, it makes sense that we share many of the same diseases as our nonhuman cousins. We aren't—after all—plants. We aren't at risk for catching aphids. Many of the major pandemics we've been plagued with were acquired from nonhuman animals, such as tuberculosis (from cattle), influenza (from pigs and birds), whooping cough (from pigs and dogs), and smallpox (from cattle). Even HIV, the virus that causes AIDS, is believed to have been first transmitted to humans through the butchering and consumption of infected chimpanzees.

The development of vaccines provided us with immunity to certain diseases, and the word itself reveals the origin of these zoonotic infections. At its root is the Latin word *vacca*, meaning "cow," referring to the cattle diseases against which the vaccines were meant to protect humans.

Although eating a plant-based diet and keeping a vegan home virtually reduce the chance of contracting foodborne illnesses, it will never be eliminated while the animal agriculture industry exists, tainting vegetables and contaminating plants.

So next time you hear a media outlet blaming produce for the next outbreak of a foodborne illness, you may want to remind people that it is our consumption of animals—not plants—that exacts a high price for both the consumed and the consumer. Write a letter to the editor to make this important message heard.

THE MISFITS
DIRECTED BY JOHN HUSTON

The many legends about the drama of the *making* of this 1961 poignant film tend to eclipse the drama of the film itself, written by Arthur Miller and directed by John Huston.

Roslyn Taber (skillfully played by Marilyn Monroe) is in Reno, Nevada, to file for divorce. Soon after she finishes with the court proceedings, she meets three men who very rapidly—and quite understandably—fall in love with her:

* Guido Racanelli (Eli Wallach), an ex-mechanic, former WWII pilot, and self-pitying widower

* Gay Langland (Clark Gable), an aging, washed-out "real-life" cowboy, embodying the rugged individualism of the American West

* Perce Howland (Montgomery Clift), a reckless, worn-out, injured "rodeo cowboy"

Misfits themselves in an emerging modern world, the trio of men find in Roslyn an unexpected bright light in their lives. In her, flickers life and hope for them, but she has played that role before and wants more than anything to be loved—not as a savior or a symbol for a man but simply as a woman. Although Gay is old enough to be her father, she falls in love with him, much to the dismay of Guido.

Desperate to hold on to the past, determined to demonstrate their virility, and interested in making a quick buck, the three men decide to round up a herd of wild "misfit" horses to sell to be slaughtered for dog food. They venture into the desert, and though Roslyn knows they'll be rounding up horses, she has no idea why. The conversation that leads to her realization reflects both the excuses we make that enable us to do to animals what we please as well as the clarity of those who know it's simply not right.

Gay's dog is trembling, and when Roslyn goes to comfort him, he nervously snaps at her. Gay yells at his dog, but Roslyn rushes to his defense, "Oh don't, Gay. He couldn't help it. Has he ever been kicked by one of the horses?"

Guido replies, "It's not the horses he's afraid of. It's us."

Gay snaps, "What are you talking about? I never mistreated that dog, and you know it."

Guido: "It's only common sense. He knows there are wild animals up there. Dogs were wild too, once. He's just remembering when. He's been up here enough times to know what's going to happen. He's just scared he's gonna end up dead, too."

At this moment, Roslyn begins to realize that the horses will be killed for dog food and feels sick.

The next day, as they pursue the horses and round them up, Roslyn refuses to make it easy for them and speaks on behalf of the horses as loudly as she can. In one of the longest and most heartrending climaxes on film, Roslyn tries everything to stop them, hysterically screams at them, and calls them murderers. She successfully persuades Perce to release the horses that have already been captured, which infuriates Gay and culminates in a struggle between Gay and the stallion leader—a final emblem of the Old West that Gay finally accepts is dead.

The Misfits is a beautifully shot, powerfully written, and brilliantly acted film that reflects the brightest and darkest of the human condition.

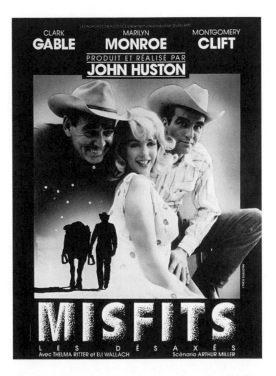

JACKY, THE CHIMPANZEE—RESCUED AFTER THIRTY YEARS

Jacky spent at least thirty years of his life in a small, barren cage at a resort hotel in Limbe, Cameroon. He grew from infancy into adulthood, then to middle age, in total privation. By the 1990s, Jacky was known around town as the "mad" chimpanzee, meaning he was insane. He showed his anguish in stereotypical behaviors—rocking frenetically back and forth or pounding the top of his head with one fist while he held his other hand in his open mouth—and he was very aggressive toward humans. Whether or not he was insane, Jacky definitely was angry.

No one was sure if he could be socialized with other chimpanzees. But on September 1, 1999, Jacky became one of the first three residents of the sanctuary. During the following three years, he astonished us all. Within the continuously enlarging chimpanzee family at the rescue center, Jacky was gentle with the adult females and gently playful and loving with the juveniles. With the support of the chimpanzee women, Jacky became the alpha male of his family and learned to play this most important role very well.

Then, in December 2002, I determined that Jacky had cataracts. During this time, he stopped climbing trees, and on the ground he was always with his alpha female Nama, following closely behind her wherever she went. I was very concerned about Jacky's safety in the forest, but I was reluctant to lock him in the satellite cage alone.

Then one afternoon in April 2003, Jacky got separated from Nama in the forest. His vision was so poor that he couldn't find his way out of the dark forest. He thrashed around screaming in desperation until he finally emerged from the forest with scratches and scrapes all over his face. In panic, he ran into the electric fence three times trying to find his way back to the comfort of the satellite enclosure, where he and all the other chimpanzees sleep. Jacky's vision had deteriorated in such a short time.

After this terrible day, I couldn't let Jacky outside. Each day he stayed alone as the other chimpanzees went out to the forest, and soon he became completely blind. It broke my heart to see him become increasingly frustrated and resume his old behaviors. I had begun looking for an ophthalmologist to come to Cameroon on a volunteer basis to remove Jacky's cataracts, but my request was turned down over and over.

Then, in July 2003, world-renowned ophthalmologist Dr. Jim Tidwell took some of his vacation time to perform cataract surgery on Jacky. On January 1, 2004, Dr. Tidwell gave Jacky artificial lenses that were made for humans, restoring what he believes to be perfect vision. Certainly, a few of the most joyful moments in my life came on that day after the successful surgery, as I watched Jacky gaze in wonder at trees, birds, and my face as if he were seeing it all for the first time. The little boy chimps who had been stealing Jacky's food from under his nose got quite a surprise that day, too.

On April 1, 2004, Jacky and his family of twenty-six chimpanzees were moved to their new enclosure, which encompasses 20 acres (8 ha) of beautiful, lush forest. Jacky's experience with blindness seems to have given him a deeper sense of responsibility. He has earned the deep respect and love of all of us who know him well, both chimpanzee and human.

—*Dr. Sheri Speede, founder of Sanaga-Yong Chimpanzee Rescue Center, Cameroon, Africa*

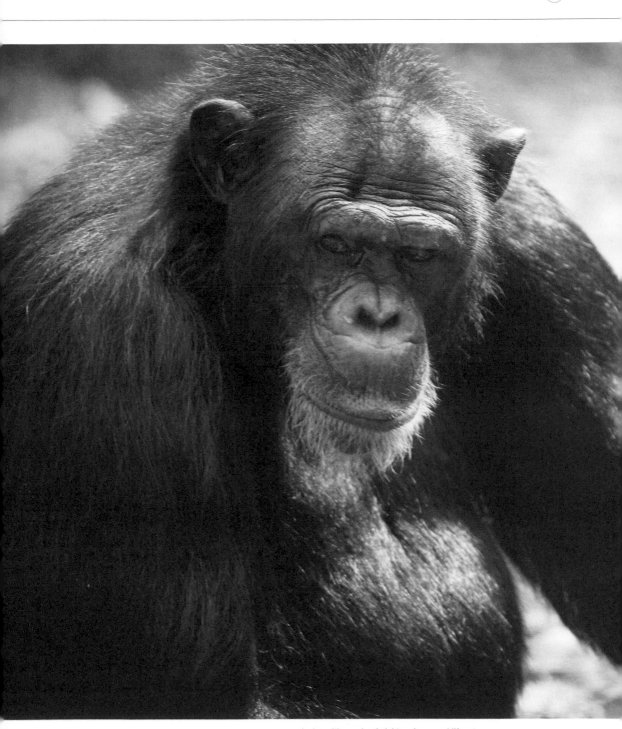

Jacky, with regained sight and renewed life, at
Sanaga-Yong

Photo courtesy of Sanaga-Yong Chimpanzee Rescue Center

CAULIFLOWER AND QUINOA MASH

A hearty and simple side, this protein-rich dish can be whipped up in a flash.

- 1 tablespoon (15 ml) water or oil, for sautéing
- 2 yellow onions, finely chopped
- 2 cups (146 g) quinoa, rinsed
- 4 to 5 cups (940 to 1,175 ml) vegetable stock
- 1 head cauliflower, cut into medium-size florets
- ½ teaspoon salt

Heat the water in a 3-quart (2.7 l) saucepan. Add the onions, and sauté until translucent, about 5 minutes. Add the quinoa, stock, cauliflower, and salt.

Cover, and cook until the quinoa has absorbed all the water and cooked through, about 15 minutes. Mash the mixture together with a potato masher to the desired consistency. The cauliflower will mash down quite a bit, but keep in mind the quinoa will still hold its shape and texture and not become a purée.

Yield: 4 to 6 servings

*Soy-free, oil-free if using water to sauté, wheat-free

PINTO BEANS

The pinto bean (literally means "painted bean" in Spanish) is named for its mottled skin (think of a "spotted" Pinto horse), which is much more noticeable when the bean is dried. It's most often eaten whole in broth or mashed and refried, especially as a burrito filling.

As with all other beans, pintos are high in protein, high in fiber, and low in fat, making them a healthful addition to salads, soups, tortillas, and casseroles. Here are a few other serving ideas:

* Pintos make a great addition to chili instead of (or with) kidney beans.

* Soft like white beans, pinto beans' texture is conducive to pâtés, purees, and dips. Make a dip by pureeing pinto beans with dried sage, dried oregano, garlic, and black pepper. Use as a crudité dip or sandwich spread.

* Add pinto beans and chopped tomatoes to a tortilla spread with hummus. Broil in the oven for 1 minute. Top with chopped avocado and cilantro.

* Heat pinto beans with cooked rice, shredded kale, chili powder, and cumin. Season with salt, and enjoy with tortilla chips and salsa.

* Pair pinto beans with whole corn and corn bread.

> Traditionally, lard (animal fat) is used for cooking refried beans. Whenever you're ordering them from a restaurant, simply ask the server if they use lard. If so, order whole beans instead.

HOW DO YOU RESPOND TO, "IF YOU WERE ON A DESERTED ISLAND, WOULD YOU EAT MEAT/CHEESE/EGGS?"

The excuses we make for to eating animals are numerous. Some of them manifest themselves in hypothetical scenarios, such as this one:

"So, you're on a deserted island. You've been there for weeks, and you're not going to get rescued. You have to eat animals in order to survive. What would you do?"

The answer? For now, I will live my life here on this planet, in this reality, and not eat a single animal. Then, some far-off day, if I find myself on that hypothetical island, I'll cross that bridge.

Some hypothetical questions lose sight of what being vegan is all about. We can hope that the people asking these questions are also interested in a genuine dialogue, not just verbal exercises.

We rely on hypotheticals and misinformation to justify real-life situations because we want to hold on to a perception of ourselves that may or may not be true. Few of us want to consciously contribute to violence or suffering. But, there just isn't any way around it when we eat animals. And if we can't tell ourselves the truth about what we're supporting, then we need to ask ourselves what we're avoiding.

EATING HEALTHFULLY ON THE GO

These meals are quick, easy, familiar, filling, and compact. Buy reusable containers and/or insulated cooler bags for transporting sandwiches.

* **Nut Butter and Jelly**: I don't care how old you are, this is a great sandwich to include in your rotation. The old standby of peanut butter with preserves will be the least expensive, but try almond or cashew butter, too.

* **Add a few apple or banana slices** or grated carrots or, spread the nut butter on a tortilla, top with sliced banana, and roll up and eat.

* **Vegetarian "Lunchmeats"**: There are a number of vegetarian lunchmeats available. Spread on some eggless mayonnaise such as Nayonnaise, Vegenaise, or Wildwood's Garlic Aioli. Or mustard, relish, or ketchup. Add lettuce and tomatoes.

* **Sloppy Col**: Instead of Sloppy Joe, why not try a Sloppy Col? Spread hummus and/or avocado on slices of Italian bread or Italian rolls. Add roasted red peppers, alfalfa sprouts, arugula or lettuce, shredded carrots, and shredded beets.

* **Burritos**: Just roll up your favorite beans in a tortilla with rice, salsa, avocado, shredded lettuce, and nondairy sour cream. Roll it, wrap it, and carry it out.

* **Portobello Sandwich**: Marinate portobello mushrooms in tamari soy sauce and fresh herbs such as sage, tarragon, and basil. Sauté for 15 minutes until they're tender and easily pierced with a fork. Add to a hearty roll with vegan aioli.

THE FOUR STAGES OF CRUELTY
BY WILLIAM HOGARTH

The Four Stages of Cruelty is a series of four engravings created and published in 1751. Their creator was William Hogarth, an English painter, social critic, and editorial cartoonist who lived from 1697 to 1764.

Believing as he did that violence toward animals bred violence toward humans, Hogarth illustrates this through his fictional character Tom Nero, whom we watch develop from a cruel child into a criminal adult. Each print in the series depicts various acts of sadomasochism toward animals, culminating in the same acts being perpetrated against Nero in his own execution and death.

Concerned about acts of brutality against animals he regularly witnessed on the streets of London, Hogarth created the series, whose images are accompanied by text, as a moral instruction against animal cruelty. Pulling no punches, the scenes are as disturbing today as they would have been to an eighteenth-century audience.

The First Print

In the first print, Nero (whose name would most certainly have evoked the Roman emperor who allegedly had his mother executed), is shown inserting an arrow into a dog's rectum, along with the help of some other boys, while another boy begs them to stop, bribing them with some food.

Other scenes of barbarism include:

* Two boys burning the eyes out of a bird with a hot poker

* A boy tormenting a dog by tying a bone to his tail

* A pair of cats hung by their tails to a lamppost

* A cockfight

* A dog disemboweling a cat, at the urging of a cheering boy

* A cat—with false wings tied to his sides—thrown from a high window

The Second Print

In the second plate, Tom Nero is now a young man who works as a driver of a horse-drawn coach—an imprudent occupation for one who abused animals as a child. He is shown beating his horse so severely that he has put out his eye, ostensibly because the horse collapsed under the weight of an overloaded carriage. The men emerging from the carriage ignore the cruelty, while blood runs from the emaciated animal. Other acts of cruelty against animals—and now people, too—abound.

As in the first plate, only one person shows concern. Barely noticeable, a man writes down Nero's coach number in order to report him.

The Third Print

The third print shows Tom Nero as a full adult, whose cruelty to animals has now degenerated even further into theft and murder of people. The scene depicts Nero being subdued at the scene of the murder of his lover. Many elements in the scene reflect violence, including the gun and knife found on Nero's person, and an overall feeling of doom permeates the image, including the fact that the murder takes place in a graveyard.

The Fourth Print

In the fourth print, which Hogarth named *The Reward of Cruelty,* evidence suggests that Nero has been tried and executed for murder and is now in the hands of surgeons, who mutilate his body much the way he mutilated the body of his victims.

In 1801, Hogarth wrote:

> There is no part of my works of which I am so proud, and in which I now feel so happy, as in the series of *The Four Stages of Cruelty* because I believe the publication of them has checked the diabolical spirit of barbarity to the brute creation which, I am sorry to say, was once so prevalent in this country.

The Four Stages of Cruelty: First Print
by William Hogarth

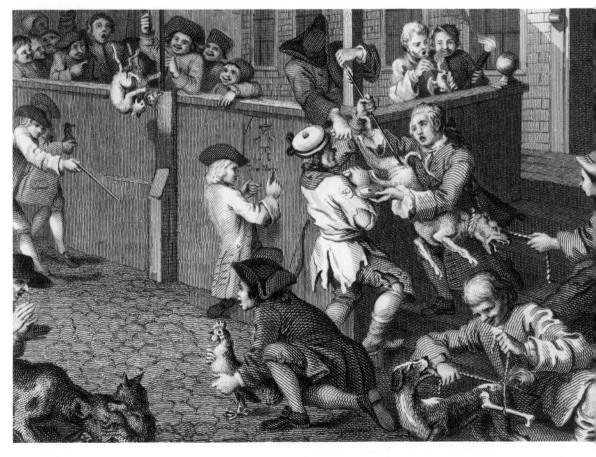

A CALL TO VEGANISM

I was a typical meat-eater for all of my life until my early forties. I loved how meat tasted, and I loved the texture. Although I adored animals, I was raised to eat meat and didn't question it.

Not very long ago, I read *Dominion: The Power of Man, the Suffering of Animals, and the Call to Mercy* by Matthew Scully. I was stunned; I had no idea the extent of our cruelty or the pain caused to animals from the meat production industry. Scully's call to vegetarianism spoke to me, and I began the path immediately.

However, it was hard. I have never been good at putting limits on myself, but I made progress. I bought good vegetarian cookbooks and attended cooking classes and I learned to make delicious meals, and so I became a *part-time* vegetarian—not perfect, but I was 90 percent there.

Needless to say, I never spoke my truth, except to my fantastic husband, who was initially very supportive and is now also vegetarian. However, I was sure I could never be a vegan because I love cheese. I am sure that would have been the extent of my vegetarianism had I not found the *Vegetarian Food for Thought* podcast. Many of the episodes bring the book *Dominion* back to life and the horrors we humans bring upon animals, even those of us who claim to love them. I now see everything—and I mean everything—more clearly.

Not eating animals and their products is a joyful lifestyle full of abundance—not one of restrictions. As I head down the path of veganism, I'm excited like I never have been before. I am joyful . . . while speaking my truth in a pleasant, positive way.

—*Patty in Georgia (U.S.)*

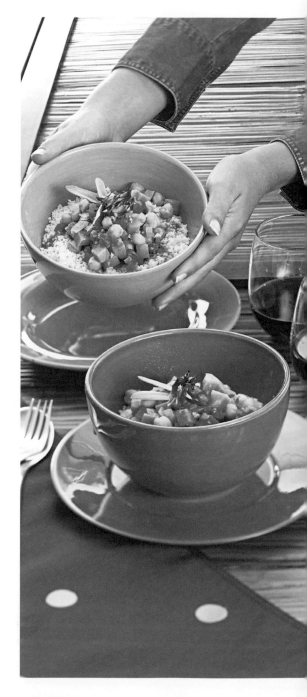

CREAM OF MUSHROOM SOUP

Thank you to Compassionate Cooks member Melissa Phillips for allowing me to share this rich and satisfying soup.

- **2 tablespoons (28 g) nondairy butter**
- **1 tablespoon (15 ml) olive oil**
- **1 large yellow onion, finely chopped**
- **1 large carrot, finely chopped**
- **3 stalks celery, finely chopped**
- **2 large oyster mushrooms, finely chopped**
- **1 pounds (455 g) white mushrooms, coarsely chopped**
- **2 teaspoons (0.6 g) dried parsley**
- **2 teaspoons (1.4 to 1.6 g) dried or fresh thyme**
- **1 ½ cups (353 ml) dry white wine**
- **4 cups (940 ml) vegetable stock**
- **1 cup (100 g) walnuts**
- **Salt and freshly ground pepper**

In a large soup pot, heat the nondairy butter and oil together over medium heat. Add the onion and cook for 5 minutes. Add the carrot and celery and cook for 5 minutes longer.

Lower the heat, and add the mushrooms, parsley, and thyme. Cook for 5 minutes. Add the wine, and increase the heat to medium-high. Bring to a boil, and cook until the liquid reduces and the alcohol cooks off. (You'll be able to smell a less noticeable alcohol smell.)

Add the stock, and stir. Reduce the heat to low and cover.

To a blender, add the walnuts and just enough hot water to cover, and let stand for 5 minutes. Blend on high speed until smooth and creamy. Ladle 2 to 3 cups (470 to 705 ml) soup from the pot into the blender, and blend until smooth. (Alternatively, you can puree the entire soup. I like the combination of smooth and chunky.)

Stir the pureed walnut mixture into the soup pot, and heat through. Add salt and pepper to taste.

Yield: 4 to 6 servings

*Wheat-free, soy-free

SHIITAKE MUSHROOMS

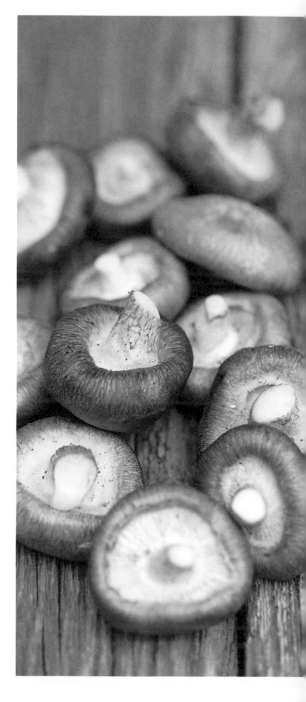

Shiitake made me the mushroom lover I am today. Also used in cancer therapy and as a treatment for high cholesterol, shiitakes are incredibly flavorful and versatile, and are used in many Asian cuisines. Dried on a large scale, they are easy to find in the most generic of grocery stores, fetching a lower price than the fresh.

In fact, because the shelf life of fresh mushrooms is extremely short, mushrooms can be preserved in a number of ways (pickled, brined, canned), but the most common means of preserving them is to dry them. To reconstitute them, you have a couple options: soak them in cold water overnight for a richer flavor and smoother texture or soak them in boiling water for 10 minutes if you're using them at the last minute.

Here are some delicious ways to prepare shiitake mushrooms:

* Sauté them with a chopped onion, minced garlic cloves, and olive oil. Cook until the mushrooms are just tender—about 10 to 15 minutes. Toss with pasta, tofu, or sautéed greens.

* Add to your favorite soups, such as vegetable, miso, or lentil.

* Make sautéed shiitake the basis for tacos or burritos.

* Marinate them in wine, and cook slowly over medium-low heat. Toss with soba noodles or pasta.

* Roast or grill them, and add to a veggie burger with caramelized onions.

* Add them to a tofu scramble.

As with all mushrooms, it's best to wipe them with a damp cloth or use them right away if you rinse them under running water. They don't keep well once they've been wet.

COMPASSIONATE LANGUAGE: **SCAPEGOAT**

A *scapegoat* is someone who is punished for the faults of another. Although scapegoats are innocent, they suffer for wrongs of another, generally to distract attention from the real culprit.

The word has its roots in the Bible when God tells Moses how Aaron is to atone for his sins. He mentions two goats, mandating that one be slaughtered as an offering and the second be allowed to escape after people symbolically lay down their sins on the Day of Atonement (Yom Kippur).

> Leviticus 16:7–10: "And Aaron shall cast lots upon the two goats; one lot for the Lord, and the other for the scapegoat."

The goat that escaped was called an *escapegoat* or *free goat* (*caper emissarius*, in Latin). When William Tindale was translating Leviticus from Hebrew into his Early Modern English, he was not familiar with a word that meant "escape" and used "scape" instead. *Scapegoat* was appropriated in the King James Version of the Bible and the word became entrenched, making it difficult to devise a compassionate alternative.

Alas, an alternative may not be necessary. In the original story, the goat has the sins of the community placed on him; he is the innocent victim. Unlike with idioms that reflect violence toward animals, the use of the word *scapegoat* reflects the ugliness of the act and the person who "scapegoats" more than it belittles goats.

REFRAMING ANGER

Learning about the atrocities enacted against animals is enough to drive the most levelheaded of us to despair, grief, and even anger. Desperate and outraged, many new activists become engulfed by their grief, which manifests itself as anger.

And why shouldn't they be angry? Corporate greed, personal convenience, and human pleasure drive the institutionalized abuse of billions of nonhuman animals all over the globe. It's considered radical to oppose this. Of course they're angry.

Anger is a real response to a devastating reality. I encourage people to identify anger for what it is, to accept it as a part of awakening, and to resist

being afraid of it, suppressing it, or labeling it as "wrong." Feeling anger is necessary; it's what we do with anger that will make or break us.

The root of the word *anger* is the same as that for anguish. Its earliest roots referred to being "painfully constricted," a "strangling, narrowing, squeezing, throttling." If you reframe anger in this context, you can see there isn't a contradiction between the peace that comes with eating nonviolently and the anger you feel as the result of so much abuse. The key is transforming anger into action. It's easy to become cynical, disheartened, and hopeless, but that doesn't do anyone any good. Become active. Dwell in the solution rather than the problem.

"DO THEY KNOW?"
BY JOHN GALSWORTHY

John Galsworthy was an English novelist and playwright who lived from 1867 to 1933. He was also a committed social activist and an outspoken advocate not only for the women's suffrage movement and prison reform but also for animal welfare.

In 1913, Galsworthy gave a speech called "Treatment of Animals" during a meeting of the London for the Animals' Friend Society to protest the cruel treatment of performing animals. John Galsworthy observed: "The degree of a people's civilization is reflected in its attitude towards animals," reminiscent of Gandhi's oft-quoted observation: "The greatness of a nation and its moral progress can be judged by the way its animals are treated."

Galsworthy was an eloquent voice for animals and left behind some lovely observations about our relationship to them and our sadness when we lose those we have loved. This is an especially poignant poem for me, as it recalls the loss of my beloved cat, Simon, who looked at me "more plainly than all the words could" and told me he must go. (Simon died on August 5, 2009.)

Do They Know?

Do they know, as we do, that their time must come?

Yes, they know, at rare moments.

No other way can I interpret those pauses of his latter life, when, propped on his forefeet, he would sit for long minutes quite motionless— his head drooped, utterly withdrawn; then turn those eyes of his and look at me.

That look said more plainly than all words could: "Yes, I know that I must go."
If we have spirits that persist—they have.

If we know, after our departure, who we were— they do.

No one, I think, who really longs for truth, can ever glibly say which it will be for dog and man— persistence or extinction of our consciousness.

There is but one thing certain: the childishness of fretting over that eternal question.
Whichever it be, it must be right, the only possible thing.

He felt that too, I know; but then, like his master, he was what is called a pessimist.
My companion tells me that, since he left us, he has once come back.
It was Old Year's Night, and she was sad, when he came to her in visible shape of his black body, passing round the dining table from the window end, to his proper place beneath the table, at her feet.

She saw him quite clearly; she heard the padding tap-tap of his paws and very toe-nails; she felt his warmth brushing hard against the front of her skirt.

She thought then that he would settle down upon her feet, but something disturbed him, and he stood pausing, pressed against her, then moved out toward where I generally sit, but was not sitting that night.

She saw him stand there, as if considering; then at some sound or laugh, she became self-conscious, and slowly, very slowly, he was no longer there.

Had he some message, some counsel to give, something he would say, that last night of the last year of all those he had watched over us?

Will he come back again?

No stone stands over where he lies. It is on our hearts that his life is engraved.

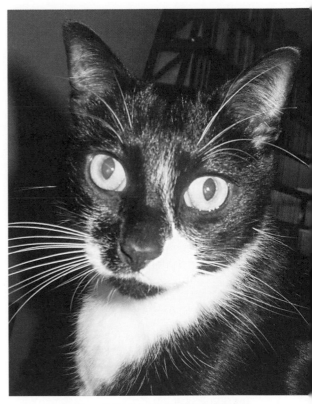

Simon, Colleen's beloved cat for sixteen years

BRUCE IN A NATION OF PIGS

Bruce grew up on a farm—alone. Sometimes a pony kept him company; sometimes it was a town of Bruce, population one. Of course, he didn't have a name then. It was just "pig" or "hog," nothing to identify him as an individual. And for years, he was deprived of nourishment. At one point, he looked like a skeleton with skin draped over him. To see an animal so enamoured of food be so painfully denied that life-sustaining nourishment is heartbreaking.

Most farmed animals never get to run free at a sanctuary. The lucky ones do so because they have advocates: people who see cruelty and refuse to look away. For Bruce, this came in the form of an anonymous woman who tried to reason with the farmer, but no luck. She called Animal Control—no luck. She took pictures and showed them *again* to Animal Control. They came out and deemed the property acceptable for farmed animals. This is when most people would give up.

But this person didn't. She researched sanctuaries and found Animal Place. Staff drove out to the property and knew right away something needed to be done. It took some convincing, but the farmer finally agreed to let Bruce come to Animal Place.

As rescues go, he was one of the easiest animals to load up and transport to his new home. He *wanted* to leave, and anyone who was nice enough to share food with him was someone he wanted to befriend. When Bruce arrived at the sanctuary he was confined to a stall. Before his eyes was a veritable feast—anything he wanted, he received. He was in heaven, but it was a quiet place, save for the sound of his smacking lips. Bruce didn't talk. No grunts of contentment, no screams of displeasure, no gracious greetings or loud departures. Just silence, and in it Bruce, still population one.

There were times when we thought he'd never talk, never seek out the contact pigs thrive on. We gave him time. We let him eat until he gained 300 pounds (136 kg). And then we let him out to be with his own kind, his own nation of pigs. He thwarted us, choosing to go off on his own, sleeping under the stars, mostly avoiding the other pigs.

Little by little, Bruce started to loosen up. It took years. He started to develop friendships and bonds with the other pigs, but he never opened up to them, never really shared his words with them.

But that's okay. Accepting each individual as a unique, feeling being means honoring each unique personality. It is the least that can be offered to these animals who have suffered so much.

—*Marji Beach of Animal Place, Grass Valley, California (U.S.)*

Bruce in his sanctuary home, Animal Place

Photo courtesy of Animal Place

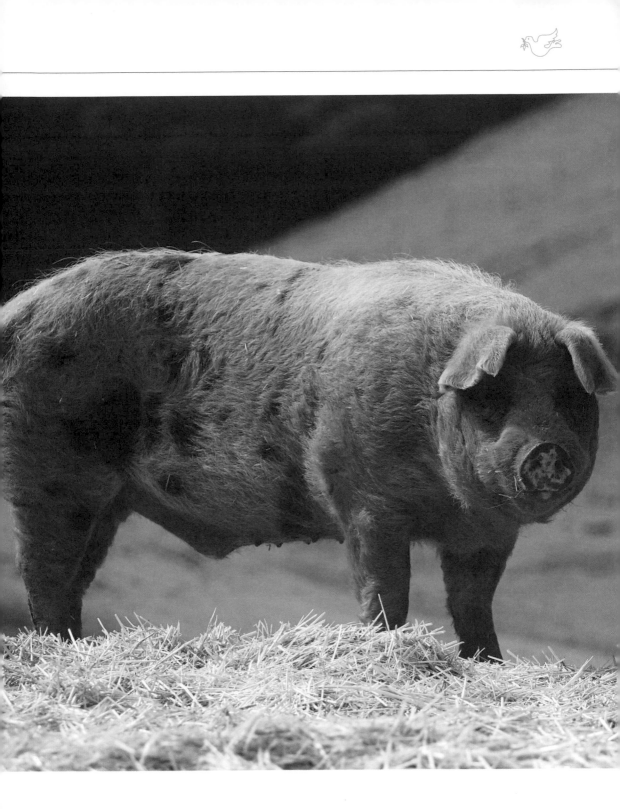

INDIAN FRIED RICE

This flavorful dish, courtesy of my friend Cadry Nelson, is a testament to the fact that "fried" need not necessarily be laden with oil.

- 1 tablespoon (15 ml) canola oil
- 2 teaspoons (4.2 g) cumin seeds
- 2 carrots, finely chopped
- 2 cups (200 g) chopped cauliflower (½ large head)
- 1 cup (130 g) frozen peas, thawed
- 1 red bell pepper, finely chopped
- 1 teaspoon (2 g) minced or grated fresh ginger
- 2 cups (330 g) cooked brown rice
- 1 tablespoon (15 ml) lemon juice
- 1 teaspoon (2 g) ground coriander
- ¼ teaspoon turmeric
- ¼ teaspoon cayenne pepper
- ½ teaspoon garam masala
- ¼ cup (60 ml) water
- Salt
- Chopped cilantro or parsley, for garnish

Heat the oil over medium heat in a large sauté pan. Test the oil by adding one cumin seed. If it pops right away, the oil is ready. Add the cumin seeds to the oil. Once they start to sizzle or pop, add the carrots and cauliflower to the pan, and stir-fry until the cauliflower starts to brown a bit and soften, about 7 minutes.

Add the peas, bell pepper, and ginger, and stir to combine. Continue cooking until all the vegetables begin to soften but remain crisp, about 5 minutes. Add the cooked rice, lemon juice, coriander, turmeric, cayenne, and garam masala and toss to combine. Add the water, and cook for about 5 minutes longer, stirring frequently.

Add salt to taste, and remove from the heat. Garnish with the cilantro, and serve.

Yield: 4 servings

*Wheat-free, soy-free

BLACK BEANS

The black bean (also called the black turtle bean) is commonly used in countries in and around the Caribbean. Black beans have a dense, meaty texture—almost earthy, like mushrooms.

* A simple way to prepare them is to open a can of beans, rinse and drain them, and heat them on the stove in about ¼ cup (60 ml) water with cumin and chili powder. While they're heating, sauté garlic, onions, and tomatoes, and then stir together with the beans. Or, add salsa or a can of fire-roasted tomatoes to the beans. Serve over brown rice or rolled in a tortilla.

* To make tacos, prepare as above, mashing the beans before you add the tomatoes/salsa, so the mixture sits in a taco shell. Add your favorite fixings, and serve.

* To make black bean quesadillas, spread hummus on a flour or corn tortilla, and place it faceup in a nonstick pan over medium-low heat. Spoon a thin layer of black beans (mashed or whole) on top of the hummus with some salsa, a couple of slices of avocado, and maybe spinach leaves or tomatoes. Just don't overfill. Add a second tortilla on top, let the bottom tortilla turn golden brown, and flip. Let the other side get golden brown, and remove from the pan. Cut into triangles with kitchen shears, and serve right away.

* Because they're easy to mash and bind well, you can use black beans to make burgers and loaves.

MORE COMPASSIONATE ALTERNATIVES TO VIOLENT BIRD IDIOMS

Stone the crows—An expression of surprise or dismay, it is most likely of British or Australian origin. Because crows tend to be disliked by farmers, it isn't a hard leap to imagine people throwing stones at them—in surprise and annoyance at their eating crops. There are other nonsensical expressions that make the same point, without referencing cruelty to crows, such as:

* I'll go to the foot of our stairs!

* Strike me pink!

* I'll be a monkey's uncle!

* If that don't take the rag off the bush!

Stop cold turkey—This expression has everything to do with "turkey meat." An idiom used mostly in the United States, it refers to someone suddenly quitting an addictive substance (or, by extension, any habit or pattern of behavior). The exact origin is unknown, but it most likely arose from another idiom: "to talk turkey," which means to talk plainly. Because "cold turkey" (meat) is a plain, uncomplicated meal, it became a metaphor for no-nonsense, direct speech. Since "talk turkey" or "talk cold turkey" was already a popular idiom, it is likely it came to mean "to quit suddenly, with no nonsense or equivocation." Alternatives? How about *cold potato*? Really, any "plain" food will do.

To call someone a **"stool pigeon"** is to call him a police informer or a criminal's lookout. Most sources indicate that this expression derives from the hunting practice of affixing a dead or replica pigeon to a stool to act as a decoy to attract other birds. "Informant," "snitch," and "whistle-blower" are phrases that work just as well, and no birds were hunted in the making of them.

SUPPORTING COMMUNITY SUPPORTED AGRICULTURE

Community Supported Agriculture (CSA) in the consumer has a direct relationship with the farmer. In exchange for a fee, a box of produce is delivered to your door or to a pickup location near by each week (or however often you decide).

The produce is locally grown, just harvested, often mostly organic, and delicious. Local Harvest is the premier resource to find a CSA near you, and they also explain well what the advantages are for grower and consumer.

When you participate in a CSA, it changes the way you cook somewhat, and it might not work for those people who keep a rigid meal plan. Because you will receive vegetables you've never cooked with before or didn't plan on, it forces you to be creative.

Many farms now enable you to opt in or opt out of certain items. For instance, you might say you don't ever want cilantro or that you want more fruit than vegetables. Some even allow you to choose exactly what you want based on available options. Many farms also offer flowers, preserves, or nuts. Often they partner with a neighboring farm to provide more variety to the CSA customers.

Most farms also include recipes for the ingredients in the box, and many of the recipes are vegetarian and can easily be made vegan with a few switcheroos.

EXCERPT FROM "THE HUNTING OF THE STAG"
BY MARGARET CAVENDISH

Margaret Cavendish, Duchess of Newcastle-upon-Tyne (1623–1673), was a poet, a philosopher, an essayist, a playwright, and a voice for the animals. Cavendish used her social influence and position as a published writer to express her animal-protection views publicly.

Her deep sympathy for animals is apparent in two poems, whose narrator describes a hunt ("The Hunting of the Hare" and "The Hunting of the Stag"), focusing on the suffering of the terrified animals rather than of the prowess of the hunters.

> The Stag no hope had left, nor help espies.
> His Heart so heavie grew, with Griefe, and Care,
> That his small Feet his Body could not beare.
> Yet loth to dye, or yeild to Foes was he,

> But to the last would strive for Victory.
> Twas not for want of Courage he did run,
> But that an Army against One did come.
> Had he the Valour of bold Casar stout,
> Must yeild himselfe to them, or dye no doubt.
> Turning his Head, as if he dar'd their Spight,
> Prepar'd himselfe against them all to fight.
> Single he was, his Hornes were all his helpes,
> To guard him from a Multitude of Whelpes.
> Besides, a company of Men were there,
> If Dogs should faile, to strike him every where.
> But to the last his Fortune he'll try out:
> The Men, and Dogs do circle him about.
> Some bite, some bark, all ply him at the Bay,
> Where with his Hornes he tosses some away.
> But Fate his thread had spun, so downe did fall,
> Shedding some Teares at his owne Funerall.

A PIG NAMED FRANKLIN

I peered through the door of the cat-sized crate at the sanctuary's newest friend: a brown-eyed, pink-skinned, 4-pound (1.8 kg) piglet whom we'd soon name Franklin.

He had been found him lying against a wall at a pig farm. Tossed there by the farmer who knew he was too small to thrive, he was shivering and would soon be dead. His siblings, slated to become bacon, pork chops, and sausage, would be allowed to nurse briefly, then subjected to a wretched life before being shipped for slaughter by six months of age.

Life, it seems, had a different plan for Franklin.

Once I whispered to him to come out, Franklin was in my lap in a nanosecond, pressing hard into my arm, my belly, my thigh with a snout the size of a quarter. His need to nurse and to root consumed him. For the next weeks and months, Franklin was fed every couple of hours, was allowed to roam the house freely, and followed me as closely as if I were his mother.

Still only the size of a golden retriever, still terrified of adult pigs, Franklin was not ready for life with the big pigs, many of whom weigh well over 1,000 pounds (454 kg). So we turned him out in the goat pasture just steps outside the main barn and in full view of all the goings-on, where, naturally, he had a tantrum of the first order.

Franklin screamed; first loud, then louder. He paced the fence until . . . he smelled sympathy.

"Can I please give him a pumpkin?" staffer Allen Landes asked.

"Oh, good grief, okay," I said. I couldn't wait to watch our little imp bite a hole in the baby pumpkin so that he could race gleefully around the field (the one that just moments ago was his prison), holding the pumpkin in front of his snout like a bulbous appendage, exclaiming, "Look, world! My new favorite treat!"

We humans were defeated once again, like we always are at this place where animals rule, where we're the bosses only in theory.

—*Kathy Stevens, founder of Catskill Animal Sanctuary, Saugerties, New York (U.S.)*

ROASTED BALSAMIC RADICCHIO

Because the vinegar is simply drizzled over the radicchio at the end, try to find an artisan-quality balsamic, as opposed to one labeled "of Modena."

> 2 large heads radicchio (about 1 pound [455 g] total), halved through the core end, each half cut into 3 wedges with some core still attached
> 3 tablespoons (45 ml) olive oil
> 1 tablespoon (2.4 g) chopped fresh thyme
> Salt and freshly ground pepper
> Balsamic vinegar, for drizzling

Preheat the oven to 450°F (230°C, or gas mark 8).

Rinse the radicchio wedges with water; gently shake off the excess water (do not dry completely). Place the radicchio in a large bowl. Drizzle with the olive oil and sprinkle with the thyme, salt, and pepper; toss to coat.

Arrange the radicchio wedges, cut side up, on a rimmed baking sheet. Roast until wilted, about 12 minutes. Turn over and roast until tender, about 8 minutes longer.

Arrange the radicchio on a platter, drizzle with the balsamic vinegar, and serve right away.

Yield: 4 servings

*Wheat-free, soy-free

See Day 218 for information on vinegars.

SEITAN

Pronounced *SAY-tan*, this wheat-based food has many names: wheat gluten, grain meat, wheat meat, gluten meat, and mock meat. Believed to have originated in China where Buddhists eschewed the consumption of animal flesh, seitan was developed as an alternative to duck meat.

Seitan has been eaten in Asia for centuries, though the exact moment of discovery remains a mystery. Legend has it that seventh-century Chinese Buddhist monks were searching for a

chewier meat alternative that wasn't tofu. As they were making a simple dough out of wheat flour and water, they noticed that the starch rinsed off. The more they kneaded, the more the starch came out. After considerable kneading, they produced a chewy, protein-rich substance they called "wheat meat" or *mien chien*. It has also been called "Buddha's food."

Fast-forward many years to Japan, where cooks took it a step further, simmering it in soy sauce, sea vegetables, ginger, and other seasonings, and created what they called "seitan," whose etymology is unknown.

When Chinese and Japanese traversed the Pacific to North America, they brought with them their wheat-based meats. Today, it is widely available in a relatively simple state, which you can marinate yourself or add to any dish, or as a main ingredient in flavored vegetarian meats, such as Field Roast's sausages, deli slices, and meat loaf.

Sauté seitan as part of a stir-fry, grill it, bake it, barbecue it, or fry it. Flavor it however you like, and serve it up.

 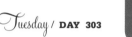

MORE COMPASSIONATE ALTERNATIVES TO VIOLENT BIRD IDIOMS

Several of our common idioms about birds would be best put to rest in favor of kinder, gentler language.

* Your **"goose is cooked"** if you're ruined, damaged, or in trouble. For instance, if you borrow money you can't pay back, "your goose is cooked." How about *your cookies are burned* instead?

* If something is **"as easy as duck soup,"** you can say it is *as easy as boiling water.*

* Instead of warning people not to **"put all your eggs in one basket,"** you can warn them not to put *all of your berries in one bowl.*

* Instead of going on a **"wild goose chase,"** you can just pursue a *fruitless search*, because that's all it means.

* To **"eat crow"** is one that cries out for a compassionate version. To "eat crow" is to "abase oneself," and you can easily just say *to eat humble pie.*

* Something that is **"for the birds"** is "trivial" and "worthless" and is a shortened form of a vulgar saying suggesting the habit of some birds of pecking at horse droppings to find seeds. Say instead that something is simply *for the trash heap.*

THINKING MAKES IT SO

I believe the creation of the world we want starts with our thoughts. If we see abundance, that's what we will experience. If we see lack, then that, too, will be.

With so much suffering in the world, it can be hard to feel hopeful. With so many billions of animals killed for human consumption, many people are tempted to say, "Things will never change. The problem is just too large."

If that is what we think, then it will be so. If we believe that injustice will prevail, then it will.

But let me just say I don't share those thoughts, and those negative thoughts compete with my hopeful thoughts that justice will prevail.

It is because of this hope, because of the transformations I witness every day, that I remain a joyful vegan. In any given moment, I can choose this perspective or I can choose despair or fear or compromise. But I choose hope.

Don't underestimate the power of thought; it shapes our perceptions, it determines our actions, and it creates the world we envision. If I'm wrong, I have nothing to lose by thinking this way; but if I'm right, there will come a time when we look back upon our consumption of and treatment of nonhuman animals and say, "What were we *thinking*?"

"BEYOND LIES THE WUB"
BY PHILIP K. DICK

A 1952 science fiction short story, this is the provocative tale about a group of men who travel to Mars on an expedition to round up exotic animals and bring them back to Earth. When one crew member, named Peterson, boards the spaceship with a 400-pound (181 kg) piglike creature called a "Wub," his captain Franco is less interested in the Wub's apparent intelligence and more in how it might taste.

As they begin their journey back home, the crew realizes that the Wub is a sophisticated creature, capable of telepathy and possibly even mind control. Peterson and the Wub pass time discussing mythology, though Franco is fixated on killing and eating it.

When asked about his race, the Wub says they live on "Plants. Vegetables. We live and let live. That's how we've gotten along. And that's why I so violently objected to this business about having me boiled . . . How can any lasting contract be established between your people and mine if you resort to such barbaric attitudes?" But Franco kills the Wub.

The crew opposes the killing and sits sullenly around the table as Franco finishes his meal. To their amazement, he then resumes the earlier conversation Peterson had been having with the Wub, who, through death and digestion, has possessed the captain's body.

COMPASSIONATE CHRISTIAN IN JAPAN

For years, my husband and I discussed going vegan. We talked openly together about being uncomfortable and disgusted by what we knew, without knowing how we were going to tackle the obstacles of family disapproval, lack of education, and a perceived lack of choice. It seemed too big. Living vegan . . . all the time. It seemed like this huge mountain that we couldn't realistically climb.

We hit a moment two months ago, as I was preparing a Thanksgiving meal that included turkey, when it all clicked. I am an excellent cook, and I have spent a lifetime in the kitchen. As an adult I have prepared more than fifteen years' worth of holiday meals as well as home-cooked meat dishes on a daily basis. That day, as I looked at the dead bird on my counter, slathered with butter and stuffed with spices, I called my husband into the kitchen and told him it was time to put the turkey in the oven.

He could tell that something was wrong. I was standing there with my hands covered in grease, and I was revolted. For some reason, the veil between ourselves and the truth about our food had just crashed down. I couldn't distance myself far enough from the truth to eat this turkey with complacency. I confessed this to my husband; he wrapped his arms around me, and things have changed since that day.

We began living as vegans with patience, curiosity, and joy. We still make mistakes, but we're learning, and this process has already brought so much happiness and light into our home. Making the choice was like immediately being lifted to the peak of that imaginary mountain we feared. Let me tell you: The view from up here is breathtaking.

—*Amy in Okinawa, Japan*

ROASTED RED PEPPER RELISH

This is a quick-to-prepare appetizer for an unexpected guest or a great side dish for burgers or wraps.

- **2 roasted red peppers, finely chopped**
- **½ cup (50 g) finely chopped kalamata olives**
- **2 cloves garlic, pressed or crushed**
- **1 shallot, finely chopped**
- **1 tablespoon (15 ml) balsamic vinegar**
- **1 tablespoon (15 ml) olive oil**
- **2 tablespoons (5 g) chopped fresh basil**
- **1 tablespoon (4 g) chopped fresh parsley**
- **Salt and freshly ground pepper**

Combine all the ingredients in a large bowl. Store for a week in the refrigerator, or serve right away. The flavors will intensify.

Serve on toasted baguette slices or grilled polenta squares.

Yield: 1 ½ to 2 cups (375 to 500 g)

COMPASSIONATE COOKS TIP
The finely chopped roasted red peppers should yield ½ to ¾ cup (90 to 135 g).

*Wheat-free, soy-free

Originally published in *Color Me Vegan*

261

MIDDLE MEALS

The foods we choose, the meals we plan, and the way we construct our plates are cultural, personal, familial, and societal habits. Likewise, though the notion of eating three meals a day is a strongly ingrained habit, if we look around the world, we'll find that eating throughout the day is a time-honored tradition.

Brunch

Brunch, a portmanteau of *breakfast* and *lunch*, originated in the United Kingdom in the nineteenth century among the privileged elite, who had the time and money to enjoy extracurricular meals. Today, especially in the United States, it's a late-morning meal consisting of standard breakfast foods and typically enjoyed between 10:00 a.m. and 1:00 p.m.

Elevenses

Perhaps taking our suggestion to the extreme, the Hobbits who live in J. R. R. Tolkien's Middle Earth enjoy seven meals a day (breakfast, second breakfast, elevenses, luncheon, tea, dinner, and supper). Although the term may be a little outdated, elevenses (taken around 11 a.m.) refers to an actual snack time in the United Kingdom—similar to afternoon tea but eaten in the morning.

Tiffin

Related to the Old English word *tiffing*, meaning "a little drink or sip," a tiffin in India refers to a light meal eaten during the day. Prepared for working Indian men by their wives, these meals are transported using a complex system to get these tiffin boxes to their destinations. Commonly, rice is in one box, dal (a thick stew made with lentils, onions, and spices) is in another, and bread, vegetable curry, and a sweet are each in their own boxes.

Dim Sum

A Cantonese word meaning "touch the heart," dim sum consists of a variety of dumplings, steamed dishes, other sweet and savory goodies, and lots of green tea. In restaurants, customers select small dishes from passing carts, and though you can ask for vegan options, you'll have many more to choose from if you host your own brunch at home. Serve steamed green vegetables, tofu dumplings, pot stickers, steamed buns, spring rolls, and mango pudding.

PRAYER FOR HUMANS ON BEHALF OF THE ANIMALS

As an animal activist, I have learned many things about animals, but I have learned a lot more about humans. If I didn't hear from the most remarkable people every day who share their stories of transformation, it would be very challenging to hold on to any hope for humanity in general or the animal rights movement in particular. But I do have hope, and it fills my heart every day.

I wrote this prayer to remind us of who we are and what we have to learn from the animals. Many people have asked for it over the years and have used it as a way to speak on behalf of the animals.

My hope is that we can navigate through this world and our lives with the grace and integrity of those who need our protection. May we have the sense of humor and liveliness of the goats; may we have the maternal instincts and protective nature of the hens and the sassiness of the roosters. May we have the gentleness and strength of the cattle, and the wisdom, humility, and serenity of the donkeys. May we appreciate the need for community as do the sheep and choose our companions as carefully as do the rabbits. May we have the faithfulness and commitment to family of the geese, the adaptability and affability of the ducks. May we have the intelligence, loyalty, and affection of the pigs and the inquisitiveness, sensitivity, and playfulness of the turkeys.

My hope is that we learn from the animals what it is we need to become better people.

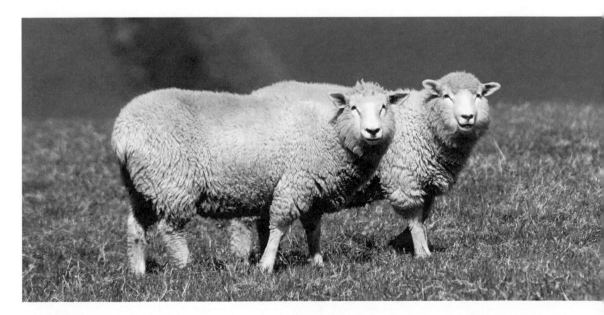

EATING ORGANIC

I'm often asked how to incorporate "organic" food into our diets without breaking the bank. First of all, the typical consumer is not paying the true cost of food. The meat, dairy, and egg industries, in particular, enjoy many government subsidies, which keep the cost of these unhealthful products artificially low and thus affordable.

The same goes for produce laden with chemical fertilizers and pesticides. Organic fruits and veggies are usually not grown on an industrial scale, so efficiencies aren't as great, and there are also significant costs involved in switching farmland from nonorganic to organic status. Growing costs tend to be higher because there is more manual labor involved, such as weeding by hand.

In other words, it's not that organic is expensive; it's the nonorganic is cheap.

To purchase organic produce means supporting a growing system that works with the Earth rather than against it. You're paying for sustainable growing methods that enrich rather than deplete the soil. When you purchase nonorganic produce that was shipped in from other countries, there are concerns about food safety, as well. The growing standards in other countries may not be the same as those in the United States or wherever you live.

As we adjust to paying the true cost of food and a nontoxic system of agriculture, it's helpful to know which fruits and vegetables are the most highly sprayed so we can make informed decisions when we simply cannot purchase everything organic. Certain produce, termed the "Dirty Dozen" by the Environmental Working Group, is so highly sprayed with toxic chemicals that many experts recommend eating them only when they're organic.

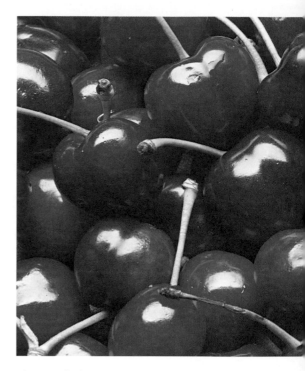

These include:

* Apples
* Cherries
* Grapes, imported
* Nectarines
* Peaches
* Pears
* Raspberries
* Strawberries
* Bell peppers
* Celery
* Kale
* Potatoes

AMORES PERROS
DIRECTED BY ALEJANDRO GONZÁLEZ IÑÁRRITU

Amores Perros is a fast-paced Mexican film whose intricate narrative tells three different stories linked by a car crash in Mexico City. Each of the three vignettes is a reflection on the relationship between cruelty to animals and violence toward humans. Whether taking place in the dirty underground dog-fighting culture or in the seemingly respectable upper middle class, animal cruelty cannot but affect the people who participate in it or witness it.

The first segment, "Octavio y Susana," reveals the extreme violence of the illegal dog-fighting industry. Because of the realistic nature of the fights and the appearance of bloody dogs, who really do look dead, many viewers and critics believed director Iñárritu staged actual dog fights and thus boycotted the movie. Even once he demonstrated that no animals were harmed in the creation of the simulated fights (the DVD includes a documentary that shows how the scenes were filmed using trained dogs), others criticized him for romanticizing the dog-fighting world.

Although some filmic depictions of violence are certainly gratuitous and are utilized only for shock value or entertainment, there is nothing romantic or entertaining about these graphic scenes. They are a reflection of reality, revealing the ugliness of this world and the depravity of the people steeped in it. Violence toward animals does not exist in a vacuum; it extends in every direction, contaminating everyone involved. Drug addiction, alcoholism, murder, crime, spousal abuse, and child abuse are all by-products of an industry marked by greed and aggression, and this is what the film depicts.

The second segment, "Daniel y Valeria," focuses on a couple whose already strained relationship—he had recently left his family for her—disintegrates when Valeria, a famous fashion model, is struck by a car and suffers a severely broken leg, confining her to a wheelchair. The car that hits her was driven by Octavio of the first segment. An innocent victim of the violent repercussions of the dog-fighting industry, Valeria reinjures her leg trying to save her dog, who has disappeared under the floorboards in her apartment. The trauma of the accident and her obsession with trying to save her dog cause Daniel and Valeria's once-loving relationship to spiral downward into a point of no return.

In the third segment, "El Chivo y Maru," the focus is on a man named El Chivo ("The Goat"), who appears briefly in the first two stories and now links them all together. A professional hit man, El Chivo, played by the remarkable Emilio Echevarría, dresses as a scruffy vagabond and pushes a shopping cart full of junk, accompanied by several homeless dogs for whom he cares.

Witnessing the car crash in which Octavio hits Valeria, El Chivo tenderly retrieves Octavio's injured and bleeding dog, Cofi, and takes him home to nurse him. Because violence has been ingrained in Cofi after so many dogfights, tragedy strikes when El Chivo leaves Cofi in the company of his six beloved dogs. In a powerful scene of forgiveness and self-awareness, El Chivo realizes he is no different than Cofi, both victims in a culture of violence.

Experiencing a transformation that is both physical and spiritual, El Chivo is the hope on which the movie ends.

NONVEGETARIAN BUDDHIST BECOMES VEGAN

I was born in Taiwan but grew up mostly in Africa and the United States. One vivid memory I have of Taiwan is of my mom taking my brother and me to the market to buy turtles. Afterward, we traveled to a river and set them free. This practice of "releasing life" is common among devout Buddhists.

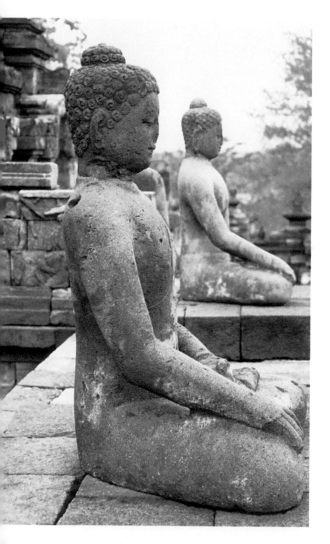

Unlike many Buddhist monks and nuns, we were not vegetarian. In fact, I hated vegetables and wanted to eat only meat. I always saw vegetarianism as a "preference" or a "healthy lifestyle choice" rather than an ethical practice. In my twenties, I would even tell my vegetarian friends (half jokingly) that I was going to write a book about how vegetarianism is bad for our planet. I think back now about how naïve I was, but I just *loved* meat.

In my early thirties, I became more interested in ethics as a secular alternative to organized religion. I started reading books on ethics, including Peter Singer's *Writings on an Ethical Life*. The book covered many issues, but there was enough in there about animal welfare to make me give "vegetarianism" a try. It lasted six months.

A few years later, Peter Singer released another book, *The Way We Eat: Why Our Food Choices Matter*. After I read it, I knew there was no going back. I had to give up meat—and all animal products—for good.

I had to learn how to cook. I bought several vegan cookbooks, rolled up my sleeves, and started cooking in earnest. I wanted to make sure that my focus was not on what I was giving up but what I'm eating. The new diet had to be *more* pleasurable, not *less*. When I began cooking for real (and not just heating up food), my meals became more tasty, more adventurous, and more healthful.

Every time I cook, eat, or shop, I am aware of the suffering I am alleviating and the liberation that is possible for myself and other animals. I know I am making a difference—that I am "releasing life" every day—and there's true joy in that.

—*Charles in Vancouver, British Columbia*

PESTO PASTA TOSS

The following recipe proves that you absolutely do not need cheese to make a fantastic pesto.

PESTO

- 3 cups (120 g) loosely packed fresh basil leaves
- 6 tablespoons (54 g) pine nuts
- 2 to 4 cloves garlic
- 1 to 3 tablespoons (15 to 45 ml) extra-virgin olive oil
- ½ teaspoon salt, or to taste

PASTA AND VEGGIES

- 1 pound (455 g) penne pasta (or any pasta of your choice)
- Bunch of chopped spinach, raw or blanched
- Fresh, seasonal tomatoes, chopped
- Fresh basil, chopped

To make the pesto, combine the basil, pine nuts, and garlic in a food processor, and blend until the ingredients are finely chopped, scraping down the sides of the bowl as necessary. Add the oil slowly and a little at a time, and process until smooth and creamy (you do not need a lot of oil—just add enough to smooth it out a little). Add the salt to taste.

Prepare the pasta according to the package directions. Drain. Toss the pasta with the pesto, chopped tomatoes, and fresh basil.

Yield: 4 servings

COMPASSIONATE COOKS TIP
Pesto freezes very well. Defrost it at room temperature for 20 minutes. To reinvigorate frozen or refrigerated pesto, add a drizzle of olive oil and stir.

*Soy-free

AGAR-AGAR

Agar is a gelatinous substance derived from red algae and known as "vegetarian gelatin,," kanten, or Japanese isinglass. The word *agar* comes from the Malay word *agar-agar*, which simply means "jelly."

Japanese cuisine tends to specialize in the use of agar, such as in a dessert called *anmitsu*, made of small cubes of agar jelly and served in a bowl with various fruits. With its soft, slippery texture, it takes getting used to in this form.

Agar works beautifully in place of animal-based gelatin, which is the boiled remains of bones, skin, and connective tissues of animals, most often cattle, pigs, horses, and fish. Labeled commercially as "agar-agar," this vegetable gelatin comes in small packages of semitranslucent white flakes. Directions for use should be on the package, but essentially, you mix the flakes with water, and boil until the solids dissolve. Once it is dissolved in water, it is essentially translucent and begins to thicken. It can be used as a thickener, but arrowroot, kudzu root, or cornstarch work better; reserve agar as a gelatin. It will definitely lend a gelatinous texture to whatever dish you use it in.

ADMITTING WHEN YOU DON'T KNOW

In addition to asking questions (see Day 51), it's important to simply admit when you don't have the answer to a question about veganism, animal rights, or nutrition. People appreciate this much more than if you try and fake an answer or if you appear to be grasping at straws just to have something to say.

Admitting that you don't know something goes a long way when talking about such an emotional and misrepresented issue and gives you more credibility than if you made up a statistic that may or may not be accurate. It's perfectly reasonable, humble, truthful, and effective to simply say:

* "That's a really good question, I'm not really sure about that. Let me find out and get back to you." (And then get back to them!)

* "I've never heard that before. I'm really curious myself now. Can you tell me more?"

* If the question/debate is about nutrition, you can say, "Ya know, I'm not an expert, but all I can tell you is that I feel better, I look better, my skin's clearer, and my heart is more open, and I just love living this way." No one can argue with that.

Always err on the side of humility and honesty.

SCAPEGOATING TRANS FATS

As if people aren't confused enough about "good fats" and "bad fats," along came the opponents of "trans fats," whose campaign to have them banned enables food companies to commend themselves for selling products that are "trans-fat-free." Trans fats have been linked to increased dietary cholesterol (and hence risk of heart disease), but they're incredibly easy to avoid by eating a diet based on whole foods.

Trans fats are essentially the result of plant fats that have been partially hydrogenated to increase their shelf life and reduce the need for refrigeration. The products that contains trans fats are convenience food, fast food, packaged food, processed food, and fried food.

But if you look at the marketing language of these products, you'd think you were eating nature's bounty. Trans-fat-free doughnuts and cookies do not a healthy choice make. And yet all the media buzz around fast-food restaurants using palm oil (not a trans fat) completely masks the real issue: once you remove the trans fat from a meal at a fast-food restaurant or doughnut shop, you're still eating artery-clogging junk.

If you are looking to eat a trans-fat-free diet and feel good about it, check out the produce section of your grocery store.

"WATCH THE ANIMALS"
BY ALICE ELLIOTT DARK

A keen observer of humans and their idiosyncrasies, contemporary American writer Alice Elliott Dark seems to know what makes people tick, as evidenced by her compassionate portrayal of the main character, narrator, and community of women who make up those who "Watch the Animals."

A woman named Diana Frick, a "moneyed blue blood" who lives in a tony community in the fictional East Coast town of Wynnemoor, is dying of cancer and asks her neighbors to care for her myriad of animals when she is gone.

We learn from the narrator, an anonymous member of the community, that Diane "was interested in animals to the point of obsession," having "chosen the company of other species over companionship with her own kind, a preference we naturally took as a rejection." Revealing her own bias, the narrator talks about the annoyance many of the neighbors felt at being asked to take on such a responsibility, especially in light of the way Diana goes about it: "People want to believe they are high-minded and generous, not greedy and bought. A good monger could have offered us the same deal in terms that would have us not only clamoring to agree to it, but also feeling grateful she'd come to us. Diana created no such feeling."

Despite their own disapproval of Diana's tactlessness, they admire her nonetheless, being animal lovers themselves: "She took [in those] animals that otherwise would have ended up euthanized at best, and she trained them and groomed them and nursed them and fed them home-cooked foods until—we had to admit—they bore a resemblance to the more fortunate of their species."

In the end, the neighbors reveal the largeness of their hearts, all of them agreeing to care for Diana's brood. They also care for Diana herself during the last days of her waning health: "She was dying and there was no time to dwell on slights or insults, no room for the luxuries of holding grudges and taking offense. She needed us at last, and her need was as good as an apology."

When they find her on a spring morning, having died the night before, it is a peaceful scene: "The only disturbing note was that the dogs were still with her—the large ones in their customary spots along the walls, and the smaller creatures arrayed around her on the bed like a wreath."

Her final words, written on a note: *Watch the dogs.*

BABE

Babe is a female African elephant who was born into a herd in Kruger National Park in South Africa in 1984. That year, park rangers decided that too many elephants were living in the park and some of them would have to be killed. Babe's mother and all of the older elephants around her were shot. The baby elephants, including Babe, were then sold to zoos and circuses around the world or taken to other parks.

Babe was packed into a tiny crate and shipped to a small circus in the United States. Upon her arrival in 1985, it was discovered the Babe— terrified and alone—had thrashed about in her crate so much that she badly bruised her head and broke her right front leg. No care was provided for Babe's painful injuries. The bruises faded and her leg slowly healed, but it remains permanently deformed.

While in the circus, at the age of one, another large elephant began to bully Babe while they stood for endless hours chained next to one another. This caused severe injury to her right hind leg. Again, no one treated the injuries. Despite Babe's obvious limp, she was forced to perform in the circus for the next eleven years.

By age twelve, she was no longer able to perform or make the circus money, so she was no longer wanted. In the first turn of good fortune in Babe's young life, she arrived at Cleveland Amory Black Beauty Ranch sanctuary on February 14, 1996. She was thin, hungry, scared, and in pain. Slowly, with the compassionate care of a loving staff, Babe began to build trust. She was fed healthy fruits, vegetables, hay, grasses, and a special elephant diet to build weight and strength. Her dry skin was bathed and oiled daily.

Over time, she began to recover from the trauma of those early years. Upon veterinary examination, however, it was confirmed that Babe's legs would always be damaged and her feet fused the way they had healed. Walking would always be difficult for her, and eventually her damaged bones and joints would degenerate more quickly than those of other elephants without her disabilities.

Babe spent her days peacefully at the sanctuary. She had her own barn with a heated floor, a pool where she could dip and cool off during hot summers, and the companionship of hundreds of other rescued animals. Babe was twenty-six years old when she succumbed to the effects of her injuries.

Although her journey was difficult, she spent years with friends who loved her and provided for her every need.

—Diane Miller of Cleveland Amory Rolling Dog Ranch, Murchison, Texas (U.S.)

Beautiful Babe

Photo by Jean-Paul Bonnelly

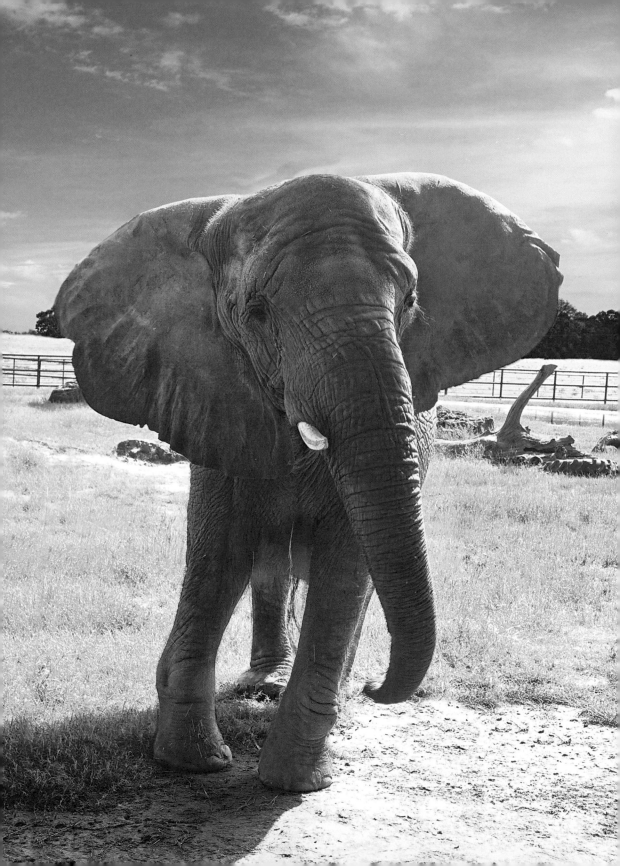

ROASTED MUSHROOMS WITH HERBS

In all the years I've been enjoying mushrooms, I never roasted them until recently. A delicious way to enjoy mushrooms, they can be cooked for as little or as long as you like, changing the texture completely.

12 ounces (340 g) cremini mushrooms, washed, stemmed, and sliced
4 ounces (115 g) shiitake mushrooms, washed, stemmed, and sliced
¼ cup (60 ml) olive oil
Salt and freshly ground pepper
¼ to ½ cup (10 to 25 g) loosely packed minced fresh herbs such as chives, thyme, marjoram, and parsley

Preheat the oven to 475°F (240°C, or gas mark 9). Line a large baking sheet with parchment.

Toss the mushrooms in a large bowl with the olive oil and a generous amount of salt and pepper. The mushrooms soak in the oil pretty quickly, so toss right away to distribute evenly and trust that the oil will come out when the mushrooms start cooking.

Place the tray in the oven, and roast for 20 minutes, then toss the mushrooms once, and return to the oven. Roast for an additional 10 minutes, or until they are dark and slightly shrunken.

Return the roasted mushrooms to the bowl. Taste, and add more salt and pepper, if necessary. Toss with the herbs, then transfer to a serving dish. Serve immediately.

Yield: 2 to 4 servings

*Soy-free, wheat-free

AZUKI BEANS

These beans have long been cultivated in Asia, originating most likely in China. They were brought to Japan sometime between the third and eighth centuries. The word *azuki* means "small bean."

Containing more fiber than any other bean (a whopping 17 grams per cup), they are widely used in Japanese cuisine—second in popularity to the soybean. Although they can be prepared and eaten whole like any other legume, they are most commonly eaten as red bean paste, especially in Japan, where the beans are boiled with sugar to make a paste and then used to create sweet treats and confections.

For special occasions in Japan, azuki is used to make a celebrated dish called *sekihan*, which translates literally into "red bean rice." Azuki beans are steamed with sticky rice and often served with *gomasio* (see Day 134), resulting in a beautiful red-pink dish.

Whole, they can be added to a green salad, used as the basis for a bean salad, or seasoned with spices and tossed with steamed kale. Canned azuki beans are available. Their small size and delicate flavor—somewhat sweet and nutty— lend themselves to Asian-style dishes.

HOW DO YOU RESPOND TO, "DON'T PLANTS HAVE FEELINGS, TOO?"

We've all heard this question. It's often asked as somewhat of a joke, and yet, the person asking often expects a serious answer.

Short answer: Plants do not have pain receptors, nerves, or a central nervous system. If you don't have pain receptors, you don't feel pain.

Bigger issue: Even though those are the facts, they often aren't enough to satisfy people. Why? Because their question is not really about the emotional lives of plants.

What they really want to know is, "If I decided to do this vegan thing, how far do I go? Where do I draw the line?"

Instead of asking that in a constructive way and seriously contemplating their need/desire to stop eating animals and their secretions, they pose the question so as to make veganism seem downright absurd. And they may succeed in distracting you from the real point, which is the suffering of animals.

What you can say is that though we may learn some things about plants in the future that we don't know right now, we know that plants don't have pain receptors and thus don't feel pain. We know for certain that human and nonhuman animals have pain receptors, nerves, and a central nervous system; they feel pain, suffer, and struggle to live when being forced to die. That's the bottom line.

All any of us can do is the best we can with the information we have here and now.

LOSING WEIGHT

If weight loss is your goal, it's simply a numbers game: 3,500 calories represents 1 pound (0.45 kg) of body fat. So, if your goal is to lose 10 pounds (4.5 kg) in 10 weeks (70 days), you must burn 35,000 more calories than you consume during that period. That amounts to an average daily deficit of 500 calories. You can do that either by eating 500 fewer calories a day or by burning 500 additional calories a day. (If you do both, then your daily deficit is 1,000 calories, and the 10 pounds [4.5 kg] will be dropped in 5 weeks instead of 10.)

Splitting up your cardio exercise throughout the day is fine (and certainly better than nothing), but one of the benefits of a sustained cardiovascular exercise is the "afterburn," which refers to your elevated metabolism after a workout. Afterburn can last anywhere from 15 minutes to 24 hours, depending on the intensity and duration of your workout, and increases the number of calories you burn.

* **Running**: Calorie burn: On average, men burn about 124 calories and women 105 in a 1-mile (1.6 km) run.

* **Hiking**: Nothing beats being in nature, and it's free! Calorie burn: A 140-pound (63.5 kg) person hiking for 60 minutes burns about 400 calories.

* **Walking**: One of the best ways to motivate you to walk more is to look to your canine friend (or walk a neighbor's dog!). According to studies, people who have dogs get more exercise than the average gym member. Calorie burn: On average, men burn about 88 calories for a 1-mile (1.6 km) walk; women, 74.

* **Cycling**: Calories burned: A 140-pound (63.5 kg) woman cycling at a moderate 12 miles (19.2 km) per hour can burn 400 calories in that time frame; a 190-pound (86.2 kg) male would burn about 540.

In terms of the second part of the equation (reducing calorie intake), you might want to track your calories to get a better idea of how many calories you're taking in to attain the calorie deficit you need to lose weight. Use any number of online calculators by searching for "calories in food." Once you log it for a bit, you'll get a good idea of the calorie content of your favorite foods.

"A VINDICATION OF NATURAL DIET"
BY PERCY BYSSHE SHELLEY

An ethical vegetarian born in 1792, Percy Bysshe Shelley was one of the most critically regarded poets of the Romantic period. Known mostly for his poetry, Shelley also wrote plays, prose, and essays. Friends with John Keats and Lord Byron (see Day 165), Shelley was married to Mary Shelley (née Godwin), author of *Frankenstein* (see Day 186) and daughter of Mary Wollstonecraft (see Day 81)—and also a proud vegetarian.

An advocate for animals, Shelley wrote several passionate essays about the necessity of showing mercy to animals and about the superiority of a plant-based diet. In 1813, in "A Vindication of Natural Diet," he wrote:

> If the use of animal food be, in consequence, subversive to the peace of human society, how unwarrantable is the injustice and the barbarity which is exercised toward these miserable victims. They are called into existence by human artifice that they may drag out a short and miserable existence of slavery and disease, that their bodies may be mutilated, their social feelings outraged. It were much better that a sentient being should never have existed, than that it should have existed only to endure unmitigated misery.

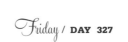

EDDIE—FROM MARKET DOG TO DOCTOR DOG

His almond brown eyes looked pleadingly into mine and, from that second, I was smitten. The sights, sounds, and smells of the animal market where he was caged in southern China were overpowering, and I cried behind the camera as I took photos.

Big dogs, small dogs, mixed breed and pure—all considered a delicacy or a snack that goes down well with beer—were caged in this market, miserable and diseased, and their terrified cries rang out. Cats, too, desperately pushed their paws through the mesh as they panted from thirst and the heat.

Every year in China millions of dogs and cats are raised and killed for their meat and their fur—but the tide is turning. Today, many emerging animal welfare groups across the country are now intelligently stating the case for companion animals in this developing country, which is finally open to change.

Today, for example, our "Doctor Dog" and "Professor Paws" animal therapy and education programs are showing why dogs and cats are our friends—not food. Through these programs, our four-legged ambassadors and their loving Chinese guardians provide patients in hospitals, disabled centers, orphanages, and homes for the elderly with a furry companion bestowing upon them unconditional love.

Back at the market, and bartering with the trader, a price was finally agreed on, and the scruffy cream-colored dog was mine. Today, Eddie is typical of a small dog with a big attitude who lights up my life and is the perfect ambassador for his breed.

—*Jill Robinson, founder of Animals Asia Foundation*

BARLEY-QUINOA PORRIDGE

Porridge is not just for Goldilocks *or* thieving bears! This is a hearty way to start the day and combines two healthful grains.

- ½ cup (100 g) uncooked hulled or pearled barley
- ½ cup (87 g) uncooked quinoa
- 4 cups (940 ml) water
- Pinch of salt
- ¼ cup (60 ml) nondairy milk (soy, rice, almond, hazelnut, hemp, or oat), plus extra
- ¼ cup (30 g) combination of dried fruits (raisins, chopped dates, cranberries, and cherries)
- ½ teaspoon ground cinnamon
- ¼ teaspoon ground nutmeg
- ¼ teaspoon ground cardamom
- 2 tablespoons (40 g) agave nectar or maple syrup

In a saucepan, combine the barley, quinoa, water, and salt. Bring to a boil, reduce to a simmer, cover, and cook for 30 to 40 minutes, until all the water is absorbed and the barley is soft. Check periodically to make sure the heat isn't so high as to evaporate the water before the grains are cooked.

Just as the grains are done cooking (or once they're cooked) and the water is absorbed, stir in the milk, dried fruits, cinnamon, nutmeg, and cardamom.

Transfer the porridge to serving bowls, drizzle with the agave nectar, and top with a few extra pieces of dried fruit. Pour some additional milk into each bowl, and serve.

Yield: 4 servings

*Wheat-free, oil-free, soy-free if not using soy milk

COCONUTS

Coconuts suffer from a bad reputation because of all the sound bites we have heard demonizing their fat content—particularly the saturated fat. Luckily, the story is beginning to be set straight and people are starting to understand the bigger picture.

It's true that coconuts contain saturated fat, and it's true that saturated fat—from animal products (namely meat, dairy, and eggs)—has been linked to heart disease. But the chemical makeup of saturated fat from coconuts is structurally different than that of animal products. The saturated fats in coconuts are mainly medium chain, and they differ in physiology and biochemistry from their "long-chain" animal-based-saturated-fat cousins.

We need fat in our diet in order for our bodies to absorb various fat-soluble nutrients. And coconuts can be one source of fat in a healthful diet; however, that doesn't mean we *have to* consume *oil*. It's important to differentiate between fat and oil. But for those times when a little oil is called for, coconut oil is a good alternative to olive or canola.

Coconut appears in our diets in many forms:

* Coconut milk—This is the sweet, thick milk sold in a can and used for rich dishes, such as Thai curries and desserts. It can also be used in place of other milks in baking, or in sweetened drinks, tea, or coffee. "Lite" coconut milk is also available and provides the same rich flavor with fewer calories.

* Coconut oil—Use in place of other plant-based oils when baking or sautéing veggies (especially for Asian-type recipes).

* Dried coconut—Available shredded or in flakes, dried coconut is best unsweetened. Add it to muffins, piecrusts, cookies, or frosting; sprinkle it on fruit salads; mix it in with oatmeal; or combine it with your favorite trail mix.

* Coconut water—This is basically the juice from a young coconut, and though it contains nutrients, it has no fat. It's one of my favorite things to drink—especially right out of the coconut—on a hot, summer day.

* Coconut meat—Once you crack open a coconut and drink the delicious, cooling coconut water, you can enjoy the flavorful, textured meat inside.

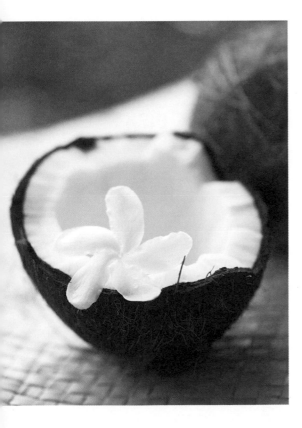

INVITING OTHERS TO TELL THEIR STORY

As important as it is to remember and tell our own stories (see Day 23), it is also effective to ask others to tell you theirs—and not just other vegans and activists. Drawing out the stories of people who are not on the same page as you will help tap into their own compassion, history, and values.

This is especially helpful when the subject is a potentially volatile one, such as hunting. For instance, if someone says he's a hunter and puts a positive spin on killing animals—serving nature or the environment, for example—instead of feeling disempowered, angry, or speechless, you could ask him how it feels to hunt. Ask, "What was it like to shoot an animal for the first time?" You will be surprised at how much people discover about themselves when asked a simple, obvious question.

This technique works in a variety of scenarios. If someone says she loves animals but she could never give up meat, instead of focusing on the "never give up meat," ask her about love of animals.

If someone says he was once vegetarian/vegan but had to stop because of health reasons, ask him to tell you about his "health issues."

Drawing out other people's stories may clarify things and shed light on other issues they weren't even aware of. And as they tell their story it may help to practice "active listening." (See Day 100.)

EATING HEALTHFULLY ON THE ROAD: 5 ONE-DISH SALADS

Whether they're based on pasta, greens, veggies, beans, or lentils, salads are so easy to prepare in advance for travel.

Corn Salad: Mix corn, chopped red onion, bell pepper, and sun-dried tomatoes with a little olive oil, some balsamic vinegar, and salt.

Bean Salad: Use a combination of canned beans, and combine with fresh herbs, lemon juice, chopped bell pepper, and seasoned rice vinegar. Add salsa, or make it heartier with a cup of cooked brown rice and avocado.

Pasta Salad: The options for pasta salads are endless. Even if you're not eating wheat or gluten, you can find rice pasta or quinoa pasta, particularly at large natural food stores.

Taco Salad: Use beans or vegetarian chicken or tofu or tempeh as your base, sauté them, add a packet of taco seasonings and water, heat, and you've got your taco salad. Pack up with tortilla chips or tortillas, along with shredded lettuce and tomatoes.

Green Salad: Choose your favorite green leafy, pile on chopped veggies, avocado, sunflower seeds, tofu, or a can of beans (rinsed and drained), and dressing (keeping the dressing separate until you're ready to assemble it).

"PITIFUL"
BY JOHN GALSWORTHY

See Day 291 for more about John Galsworthy and his commitment to being a voice for animals.

When God made man to live his hour
And hitch his wagon to a star,
He made a being without power
To see His creatures as they are.

He made a masterpiece of will,
Superb above its mortal lot,
Invincible by any ill—
Imagination He forgot!

This man of God's, with every wish
To earn the jobs of Kingdom Come,
Will prison up the golden fish

In bowl no bigger than a drum.
And though he withers from remorse
When he refuses Duty's call
He'll cut the tail of any horse,
And carve each helpless animal.

No spur to humour doth he want,
In wit the Earth he overlords,
Yet drives the hapless elephant
To clown and tumble on "the boards."

This man, of every learning chief,
So wise that he can read the skies,
Can fail to read the wordless grief
That haunts a prisoned monkey's eyes.
He'll prate of "mercy to the weak"
And strive to lengthen human breath,
But starve the little gaping beak
And hunt the timid hare to death.

Though with a spirit wild as wind,
The world at liberty he'd see,
He cannot any reason find
To set the tameless tiger free.

Such healing victories he wins,
And drugs away the mother's pangs,
But sets his God-forsaken gins
To mangle rabbits with their fangs.

Devout, he travels all the roads
To track and vanquish all the pains,
And yet—the wagon overloads,
The watch-dog to his barrel chains.

He'd soar the heavens in his flight
To measure Nature's majesty,
Yet take his children to delight
In captive eagles' tragedy.

This man, in knowledge absolute,
Who right, and love, and honour woos,
Yet keeps the pitiful poor brute
To mope and languish in his Zoos.

You creatures wild, of field and air,
Keep far from men, where'er they go!
God set no speculation there—
Alack!—We "know not what we do!"

DANCER

Dancer came to me when she was six going on seven. For the first six years of her life she had no name—just a number, as part of a large dairy herd. She was about seven months pregnant when she came to me, her great udder swinging, heavy with milk from her last calf—long gone.

Dancer had borne five, perhaps six, such babies. Like all dairy cows, from the time she was physically able to have babies, she had carried and birthed a baby a year. For 279 days each year—9 months, same as a human gestation period—she carried her baby curled high in her belly, close to her heart, while the machines sucked at her teats, extracting the milk from the baby before. One day of each year she spent giving birth and had only twenty-four hours to nurse her baby. Then they would come as they always came and seize her baby and drag it away, boys to the vealers, girls to be raised for the same servitude as their mother.

One day, an accident severed one of her teats, so Dancer was auctioned off for slaughter because she was no longer able to produce the average 25,000 pounds (3,000 gallons, or 11,356 L) of milk per year that is expected of each dairy cow. However, that day ended in good fortune for Dancer, as she—and the calf she was carrying—were spared from slaughter.

I brought her home and had calculated her due date: August 1st. And right on schedule, at dusk in the cool of the evening on August 1, Dancer gave birth to her calf and nursed her right away.

I was very proud of Dancer and saw that mother and baby were doing well. But now I had a real problem. Dancer and baby were at one end of the field surrounded by a thicket of thorns. Water and shade and sweet grass were at the other end of the field. The barn is even farther away, and August was forecast to be a scorcher.

In retrospect, the story is funny but it was serious at the time. Knowing Dancer's history, the whole notion of picking up and moving her calf was anathema. Picking up her calf would bring back all the nightmares of all her other calves. But the sun was already burning down. She and her calf had to move from her thorn fortress into the shade.

I drove to within 20 feet (6 m) of her and the calf and brought her grain. Dancer would have none of it. She tossed her head and pawed the ground and did her fighting bull act—posturing and threatening. As I approached Dancer and picked up her baby, I was much more worried about her distress than any threat to me. Dancer danced around me, threatening, making and missing passes at my body with her head. I carried her baby to the car, placing her carefully in the rear compartment.

Slowly, I started to drive toward the shade, the baby quieted, relaxed in the back, seemingly enjoying the jaunt. Not so Dancer. She ran frantically round and round searching for her baby, bellowing an awful bellow that tore my heart. But she did not seem to know to follow the car. The baby now started to fret, calling out to her.

I drove back to Dancer and opened the rear door to show her the baby. Once more I tried to drive away. Once more I drove back. The sun was roasting. I lifted the baby from the car and started out across the field with her in my arms. This worked. Dancer followed, dancing around and making soft noises to the baby, then gently butting me along to speed up the process that was getting heavier at every step. Bump. Another butt from Dancer. Stagger a few more steps. Bump again. So it went for the whole field, every rotten miserable inch of it with star thistle stuck in my sneakers and jeans.

The baby was a girl. Dancer nursed her till she was almost eighteen months old. Dancer no longer becomes frantic at the sight of cattle trucks coming on the property, bringing new arrivals. She dances with her very grown-up baby and the other cows under the light of the moon.

—Lois Flynne was the director of the Community of Compassion for Animals sanctuary in Orland, California, until she died in 2007. The sanctuary was also home to goats, pigs, dogs, chickens, turkeys, and donkeys, and three cows previously used in vivisection experiments.

GUNFLINT LODGE WILD RICE, HERB, AND DRIED CRANBERRY STUFFING

Courtesy of Compassionate Cooks' friend Lisa Puklich, this recipe is a vegan version derived from an original recipe of Lisa's grandmother, who recently died at ninety-eight years young. It's a pleasure to memorialize her grandmother this way.

1 tablespoon (14 g) nondairy butter, such as Earth Balance
1 large yellow onion, diced
5 stalks celery, diced
½ teaspoon minced garlic
3 tablespoons (45 ml) dry white wine
1 teaspoon (1.6 g) dried tarragon
½ teaspoon rubbed sage
¼ teaspoon dried thyme
1 tablespoon (20 g) maple syrup
8 cups (400 g) dried cubed bread
1 cup (165 g) cooked wild rice
½ cup (60 g) dried cranberries
½ to ¾ cup (120 to 180 ml) or more vegetable stock
Freshly ground black pepper
3 tablespoons (12 g) chopped fresh parsley

Preheat the oven to 350°F (180°C, or gas mark 4).

Melt the butter in a large sauté pan over medium heat. Add the onion, celery, and garlic, and sauté until the onions are translucent. Add the wine, and bring to a boil. Cook until reduced, about 1 minute.

Add the tarragon, sage, thyme, and maple syrup, and stir to combine. Remove from the heat.

In a large bowl, toss together the dried bread cubes, cooked wild rice, and dried cranberries. Add the vegetable and herb mixture to the bowl, and toss to combine. Add enough stock to moisten the stuffing, continually tossing and adding more liquid to reach the desired texture. Season to taste with black pepper and mix in the parsley.

Place the stuffing in a shallow casserole, and bake for 25 to 35 minutes, or until heated through and a little crusty on top.

Yield: 6 to 8 servings

Soy-free if using soy-free Earth Balance

MISO

A traditional Japanese food, miso is created by fermenting rice, barley, and/or soybeans with salt. A thick paste sold in tubs, miso is used to create soups, dressings, sauces, and spreads, and it is a staple I believe no refrigerator should be without. It provides instant flavor—and nutrition—wherever you add it. Typically salty, it is at once sweet and earthy and comes in a variety of "flavors," depending on how long it was fermented for.

Though they can most certainly be used interchangeably, it's helpful to know the differences between them so you can modify the amounts called for in recipes as needed.

White miso is made from soybeans that have been fermented with a large percentage of rice and has a sweet taste. Best used in salad dressings and light sauces, it can also be used to make miso soup. In the store, it may be called *light miso.*

Yellow miso is usually made from soybeans that have been fermented with barley and sometimes a small percentage of rice. It has a mild, earthy flavor and is also favored for its use in sauces, marinades, dressings, and soups.

Red miso is a dark, rich paste and is typically made from soybeans fermented with barley, though with a higher percentage of soybeans and for a longer fermentation period. Ranging in color from red to dark brown, it may be called *dark miso.* Its deep flavor can overwhelm mild dishes, but a little goes a long way, and it's perfect for hearty soups, glazes, and marinades. One teaspoon (5 g) of dark miso is roughly equivalent to 2 teaspoons (10 g) of the lighter varieties.

Use miso paste to create a base broth, and add soba, udon, or rice noodles; shiitake mushrooms; spinach; and tofu. When adding miso to a soup or stock, it's best to first whisk it in a small bowl with a small amount of water before adding it to the pot. This ensures that it is thoroughly dissolved.

Other ways to use miso as an ingredient:

* Peel back the husk on whole corn, spread the kernels with light miso, reposition the husk, and grill the whole ear of corn.

* Marinate tofu in light miso paste and tamari soy sauce, and grill or sauté.

* Use light miso paste in place of tahini (sesame butter) when making hummus.

* Use light miso as a replacement for fat (nondairy butter or oil) in creamy soups.

* Purée light miso with tofu and lemon juice to make a nondairy sour cream.

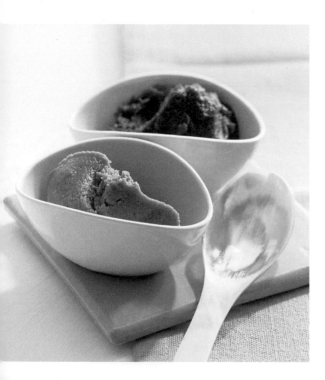

HOW DO YOU RESPOND TO SNARKY COMMENTS?

Questions such as "Do you miss meat?" and "Are you hungry a lot?" could be an opportunity for discussion about food, nutrition, practical aspects of being vegan, and so on. But questions such as the ones below are clearly designed to belittle your concern for animals and to try and catch you at being imperfect and hypocritical. Knowing when to respond and when to just smile is essential.

* If someone says, "If animals aren't supposed to be eaten, then why are they made out of meat?" you could say (with a smile), "You could say the same thing about humans."

* If someone says, "I guess you think you're better than me," you could say (with a smile), "Clearly!" Just keep it light.

* If someone says, "Mmmm. This burger tastes so good. Are you sure you don't want any?" you could say, "No, thanks. I already had one today."

* If someone says, "Don't you care about plants?" you could say, "I'm not vegan because I like animals; I'm vegan because I hate plants." With a smile.

Once you have a playful response, and they're interested in more that you have to say, you can continue. If you joke that you're clearly better than they are, you can then say, "Look. I'm just doing the best I can. I'm not better than anybody—except maybe the person I used to be." A genuine laugh or smile in response to passive-aggressiveness is also better for all your relationships.

When you rise to engage in the best part of other people's nature, they tend to respond with the best part of themselves.

KEEPING A COMPASSIONATE BATHROOM

Although it's not required to test products and ingredients on animals, it's done anyway. Why? The best answer I can offer, though it might not be satisfactory, is "because we can." That's really what it comes down to. We test on animals because we can. I believe we also test on animals simply because it became the accepted way of doing things. For now.

The good news is that there are more than 300 manufacturers of cosmetics and household products that have shunned animal tests and taken advantage of the more humane, more effective, and more scientifically sound nonanimal tests.

Look for the internationally recognized Leaping Bunny logo, which is assurance that the cosmetic, personal care, and/or household product company that features that logo has not subjected their product or the ingredients in their product to new animal testing.

It's also important to note that even if the Leaping Bunny logo is on the package, it doesn't mean that the product is "vegan." In other words, some companies may boast the fact that they don't test on animals but still include animal products in the item. You can determine this by reading the ingredients.

A way to tell whether a product is vegan and cruelty-free is to look for the Certified Vegan logo. Administered by Vegan Action, you'll find this symbol on food, clothing, cosmetics and other items that contain no animal products AND are not tested on animals. Visit vegan.org to see exactly what this symbol looks like. It's a great way to have a quick visual reference without having to read the ingredients list.

Finally, keep in mind, just because a product doesn't have these logos on it, it doesn't mean it's not vegan or cruelty-free. Companies are adding these logos all the time, and it will take time before every single product on the market carries these symbols.

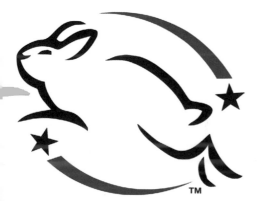

"GOOD-NATURE TO ANIMALS: A HYMN FOR CHILDREN"
BY CHRISTOPHER SMART

While confined in a mental institution, Christopher Smart (1722–1771) created his best-known work, the long poem *Jubilate Agno*, in which he writes an homage to his cat Jeoffry—the only company he kept during that time. (See Day 254 for an excerpt.) Animals, nature, and religion are prominent in his poetry, and he wrote several hymns to children, encouraging them to be moral and good. In "Good-Nature to Animals," he explains—in verse form—why they should be kind to animals.

> The man of Mercy (says the Seer)
> Shows mercy to his beast;
> Learn not of churls to be severe,
> But house and feed at least.
>
> Shall I melodious pris'ners take
> From out the linnet's nest,
> And not keep busy care awake,
> To cherish ev'ry guest?
>
> What, shall I whip in cruel wrath
> The steed that bears me safe,
> Or 'gainst the dog, who plights his troth,
> For faithful service chafe?
>
> In the deep waters throw thy bread,
> Which thou shalt find again,
> With God's good interest on thy head
> And pleasure for thy pain.

> Let thine industrious silk-worms reap
> Their wages to the full,
> Nor let neglected dormice sleep
> To death within thy wool.
>
> Know when the frosty weather comes,
> 'Tis charity to deal
> To wren and redbreast all thy crumbs,
> The remnant of thy meal.
>
> Tho' these some spirits think but light,
> And deem indifferent things,
> Yet they are serious in the sight
> OF CHRIST, the King of Kings.

ISRAELI KIBBUTZNIK DAIRY WORKER TURNED VEGAN

For ages I was a kibbutznik (a member of a collective Israeli farm). On the kibbutz, I worked in our commercial dairy, doing veterinary chores, milking our approximately 500 cows three times a day, and feeding them. Once a week, I made the five-hour bus ride to Tel Aviv. On one fateful trip, a little boy sitting next to me who had been looking out the window turned to me in tears, asking why the men were hitting the mama cow. I looked out the window to see men separating a calf from his mother, and she wasn't happy about it.

In that moment, the little boy's compassion made the scales fall off my eyes. I'd been a vegetarian for twenty-five years. I knew all my dairy cows by name, played them music in the milking parlor, and never used the electric prod. And yet, I was sometimes that man taking a baby from his mother.

I quit the dairy that day and began to run the collective kitchen of the kibbutz. I ordered the food, planned and prepared all meals for dozens of members and friends, and cleaned up. I figured I didn't have to announce that the kitchen was now serving only vegetarian fare; I only had to make the meals delicious, satisfying, and healthful. After the first month, I had forty-eight vegetarians [from only one to start] on my hands and I was dreaming in recipes!

I woke up one morning and became vegan. A month later, my plate was free of animal products, and gradually, the rest of my life has followed. Now, each year, I celebrate my vegan "birthday" by cooking a meal for my friends and asking them each to bring one dish, for which I provide recipes and lots of hand-holding as needed.

I am now informed, my ears and eyes are open to things I hadn't previously considered, and, by example, I am able to share the message of compassion in a thoughtful, effective way.

—*Itai in Tel Aviv, Israel*

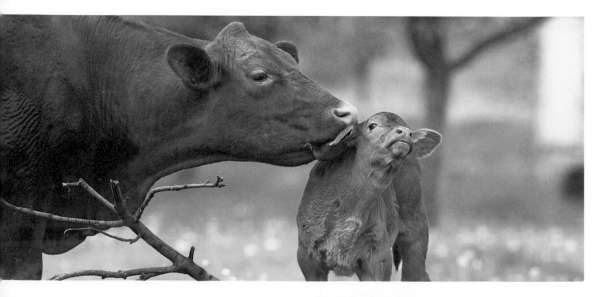

CHOCOLATE BREAD PUDDING

Although the bread requires some time for the chocolate to soak in, this is one of the easiest and richest desserts you'll ever make.

> 1 loaf Italian bread, day-old or fresh
> 3 cups (705 ml) nondairy milk (soy, rice, almond, hazelnut, hemp, or oat), divided
> ¾ cup (150 g) granulated sugar
> Pinch of salt
> 8 to 10 ounces (225 to 280 g) nondairy semisweet chocolate chips
> 1 small ripe banana
> 1 tablespoon (15 ml) vanilla extract

Cut the bread into ½-inch-thick (1.3 cm) slices and remove the crusts, taking care to preserve as much of the main part of the bread as possible. Cut the bread into ½-inch (1.3 cm) cubes, which will amount to 6 or 7 cups (300 to 350 g).

In a large saucepan, combine 1 cup (235 ml) of the nondairy milk, the sugar, and the salt. Bring to a boil over medium-high heat, stirring constantly. Remove from the heat and add the chocolate chips. Let the mixture stand for a few minutes, then stir until smooth.

In a large bowl, mash the banana, then combine with the remaining 2 cups (470 ml) milk and the vanilla. (You may use a food processor or an electric hand mixer for the best results.) Add this mixture to the chocolate mixture, then stir in the bread cubes. Let this stand for 1 to 2 hours so that the bread thoroughly absorbs the chocolate sauce. Stir and press down the bread periodically.

Preheat the oven to 325°F (170°C, or gas mark 3).

Generously butter a 9-inch (23 cm) square baking pan. Pour the bread mixture into the dish and smooth the top. Bake in a water bath for 55 to 65 minutes. Let cool for 30 minutes before serving.

Yield: 8 to 10 servings

*Soy-free if not using soy milk

Originally published in *The Joy of Vegan Baking*.

TAHINI

Tahini is like peanut butter, only it's made from ground sesame seeds and not ground peanuts. Typically, the seeds are hulled and roasted, though raw tahini is widely available.

From the Arabic word meaning "to grind," tahini originated in ancient Persia (modern-day Iran) and was quite literally called "holy food." Used in a variety of traditional Middle Eastern dishes, tahini is the second most important ingredient in hummus (next to the chickpeas).

Middle Eastern cuisines have perfected its culinary uses, making tahini-based sauces, using it as a condiment, including it as a garnish, using it as a thickener, adding it to soups, and even making desserts, such as traditional halva, with it. It can also be used in:

* Dips: Variations abound. The most obvious tahini-based dip is hummus (chickpeas, garlic, lemon juice, tahini, cumin, and oil or water for thinning). Baba ghanoush is made from mashed roasted eggplant, along with tahini,

and only your imagination will limit the many other possibilities.

* Sauces: A simple sauce made from tahini, lemon juice, and water can be poured on falafel (as tzatziki sauce), paired with any steamed or roasted vegetable, or tossed with noodles, preferably soba.

* Salad dressings: Prepare the simple sauce above (keeping it thicker than you would for a sauce) and add nondairy plain yogurt or miso (see Day 337).

* Vegetable purees: Don't just top veggies with tahini—add it to vegetable purees (such as mashed potatoes or carrots), where it will lend creaminess and tang.

* Soups and stews: Tahini thickens and enriches soups and stews.

* Desserts: Mix tahini with agave nectar or date juice. Serve with pieces of bread that are dipped into this sweet concoction.

EAT LIKE A PIG

Pigs naturally regulate their intake and do not overeat even when given access to unlimited food—though they can find food wherever it is because their snouts enable them to dig for roots and mushrooms.

The pork industry, however, gives pigs a drug called Hog-Crave, which causes pigs to overeat so that they will grow faster and will be more

profitable to those who kill them. Commercial pig food is laced with growth hormones and antibiotics, which cause them to grow quickly.

When we think of pigs, see the huge domestic pigs that are bred and killed for human consumption. It's easy to forget that humans created these overweight creatures. If you took a day-old domestic piglet from a modern-

EAT LIKE A PIG

day operation and raised him on natural food (without growth hormones) he'd still grow *huge* because of how we've genetically changed him over time to do so. Pigs weigh about 2½ pounds (1.1 kg) at birth and are slaughtered when they weigh 250 pounds (111 kg)—at six months young. Domestic pigs who are spared the fate of the frying pan often have debilitating back and hip problems because their skeletons cannot support their weight. They're not fat pigs; we're mad scientists.

There are many ways we can express our gluttonous ways without disparaging pigs. I don't "eat like a pig," though I might "eat like a glutton." Instead of "pig sty," we might simply say "mess." Rather than "sweat like a pig," how about "sweat like a human"? (Contrary to popular belief, pigs do not have functional sweat glands.)

Wednesday / **DAY 346**

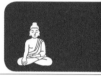

CREATING HANDMADE HOLIDAY GIFTS

Gifts that cause no harm to any living creature truly reflect the meaning of the holidays.

Pocket Full of Posies

Posies are little bouquets of flowers or herbs that make lovely gifts, particularly when the flora comes from our own gardens. Any flower works, but posies made of bay leaves, sage, rosemary, and lavender are particularly fragrant.

Au Naturel Greeting Cards

Walk in the woods to gather leaves, pinecones, seeds, and other decorative debris. Decorate recycled cardstock paper with these pretty items, or buy an inkpad and use the leaves as stamps.

Timeless Treats

Fill old-fashioned cookie tins with gingerbread people, sugar cookies, and pecan balls. Fill Mason jars with carmelized nuts and decorate with and elegant ribbon. Bake a pie and include the recipe along with a pie plate and tea towel.

Creature Comforts

Don't forget the beloved animals of friends and family. Great homemade gifts for cats include dried catnip tucked into a kitty-themed sock or a fresh catnip plant in a hand-painted pot. For the pooch, bake some homemade veggie treats.

ESSAYS BY PLUTARCH ABOUT EATING ANIMALS

Although we tend to think that "vegetarianism" as a response to suffering is a new idea—born of the "hippie" days of the 1960s and '70s—it goes back as far as recorded history allows us to see.

At the heart of our ethical dilemma over eating animals isn't *how* we treat those we breed and kill but *that* we breed and kill them in the first place—merely for our own convenience and gustatory pleasure. Factory farming is simply a perverse extension of our anthropocentric worldview.

Greek historian and essayist Plutarch observed this as far back as the second century (he lived from about 46–120 CE), recognizing the violence inherent in taking the life of someone who would otherwise choose to live. This can't but affect us on a profoundly fundamental level—deep within our heart and mind. If it didn't, we wouldn't have to make the sundry excuses and justifications we do in order to feel better about this physiologically unnecessary and psychologically harmful habit.

In an essay called "On Eating Flesh," which sounds like it could have been written yesterday, Plutarch provides his answer. Here is an excerpt:

You ask me why Pythagoras abstained from eating the flesh of beasts, but I ask you, what courage must have been needed by the first man who raised to his lips the flesh of the slain, who broke with his teeth the bones of a dying beast, who had dead bodies, corpses, placed before him and swallowed down limbs which a few moments ago were bleating, bellowing, walking, and seeing? How could his hand plunge the knife into the heart of a sentient creature? How could his eyes look on murder? How could he behold a poor helpless animal bled to death, scorched, and dismembered? How can he bear the sight of this quivering flesh? Does not the very smell of it turn his stomach? Is he not repelled, disgusted, horror-struck, when he has to handle the blood from these wounds, and to cleanse his fingers from the dark and viscous bloodstains?

The fare itself is truly monstrous and prodigious; you ought rather, in my opinion, to have inquired who first began this practice, than who of late times left it off.

And truly, as for those people who first ventured upon eating of flesh, it is very probable that the whole reason of their so doing was scarcity and want of other food; for it is not likely that their living together in lawless and extravagant lusts, or their growing wanton and capricious through the excessive variety of provisions then among them, brought them to such unsociable pleasures as these, against Nature. Yea, had they at this instant but their sense and voice restored to them, I am persuaded they would express themselves to this purpose.

But whence is it that a certain ravenousness and frenzy drives you in these happy days to pollute yourselves with blood, since you have such an abundance of things necessary for your subsistence? Why do you belie the earth as unable to maintain you? You are indeed wont to call serpents, leopards, and lions savage creatures; but yet yourselves are defiled with blood, and come nothing behind them in cruelty. What they kill is their ordinary nourishment, but what you kill is your better fare.

For we eat not lions and wolves by way of revenge; but we let those go, and catch the harmless and tame sort, and such as have neither stings nor teeth to bite with, and slay them; which, so may Jove help us, Nature seems to us to have produced for their beauty and comeliness only.

O horrible cruelty! It is truly an affecting sight to see the very table of rich people laid before them, who keep them cooks and caterers to furnish them with dead corpses for their daily fare.

Greek historian Plutarch
Courtesy of Mary Evans Picture Library/Alamy

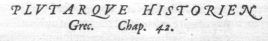

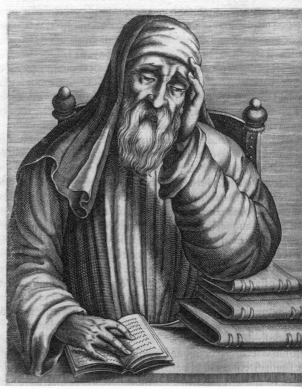

FROM SKEPTIC TO VEGAN

I was always a picky eater when it came to meat, but of course I ate it, because that was just what you did! It wasn't until my mid-twenties when my best friend, Erin, transitioned to a vegan lifestyle and began sharing the virtues of it with me that I had my awakening.

Erin always had a way of somehow knowing what was best for me long before I ever did. Soon after she went vegan, she started sharing with me how it had changed her life and encouraged me to seriously consider the idea of for myself. Naturally, I was skeptical because, I thought then, veganism is just far too extreme a lifestyle.

I would throw countless "What about this?" and "What about that?" questions at her, and she was able to volley each of them right back at me with logical answers with which I couldn't disagree.

She was relentless in her insistence that it would be one of the best decisions I would ever make. I made a deal. I promised that I would be vegan for one week if she would stop pestering me. I knew that it would be a disastrous week, that I could go back to my normal life at the end, and that then I could say, "I told you so."

This Vegan Week required some research, which was eye-opening. I had always known, on some level, what happens to animals on their journey to my dinner plate, but I had no idea of the magnitude. The things I learned horrified me. I could no longer ignore the facts and just pretend that these things weren't happening.

At the end of my Vegan Week, not only had I experienced far more varied and delicious food than I had ever expected to, but I also felt like a completely new person, both physically and spiritually. Knowing what I know now, I just could not see how I could possibly choose anything other than a vegan lifestyle. It was the only option.

I have never once felt like I'm missing out on something or that I had to "give up" something. I only feel like I've gained. Each day that I live as a vegan, my belief that I made the right decision grows stronger.

And Erin was right: It really is the best decision I've ever made.

—*Nick in New York, New York*

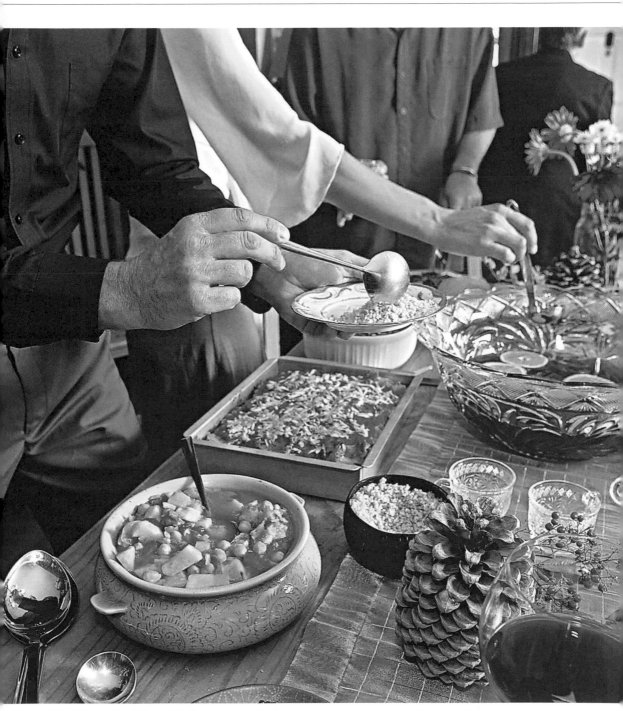

Photo courtesy of Cheri Larsh Arellano

TEMPEH SCRAMBLE

A quick breakfast or brunch, this scramble relies on the nutty fermented soybean cake rather than the oft-used tofu.

8 ounces (225 g) tempeh
1 tablespoon (15 ml) olive oil
1 bunch kale or chard, finely chopped
1 small red onion, chopped
1 small red, orange, or yellow bell pepper, chopped
1 stalk celery, finely chopped
1 carrot, finely chopped
3 cloves garlic, minced
1 teaspoon (2.5 g) ground cumin
1 teaspoon (2.5 g) paprika
1 teaspoon (1 g) dried oregano
1 teaspoon (6 g) salt
½ teaspoon red pepper flakes
3 scallions, finely chopped (green and white parts)
2 tablespoons (8 g) chopped fresh parsley
Juice of ½ lemon

Cut the tempeh cake into fourths, and steam for 10 minutes. This tenderizes the tempeh and cuts some of its bitterness. Let cool, and crumble into a bowl.

Meanwhile, heat the oil in a large sauté pan over medium heat. Add the kale, onion, bell pepper, celery, carrot, and garlic, and cook until the vegetables are glossy and softened, about 5 minutes. Add the cumin, paprika, oregano, salt, and red pepper flakes, and toss to combine thoroughly.

Add the tempeh and scallions, and cook for about 7 minutes longer, or until the tempeh is hot and thoroughly combined with the other ingredients. Add more salt, if necessary.

Just before removing from the heat, add the parsley and lemon juice, and toss to combine. Serve right away, or store in refrigerator to heat up the next day.

Yield: 4 servings

*Wheat-free

BARLEY

Cultivated 10,000 years ago in the Near East and Europe, barley is the oldest of all the grains. Once a major source of food for humans, it is used today primarily as food for "livestock" and for making malt for beer. In fact, it is likely that the word *beer* comes from the old Germanic word for barley.

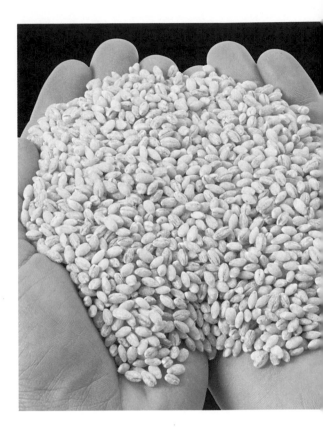

With its nutty flavor and chewy texture, barley is an excellent addition to many dishes, though it is sold in a variety of forms:

* Scotch barley has its bran (outer layer) still intact.

* Pot barley has part of its bran removed.

* Pearled barley has its hull and bran totally removed.

Because it cooks faster and is less chewy than the grains that still contain their bran, pearl barley tends to be consumed more than the others, but it is also the least nutritious of the three. If you're looking to retain some of the nutrients, look for Scotch or pot, which might also be called *hulled* barley. But even without the bran, pearled barley is still nutritious: 1 cup (157 g) of cooked pearled barley provides 12 percent of the Daily Value of iron, 24 percent of the Daily Value of dietary fiber, and 6 grams of fiber. That same 1 cup (157 g) contains only 193 calories.

Today, barley is prepared in much the same way it was in ancient times—added to soups, used to make porridge, or served as rice would be—and as an accompaniment to stir-fries. You can make cold barley salads with raw veggies, herbs, and olive oil, as well as sweet barley water that benefits from the addition of lemon juice and agave nectar.

WHAT DO YOU SAY TO, "EATING ANIMALS IS SANCTIONED BY GOD"?

Many advocates are reluctant to have conversations with people about religion and animal rights, especially if they have little knowledge of the Judeo-Christian Bible and its teachings.

I'm certainly not a scholar of world religions, but I do know that one thing they all have in common is their call to compassion. Appealing to the values we all share and the universal principles we all strive by is a much more effective approach than getting into the nitty-gritty details of religious tenets.

One conversation I had with a gentleman started with him telling me that he and his family were Christian and followed the laws in the Bible that mandate against eating "unclean" animals, such as pigs. In a very sympathetic voice, I said, "Too bad *all* animals weren't considered 'unclean.' Then none of them would be eaten." Catching my drift, he smiled.

The conversation continued, as he told me that he believed what the Bible told them regarding animals—that humans are entitled to eat them. Again, very respectfully and sympathetically, I said that it works out pretty well for humans that the Bible says it's okay to eat animals. I said I bet it would be a different story if the animals wrote that book. Again, he smiled and nodded and said that I had a good point.

Appealing to his faith in the Bible, I asked him if it was true that the Garden of Eden was considered the most ideal place and state for humans to exist. I asked, "Isn't *that* what God intended for humans—to be at peace and in harmony with nature and other animals—to avoid violence as much as possible?" He said that it was true.

Too often, these conversations either don't happen at all or they become full of strain and argumentation because people perceive themselves on opposite sides of the issue. However, my goal is not to have a debate but rather find points upon which we can agree. The more we can find common ground, the more effective advocates we will be.

SETTING INTENTIONS AND GOALS

I love the transition period from the end of one year to the next, and I make a ritual of it. I sit down with paper and pen and write my intentions for the next year and reflect on the intentions of the last. Crossing the threshold from one year to the next is magical—quite sacred, really—and I revel in this time.

At the beginning of each New Year, many people take the opportunity to reflect on the previous year and make plans and promises for the next. Recently, however, it's become somewhat hip to declare that you don't make New Year resolutions and to cynically shrug them off.

I suspect this reaction is in response to the disappointment many people feel from the times they set up expectations, only to have them dashed. With the cumulative memory of broken resolutions all too near, many people feel it's safer to make no resolutions at all than to make them and feel like a failure when they don't or can't follow through.

Although I understand not wanting to set yourself up for failure, I do think there is something very powerful in declaring what you want— saying it out loud and writing it down. If you believe that we have the power to manifest what we desire—and I do—then we must *articulate* the desire first. If we hold back saying what we really want, then it's as if we're not really that serious about it; thus, we are less apt to attract it to us.

On a purely practical level, creating goals (or resolutions) is the first step in achieving them. We have to know what we want before we can begin our pursuit. This is the power of intention.

When practicing the power of intention, we can start small. In fact, by recognizing each night's sleep as a transition period, a smaller-scale threshold, you can perform this ritual of setting your intentions and goals each day upon waking. As I lie in bed each morning, in my mind, before I rise, I create my intentions and goals for the day.

For instance, my *intentions* for a day might be:

* Speak with kindness and integrity.

* Be a voice for animals.

* Eat in such a way that reflects my desire to be healthy and energetic.

My *goals* for a day might be:

* Write one chapter of my book.

* Write the next podcast episode.

* Run 6 miles (9.6 km).

The best way to differentiate between intentions and goals is to say that goals are measurable; intentions are not. Intentions create a framework of consciousness as I go about my day, whereas goals are very tangible.

"FOR I WILL CONSIDER MY CAT JEOFFRY," EXCERPT FROM *JUBILATE AGNO*
BY CHRISTOPHER SMART

Known as an alcoholic, a madman, and a mystic, Christopher Smart (1722–1771) was a popular poet and magazine columnist who wrote about religion, language, nature, and gender. He was incarcerated in an insane asylum from 1756 to 1763, during which time he wrote his long free-verse manuscript *Jubilate Agno* ("Rejoice in the Lamb"). Thirty-two pages of the original manuscript survive, and it was finally published for the first time in 1939.

Jubilate is filled with references to and celebrations of animals, but it is his cat Jeoffry who gets center stage and takes up seventy-four lines of praise (of which this is only an excerpt). During his confinement, Jeoffry was Smart's only companion; he was otherwise left alone.

> For I will consider my Cat Jeoffry.
> For he is the servant of the Living God duly and
>   daily serving him.
> For at the first glance of the glory of God in the
>   East he worships in his way.
> For this is done by wreathing his body seven
>   times round with elegant quickness.
> For then he leaps up to catch the musk, which is
>   the blessing of God upon his prayer.
> For he rolls upon prank to work it in.
> For having done duty and received blessing he
>   begins to consider himself.
> For this he performs in ten degrees.
> For first he looks upon his forepaws to see if they
>   are clean.
> For secondly he kicks up behind to clear away
>   there.
> For thirdly he works it upon stretch with the
>   forepaws extended.
> For fourthly he sharpens his paws by wood.
> For fifthly he washes himself.
> For sixthly he rolls upon wash.
> For seventhly he fleas himself, that he may not be
>   interrupted upon the beat.
> For eighthly he rubs himself against a post.
> For ninthly he looks up for his instructions.
> For tenthly he goes in quest of food.
> For having consider'd God and himself he will
>   consider his neighbour.
> For if he meets another cat he will kiss her in
>   kindness.
> For when he takes his prey he plays with it to
>   give it a chance.
> For one mouse in seven escapes by his dallying.
> For when his day's work is done his business
>   more properly begins.
> For he keeps the Lord's watch in the night
>   against the adversary.
> For he counteracts the powers of darkness by his
>   electrical skin and glaring eyes.
> For he counteracts the Devil, who is death, by
>   brisking about the life.
> For in his morning orisons he loves the sun and
>   the sun loves him.
> For he is of the tribe of Tiger.
> For the Cherub Cat is a term of the Angel Tiger.
> For he has the subtlety and hissing of a serpent,
>   which in goodness he suppresses.
> For he will not do destruction, if he is well-fed,
>   neither will he spit without provocation.
> For he purrs in thankfulness, when God tells him
>   he's a good Cat.
> For he is an instrument for the children to learn
>   benevolence upon.
> For every house is incomplete without him and a
>   blessing is lacking in the spirit.
> . . .

For his tongue is exceeding pure so that it has in
purity what it wants in music.
For he is docile and can learn certain things.
For he can set up with gravity which is patience
upon approbation.
For he can fetch and carry, which is patience in
employment.
For he can jump over a stick which is patience
upon proof positive.
For he can spraggle upon waggle at the word of
command.
For he can jump from an eminence into his
master's bosom.

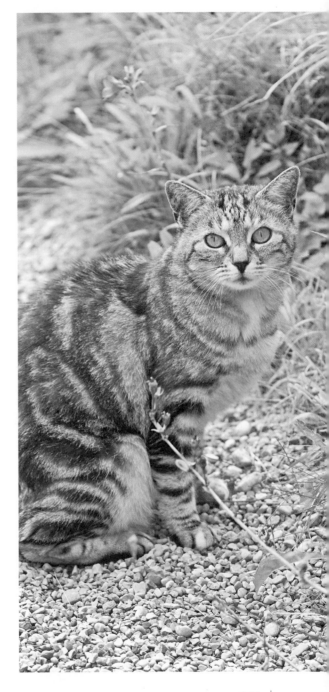

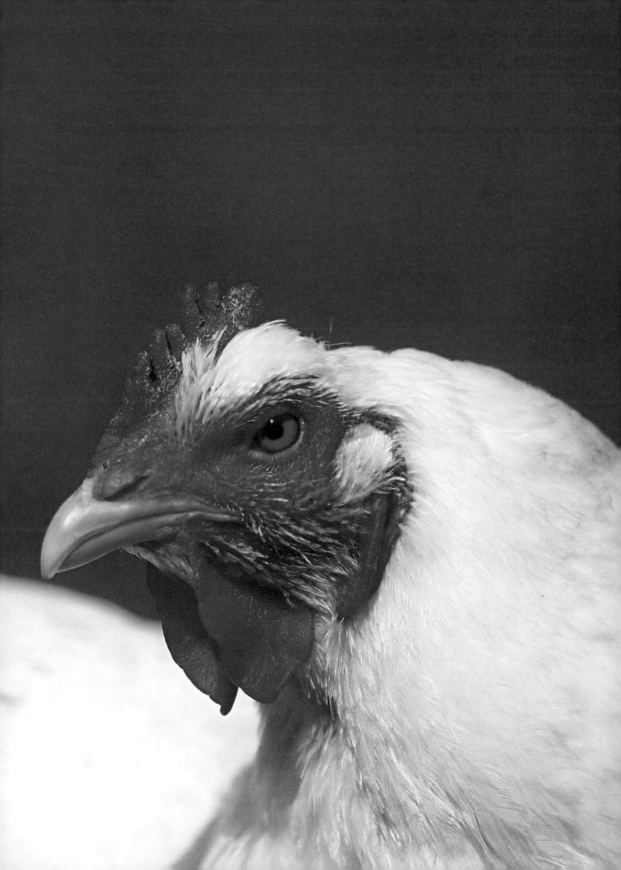

TAYLOR, THE HEN

Taylor's fate was supposed to have been that of 9 billion other birds: the slaughterhouse.

Taylor was one of 500 chicks headed to a facility in California. En route, workers at a local airport noticed that some of the chicks were dead and many appeared unhealthy. The local shelter was called and the chicks confiscated. Fifty died before arriving at the shelter and more than 100 wouldn't survive the first week. Even though chicks are incredibly sensitive babies and changes in temperature can spell disaster, it is legal to ship them through the mail for up to 72 hours without proper nourishment or even water.

Taylor's fate changed overnight; she and twelve others arrived at Animal Place; almost all were placed at other sanctuaries.

Taylor is now a hen, and a singer, a crooner, and a speaker on all subjects large and small.

One day, as she sat on my lap, she arched her speckled neck, reached up, and tugged on a strand of hair—tug, yank, pull. Ouch! My yelp gave her pause, and she cooed like a hen does to a miffed chick. It's a sweet sound, full of maternal love. When you hear this sound, your temper fades. A hen's maternal love lasts only so long, and soon she will change her tone and reinforce her message with a swift peck to the head. Mothers can be tough.

I know Taylor's sweet spot. When I scratch along both sides of her neck, her eyes close, and she makes these indescribably precious sounds. If she were a dog, she would be kicking her hind foot in wild abandon.

There is no ignoring her contented sighs and clucks of appreciation. Taylor is clearly a being who thinks, feels, and experiences the life around her.

The more you get to know another species, the harder it becomes to excuse their exploitation and abuse. Chickens are not dumb. They are not immune to pain. Their movements are not pointless reflexes, random responses to their environment. They think and plot and make decisions.

They are intelligent, emotional beings who can and do suffer. Their desires are not much different than mine or yours: They want to live, seek out that which makes them happy, avoid pain, make friends, eat until they are full, and spend time with their family and loved ones.

—Marji Beach of Animal Place, Grass Valley,
California (U.S.)

Taylor at Animal Place
Photo courtesy of Animal Place

ROASTED PLUM TOMATOES WITH GARLIC

Fresh in-season tomatoes work best, but this recipe is also a great way to use tomatoes that are starting to soften. I urge you to use fresh herbs for this—not dried!

> 8 plum (Roma) tomatoes, halved
> 12 cloves garlic, unpeeled
> ¼ cup (60 ml) olive oil
> 5 bay leaves
> 3 tablespoons (12 g) finely chopped fresh oregano
> 2 tablespoons (5 g) finely chopped fresh basil
> Salt and freshly ground pepper
> Rosemary sprigs, for garnish

Preheat the oven to 450°F (230°C, or gas mark 8). Lightly oil an ovenproof dish into which the tomatoes fit snugly. Place the halved tomatoes in the dish (cut side up), and push the garlic cloves between them.

Brush the tomatoes with the olive oil, randomly stick the bay leaves in between the tomatoes, and sprinkle with salt and pepper.

Bake for 45 minutes, until the tomatoes have softened and charred around the edges. Sprinkle the fresh minced herbs all over the tomatoes, season with salt and pepper, if desired. Garnish with some rosemary sprigs for a pretty presentation.

Yield: 4 servings

*Wheat-free, soy-free

Originally published in *Color Me Vegan*

FOOD LABELS

Although the intention behind the many labels on our food is to educate the consumer, many people are confused and many of the labels have lost their impact. We can only do the best we can with the information we have, so here is a short guide to the labels I pay attention to when making purchases:

Fair Trade: This label indicates that the farmers and farm workers have been paid a fair price for the food (or goods) they produce, are vested in their farms, and can deal directly with importers and not unnecessary middlemen. Common foods with this label: bananas, coffee, tea, cocoa.

Non-GMO: Indicates the fact that ingredients or whole products do not contain genetically modified organisms, which are created in a laboratory through the process of taking genes from one species and inserting them into another. Always choose corn, soy foods, and canola oil that are non-GMO. According to current standards, if something is labeled organic, it is non-GMO.

Organic: Grown without the use of conventional nonorganic pesticides, insecticides, and herbicides, though certain non-organic fertilizers are still used. See Day 311 for the most highly sprayed produce. Keep in mind that in animal products, "organic" reflects the absence of hormones and antibiotics in the feed of the animals. It says nothing about how the animals are treated or slaughtered.

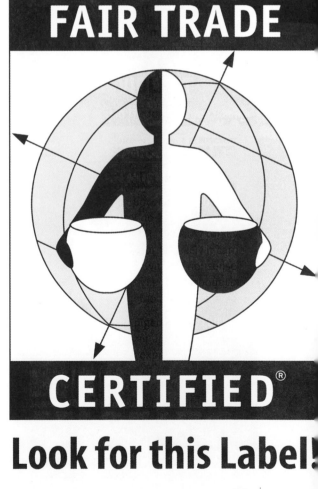

FAIR TRADE

CERTIFIED®

Look for this Label!

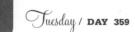
COMPASSIONATE ALTERNATIVE: **NO ROOM TO SWING A CAT**

The expression "There's no room to swing a cat" dates back to 1665 and may also refer to the cat-o'-nine-tails. (A "cat-o'-nine-tails" was a kind of multitailed whip made of leather and used to implement punishment, especially in the Royal British Navy.)

The idiom expresses the idea that you are in a confined space and have no room, which lends some plausibility to the theory that it refers to flogging a sailor in a small space, such as in the tight quarters of a ship. But no one is sure of the true origin of the phrase, whether it's referring to actually swinging a cat or flogging a person, and we have liberty to change it. Let's try, "There's no room to swing a chair." Although improbable, it provides the visual you need and makes your point. Better yet, "There's no room to dance" or "There's no room to tango."

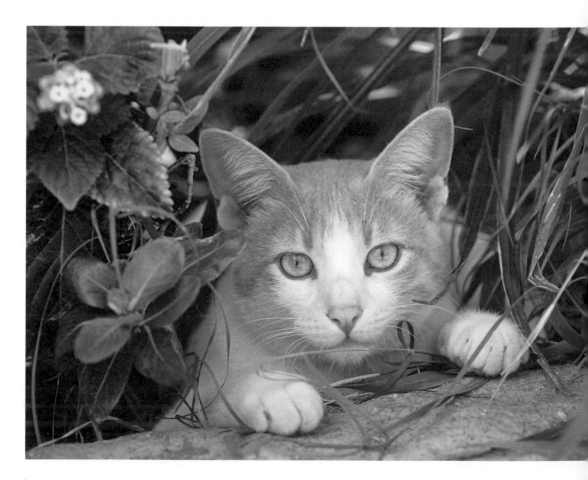

COPING WITH THE LOSS OF A COMPANION ANIMAL

Many of us have the privilege of living with and loving companion animals, which inevitably means dealing with their loss.

Facing the inevitable is perhaps the most difficult part of the process—knowing that it might be up to us to make a decision that, though it might be the end of their suffering, leads to the beginning of our own.

Many things helped me through the process of decision-making and grief.

* When facing the end, I chose not to be afraid of it. Death is part of life, and I didn't want my human fear of it to affect the transition for my cats.

* I trusted what my cats were showing me. They guided me through the process more than the other way around.

* I was able to have my dear veterinarian come to our home to aid the transition process. Many vets offer at-home euthanasia.

* I created a vigil, during which time I lit candles, gathered photos, told stories, recounted cherished memories, and collected mementos.

* I created a photo and video slide show of my departed cats to memorialize them and shared it with friends and family.

* I had a paw print created of each of my departed cats, which sit near the cedar boxes I have their ashes in, each of which is engraved with my special names for them.

* I made a donation in their names to cat rescue organizations.

* I let myself cry.

* I continue to tell their stories and let friends and family know that it's not only okay to talk about it, but it's necessary—not only to heal through the grief but to memorialize the individuals themselves.

* Painful though it is, I have come to accept the grief of their passing, because it pales in comparison to the joy I experienced in their lives.

EXCERPT FROM "SHOOTING AN ELEPHANT"
BY GEORGE ORWELL

Born Eric Arthur Blair in 1903, George Orwell is best known for his novel *Nineteen Eighty-Four* (1949) and novella *Animal Farm* (1945), though he wrote numerous essays, articles, and reviews as a journalist.

Orwell joined the Indian Imperial Police in Burma in 1922 and returned to England in 1927 to pursue a career in writing. Back home, he wrote a disturbing account about his experience of killing an elephant.

As soon as I saw the elephant I knew with perfect certainty that I ought not to shoot him ... And at that distance, peacefully eating, the elephant looked no more dangerous than a cow ... I decided that I would watch him for a little while to make sure that he did not turn savage again, and then go home ... I watched him beating his bunch of grass against his knees, with that preoccupied grandmotherly air that elephants have. It seemed to me that it would be murder to shoot him.

I shoved the cartridges into the magazine and lay down on the road to get a better aim. The crowd grew very still, and a deep, low, happy sigh, as of people who see the theatre curtain go up at last, breathed from innumerable throats. They were going to have their bit of fun after all ... I aimed several inches in front of [his earhole], thinking the brain would be further forward.

When I pulled the trigger I did not hear the bang or feel the kick—one never does when a shot goes home—but I heard the devilish roar of glee that went up from the crowd. In that instant, in too short a time, one would have thought, even for the bullet to get there, a mysterious, terrible change had come over the elephant. He neither stirred nor fell, but every line of his body had altered. He looked suddenly stricken, shrunken, immensely old, as though the frightful impact of the bullet had paralysed him without knocking him down.

At last, after what seemed a long time—it might have been five seconds, I dare say—he sagged flabbily to his knees. His mouth slobbered. An enormous senility seemed to have settled upon him. One could have imagined him thousands of years old. I fired again into the same spot. At the second shot he did not collapse but climbed with desperate slowness to his feet and stood weakly upright, with legs sagging and head drooping. I fired a third time. That was the shot that did for him. You could see the agony of it jolt his whole body and knock the last remnant of strength from his legs. But in falling he seemed for a moment to rise, for as his hind legs collapsed beneath him he seemed to tower upward like a huge rock toppling, his trunk reaching skyward like a tree. He trumpeted, for the first and only time. And then down he came, his belly towards me, with a crash that seemed to shake the ground even where I lay.

I waited a long time for him to die, but his breathing did not weaken. Finally I fired my two remaining shots into the spot where I thought his heart must be. The thick blood welled out of him like red velvet, but still he did not die. His body did not even jerk when the shots hit him, the tortured breathing continued without a pause.

He was dying, very slowly and in great agony, but in some world remote from me where not even a bullet could damage him further. I felt that I had got to put an end to that dreadful noise. It seemed dreadful to see the great beast lying there, powerless to move and yet powerless to die, and not even to be able to finish him. I sent back for my small rifle and poured shot after shot into his heart and down his throat. They seemed to make no impression. The tortured gasps continued as steadily as the ticking of a clock.

In the end I could not stand it any longer and went away. I heard later that it took him half an hour to die.

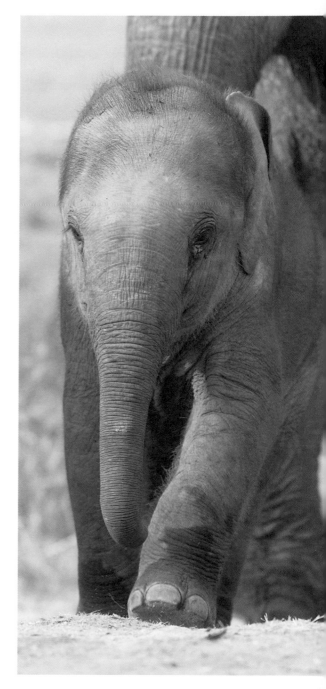

THE MIRACLE HORSES

As a child, Cleveland Amory read Anne Sewell's novel *Black Beauty* and dreamed of a place where horses could run free. His legacy, Cleveland Amory Black Beauty Ranch in Murchison, Texas, is home to almost 250 rescued horses.

Prior to their rescue, a special pair of horses, Mari Mariah and her daughter, Josie Sahara, had just days earlier been sold for slaughter and were inside the plant awaiting their certain death.

They were destined to become table food in France or Belgium, where horse meat is considered a delicacy. But Mari Mariah and Josie Sahara, along with twenty-eight other fortunate animals, are perhaps the first group of horses to have been inside a slaughter plant and survived so their story can be told.

The lives of these horses were spared in response to a federal lawsuit filed by the Fund for Animals and its partner organizations. The court struck down a scheme by the U.S. Department of Agriculture, which kept three foreign-owned horse slaughter plants operating after Congress had cut the funds for inspections of horse meat.

When news of the court decision reached the last operational slaughterhouse in the United States, it was shut down immediately. Suddenly, hundreds of horses inside the slaughterhouse were spared. Unfortunately, the reprieve was short-lived. Trucks appeared, horses were loaded, and the wheels turned north and south toward the horse slaughterhouses in Canada and Mexico.

Thirty of the spared horses went into the custody of the Humane Society of the United States and were deemed the "Miracle Horses." These were not old and lame horses, as the slaughter boosters often claim; most were young, healthy, and energetic.

The horse rescue community came out in spades to volunteer, offer assistance, and give advice and support. Adopters stopped by the stockyard to inquire about one special horse or another. Horse sanctuaries and rescues opened their doors. Some horses were immediately adopted out; others went to rescue organizations so they could recover from their time in the slaughter pipeline before finding their permanent family.

Mari Mariah and Josie Sahara had endured the ordeal together, and to separate them would be to break both a family and their spirits. They moved together, ate in sync, trotted in step, always aware of the other, and would whinny if either were out of sight. Their permanent home would be Cleveland Amory Black Beauty Ranch, where they would never be separated and would live free for the rest of their lives.

—*Diane Miller of Cleveland Amory Black Beauty Ranch, Murchison, Texas (U.S.)*

Rescued horses who will live our lives at Black Beauty Ranch

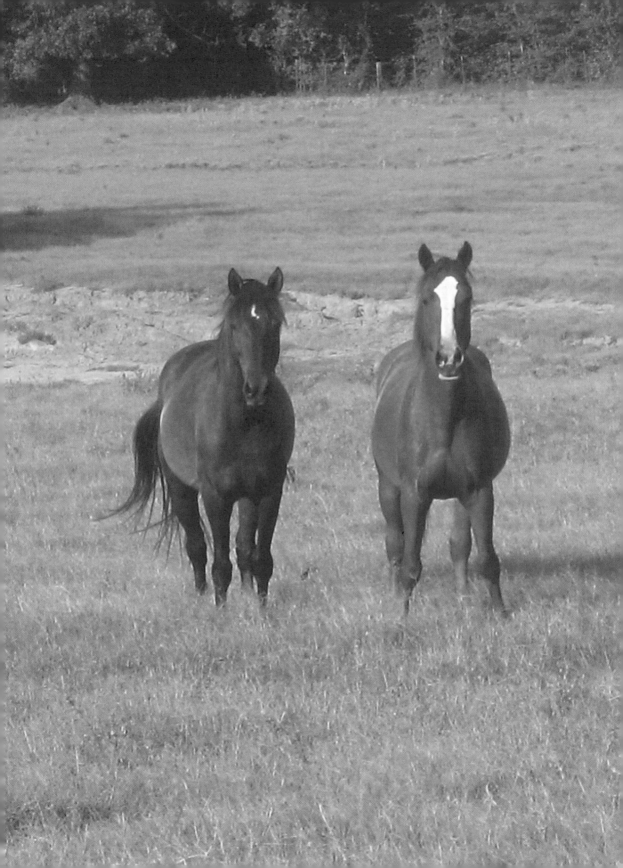

SCOTCH BROTH

This traditional Scottish soup is served as a main winter meal and often on New Year's Eve.

- 3/4 cup (200 g) pearled barley
- 3/4 cup (225 g) green split peas
- 3/4 cup (192 g) red lentils
- 1 large leek, washed well and roughly chopped
- 1 yellow onion, roughly chopped
- 2 or 3 yellow potatoes, diced
- 3 carrots, grated or shredded
- 8 to 9 cups (1,880 to 2,115 ml) vegetable stock, depending on thickness required (store-bought or homemade)
- 1 teaspoon (6 g) salt (or to taste)
- Freshly ground pepper
- 2 tablespoons (8 g) chopped fresh parsley, for garnish (optional)

Soak the barley, split peas, and lentils for 1 hour in a bowl with enough water to cover. After soaking, rinse the barley, peas, and lentils and add them to a large soup pot, along with the leek, onion, potatoes, carrots, stock, salt, and pepper.

Bring to a boil, then reduce the heat and simmer until the split peas, barley, and veggies are tender.

Ladle into individual bowls, and sprinkle the parsley on top of each serving.

Yield: 10 to 12 servings

SERVING SUGGESTIONS AND VARIATIONS
Other traditional veggies in Scotch broth include turnips, cabbage, and kale.

*Oil-free, wheat-free, soy-free

Originally published in *The Vegan Table*

PORRIDGE

Porridge has been a traditional food for thousands of years in much of northern Europe. The word *porridge* is actually derived from the Old French word *poree*, which meant "leek soup." The porridge we think of today has nothing to do with leeks and everything to do with grains—any kind of grain. A porridge is essential a gruel, and the word *gruel* has origins in the word *grain*. In fact, a loose definition of porridge is any soft dish made of boiled grains with the addition of milk to make it creamy—to make it gruel-like.

Often eaten for breakfast and sweetened with sugar, cinnamon, and fruit, porridge has been the traditional breakfast food in Scotland for ages. Before leavened bread (and ovens) became common fare in Europe, porridge was the primary way to prepare grains for the table. The Scots' favorite grain for their porridge is the reliable oat, and they take their porridge making very seriously. They even hold a World Porridge-Making Contest each year.

Traditionally, Scottish porridge is made with steel-cut oats, though in England and the United States it is made with rolled oats. Other countries that use oats as the basis of their porridge include:

* Russia, whose *owsianka* is made with oats, hot milk (in our case, nondairy!), and sugar

* Brazil, whose *mingau de aveia* is oatmeal boiled in milk

Corn—or *maize*—is also a popular grain from which to make porridge.

* In the United States, there are grits (which is made from ground hominy).

* In Mexico, there is *atole* (corn flour, water, and milk), served as a drink or thick gruel.

* In El Salvador, *shuco* is made from ground black, blue, or purple corn flour, ground pumpkin seeds, chile sauce, and cooked kidney beans.

* In Italy, polenta is a staple food made of cornmeal and milk.

Some countries make their porridge from wheat—you've most likely heard of cream of wheat or farina; some from potatoes, such as in Norway, where potatoes are cooked and mixed with milk and barley. Rice porridge is popular in Greece, Indonesia, China, Japan, and many Southeast Asian countries, and barley porridge is a staple in Tibet.

RESOURCES AND RECOMMENDATIONS

Related to entries in this book, here are additional recommended resources for you to check out.

FOR THE LOVE OF FOOD

Visit localharvest.org to find farmer's markets and Community Supported Agriculture near you.

Try La Yapa Organic for fantastic, organic, fair-trade quinoa (layapaorganic.com).

Visit vegfund.org to apply for grants for vegan food at advocacy events.

My favorite tea can be ordered online at teance.com. Visit their beautiful tea room in Berkeley when you're in the area. Other teas I recommend are from farleaves.com and samovartea.com.

Attend a Japanese Tea Ceremony at the San Francisco Zen Center sfzc.org.

Make charitable donations, create a charitable wedding registry, or send charity gift certificates at justgive.org.

OPTIMUM HEALTH

Visit, compassionatecooks.com/supplements for my recommended multivitamins and supplements.

Connect with other like-minded folks at these national conferences:

* HSUS, takingactionforanimals.com

* Farm Animal Reform Movement, arconference.org

* North American Vegetarian Society, vegetariansummerfest.org

* World Vegetarian Congress/International Vegetarian Union, ivu.org

Connect with other like-minded folks at various grassroots channels:

* vegandrinks.org

* meetup.com

My favorite line of hair products: Unite and Pureology

Becoming Vegan by Brenda Davis and Vesanto Melina is *the* bible of vegan nutrition, and their new book *Becoming Raw* will demystify the questions around raw diets.

In terms of calorie-burn monitors, the best and most heavily studied device is an armband sold as GoWear fit by BodyMedia and as the bodybugg by 24 Hour Fitness.

ANIMALS IN THE ARTS

Check out the work of these amazing animal activists/artists/writers.

Sue Coe: Coe has published many books, including *Dead Meat* and *Sheep of Fools*.

Sunny Taylor: View Taylor's artwork at her website, sunaurataylor.org.

Gale Hart: Visit whynoteatyourpet.com: Art That Gives Animals a Voice.

Michele Amatrula: Amstrula is an animal portrait artist who captures the personality and soul of her subjects (amatrulapetportraits.com).

Shad Clark: Clark is a filmmaker, fellow writer, and good friend. Visit shadclark.com to view his complete oeuvre and read "Little Boy Pig" as an ebook or Kindle edition.

Derek Goodwin: Goodwin is a talented photographer who photographs a lot of sanctuary animals (derekgoodwin.com).

STORIES OF HOPE

There are many animal sanctuaries around the world. I'm including only a handful here.

animalplace.org
farmsanctuary.org
casanctuary.org
thedonkeysanctuary.ie
sashafarm.org
peacefulprairie.org
animalsanctuary.org

blackbeautyranch.org
pigspeace.org
pasadosafehaven.org
pawsweb.org
elephants.com
chimphaven.org

animalsasia.org
animalsanctuaries.co.uk
rollingdogranch.org
saveabunny.org
ida-africa.org
blindhorses.org

Read the entire account in Cleveland Amory's own words in *Ranch of Dreams: A Lifelong Protector of Animals Shares the Story of His Extraordinary Sanctuary.*

To find out exactly which companies don't test on animals, visit caringconsumer.com or aavs.org.

BLOGS, PODCASTS, AND MAGAZINES

runtodisney.com
veganrunningmom.com
cadryskitchen.com
compassionatecooks.com
vegetarianfoodforthought.com
vegnews.com
animalsvoice.com

Visit www.compassionatecooks.com for more resources, including Colleen's cookbooks, *The Joy of Vegan Baking*, *The Vegan Table, and Color Me Vegan.*

INDEX

PHOTO CREDITS

ACKNOWLEDGMENTS

Thank you to Quarry Books for giving me the freedom and opportunity to create this book and to my editor, Rochelle Bourgault, and project manager, Tiffany Hill, who were an absolute dream to work with and who made this book better every time their hands touched it.

Being part of a movement dedicated to saving human and nonhuman lives and improving the world is incredibly gratifying and most definitely humbling. I'm so grateful to do this work alongside so many compassionate individuals and organizations. It's been an absolute joy to teach for Dr. McDougall's Wellness Program for so many years. Not only are Mary and John wonderfully supportive, but their staff is a delight to work with. (Thank you for your love and patience each month, Tiffany!) More than that, the folks who come through their program—whom I have the privilege of teaching—are some of the most open, friendly, and generous people I've ever met. Their eagerness to learn and change is one of the reasons I have hope in this world.

Thank you to the number of people who have kept me sane and made my work possible these many years: Amanda Mitchell, Megan Storms, Tami Hiltz, Jennifer Stadtmiller, Juliet Lynn, Lori Patotzka, Matt Props, Megan McClellan, Jared Greer, Pam Webb, Ryan Thibodaux, Poppy Nguyen, Aaron Weinstein, Julie Flook, Stephen and Danielle Tschirhart, and Blake Wiers.

I'm blessed to have so many loving friends and supportive family members who brighten my days, especially Diane Miller, Cadry Nelson, David Busch, Kenda Swartz, Michael Scribner, Chris Marco, Tami Wall, Cheri Larsh Arellano, Mark Arellano, John Keathley, Randy Lind, Cathleen Young, Deborah Underwood, Kristin Schwartz, Shad Clark, Robin Brande, Rae Sikora, and Mom, Dad, sister-in-love, and parents by marriage.

The bulk of my time is spent in the company of my beloved feline kids, whose affection, humor, energy, and love infuse my writing and my life, and I'm certain Simon is looking over his angel of a brother Schuster, who has patiently adjusted to our newest addition, Charlie. We continue to miss Cassandra.

My best friend of 17 years and husband of almost 10, David Goudreau (a.k.a. Bello) enriches my life every day with his humor, patience, and devotion and supports me morning, noon, and night.

ABOUT THE AUTHOR

Colleen Patrick-Goudreau is the author of three cookbooks, *The Joy of Vegan Baking*, *The Vegan Table*, and *Color Me Vegan*. She is the host of the award-winning podcast *Food for Thought*, a columnist for *VegNews Magazine*, and a contributor to National Public Radio, and she has appeared on the Food Network. She is the founder of Compassionate Cooks (www.compassionatecooks.com), an organization whose mission is to serve as a voice for the more than 45 billion land and sea animals killed every year in the United States for human consumption.

Having earned a master's degree in English Literature, Colleen uses her writing and communication skills to be a voice for animals and to inspire people to live according to their own values of compassion and healthfulness. She is a sought-after and inspiring public speaker on the spiritual, social, and practical aspects of a vegan lifestyle. She lives in Oakland, California with her husband and two cats.

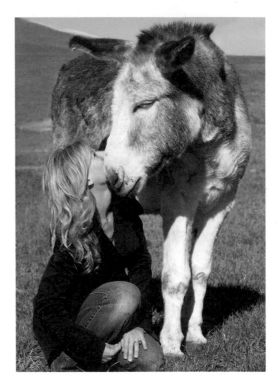